Current and Future Developments in Surgery

(Volume 1)

(Oesophago-gastric Surgery)

Edited by

Sami M. Shimi

Consultant Oesophago-gastric Surgeon, Department of Surgery
Ninewells Hospital and Medical School, University of Dundee
Dundee, Scotland, UK

General:

1. Any dispute or claim arising out of or in connection with this License Agreement or the Work (including non-contractual disputes or claims) will be governed by and construed in accordance with the laws of the U.A.E. as applied in the Emirate of Dubai. Each party agrees that the courts of the Emirate of Dubai shall have exclusive jurisdiction to settle any dispute or claim arising out of or in connection with this License Agreement or the Work (including non-contractual disputes or claims).
2. Your rights under this License Agreement will automatically terminate without notice and without the need for a court order if at any point you breach any terms of this License Agreement. In no event will any delay or failure by Bentham Science Publishers in enforcing your compliance with this License Agreement constitute a waiver of any of its rights.
3. You acknowledge that you have read this License Agreement, and agree to be bound by its terms and conditions. To the extent that any other terms and conditions presented on any website of Bentham Science Publishers conflict with, or are inconsistent with, the terms and conditions set out in this License Agreement, you acknowledge that the terms and conditions set out in this License Agreement shall prevail.

Bentham Science Publishers Ltd.
Executive Suite Y - 2
PO Box 7917, Saif Zone
Sharjah, U.A.E.
Email: subscriptions@benthamscience.org

**BENTHAM
SCIENCE**

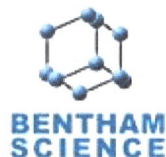

CONTENTS

FOREWORD

In this increasing age of sub-specialisation in medicine in general and surgery in particular, learning organ specific details for diagnosis and treatment is a challenge to every clinician. This e-book 'Oesophago-gastric Surgery' will therefore come as a welcome addition to the specialist literature on the subject. It has been put together, written and edited by a multi-disciplinary specialist team from Ninewells Hospital in Dundee, Scotland, who have covered the full range of oesophago-gastric conditions and their treatment. The book is meant primarily for surgical trainees, both with a general and specialist upper GI interest, as well as consultants who wish to gain up-to-date knowledge of this area. It goes into great detail in all the areas of benign, pre-malignant and malignant disease. The book is well referenced and provides very clear figures and diagrams to help the reader understand many of the complexities of treatment. While the incidence of squamous cell carcinoma of the oesophagus is falling, and of adenocarcinoma is rising, the management of the pre-malignant condition of Barrett's oesophagus has therefore, become increasingly important. The role of surgery in the management of gastro-oesophageal reflux and other benign conditions has increased significantly over the last 20 years with advances in minimally invasive surgery. This has brought the medical and surgical endoscopists into a much closer relationship than in the past, with recognition that treatment can now be tailored to the underlying condition and the patients' needs. The background pathophysiology on which both diagnosis and management are based on particularly useful and is a credit to the editorial team and the authors involved. Overall, this is a well-written, detailed and up to date e-book, which covers all the relevant areas of oesophago-gastric surgery and will be a very welcome addition to the eBook series.

Simon Paterson-Brown
Consultant General and Upper Gastro-intestinal Surgeon
Royal Infirmary of Edinburgh
Scotland,
UK

PREFACE

The natural evolution of surgical knowledge and technology meant that the traditional general surgeon concept is no longer sustainable. This has necessitated the need for sub-specialization. Along the route, the influence of volume on outcomes was established. The end result seen today is an endorsement of subspecialization by all the Surgical Colleges, professional societies and health care systems. "Super specialisation", is a separate discussion for the coming decade. The traditional textbooks on general surgery can no longer provide the core knowledge for specialist training.

This book addresses the core knowledge needs of higher surgical trainees in oesophago-gastric surgery and provides a reference manual for established consultants in oesophago-gastric surgery and other specialties. It provides a practical and user-friendly reference to all relevant topics. A comprehensive but concise approach was adopted to detail the main relevant topics. Detailed discussion of rarer topics was left for the commonly practiced Internet searches. The chapters in this book are practice based. They were written by experienced clinicians who have gone through the sub-specialisation process with full awareness of the specialist educational curriculum specified by the surgical colleges and professional societies. With this book being one of the "e-book" series, it means that busy practitioners can have instant access to this book on the Internet to refresh knowledge and gain additional insight.

I am grateful to all the contributors who have shared their knowledge enthusiastically. To our readers, we hope that you enjoy reading this book, enjoy the knowledge riches in its pages and for those who are preparing for professional examinations, we wish you success.

Sami M. Shimi
Consultant Oesophago-gastric Surgeon
Department of Surgery
Ninewells Hospital and Medical School
University of Dundee
Dundee, Scotland
UK

DEDICATION

This book is dedicated to my family who encouraged and supported me throughout the various stages of editing this book and authoring some of the chapters.

I also dedicate this book to my surgical colleagues and trainees who enlightened me with their wisdom, surgical craft and educational needs.

Finally, I dedicate this book to all my patients who entrusted me and filled my life with the joy which I derived from treating them.

"A surgeon without knowledge, creativity and skill is like a house without a roof, water or electricity."

List of Contributors

Aminah Khan Department of Surgery, Ninewells Hospital and Medical School, Dundee, Scotland, UK

Amy Sadler Department of Anaesthesia, Ninewells Hospital and Medical School, Dundee, Scotland, UK

Joanne Thomson Department of Nutrition and Dietetics, Ninewells Hospital and Medical School, Dundee, Scotland, UK

John Smith Department of Anaesthesia, Ninewells Hospital and Medical School, Dundee, Scotland, UK

Michael Wilson Department of Surgery, Ninewells Hospital and Medical School, Dundee, Scotland, UK

Robert Foster Department of Radiology, Ninewells Hospital and Medical School, Dundee, Scotland, UK

Sally Crofts Department of Anaesthesia, Ninewells Hospital and Medical School, Dundee, Scotland, UK

Sami M. Shimi Department of Surgery, Ninewells Hospital and Medical School, Dundee, Scotland, UK

Shaun McLeod Department of Anaesthesia, Ninewells Hospital and Medical School, Dundee, Scotland, UK

Shaun Walsh Department of Pathology, Ninewells Hospital and Medical School, Dundee, Scotland, UK

CHAPTER 1

Anaesthesia for Oesophago-gastric Surgery

John Smith[1], Sally Crofts[1] and **Sami M. Shimi[2,*]**

[1] *Department of Anaesthesia, Ninewells Hospital and Medical School, Dundee, Scotland, UK*

[2] *Department of Surgery, Ninewells Hospital and Medical School, Dundee, Scotland, UK*

Abstract: Major Upper Gastrointestinal (UGI) surgery encompasses a wide range of potential surgical procedures, many of which pose substantial challenges to the anaesthetist caring for the patient in the peri-operative period. Pre-anaesthetic assessment and optimisation of the patient are critical. The objectives of anaesthesia are to render the patient unaware of the surgical stimulus, to provide favourable intra-operative conditions for surgery, and to improve patient experience and outcome, particularly in cardiorespiratory function and post-operative analgesia. The specific points to consider in oesophago-gastric surgery include the position of incisions, the duration of surgery, the multi-site nature of the operations and the premorbid condition of the patients considered for surgery.

Whilst there is no substitute for experience and frequent exposure to these procedures, there are a number of specific anaesthetic issues which merit expert consideration. This chapter will explore a number of facets of patient care: from pre-operative assessment to anaesthetic technique and finally, post-operative care. Due to the high propensity of post-operative complications, particularly infections, which contribute to additional morbidity specific to oesophago-gastric surgery; a section is included on infection and antibiotic prophylaxis. In addition, multi-modal analgesia will be considered as the site of surgery for many of these patients can impact on post-operative respiration and can contribute to post-operative respiratory infections.

Keywords: Anaesthesia, Analgesia, Anaesthetic techniques, Pre-operative assessment, Cardio-pulmonary reserve testing, Premedication, Monitoring, Extubation, DVT prophylaxis, Infection and anti-microbials.

PRE-ANAESTHESIA ASSESSMENT

Introduction

Major Upper Gastrointestinal surgery poses a significant physiological challenge to any patient. It is therefore essential that a comprehensive assessment of the

---

* **Corresponding author Sami M. Shimi:** Department of Surgery, Ninewells Hospital and Medical School, Dundee DD1 9SY, Scotland, UK; Tel: +44 1382 660111; E-mail: s.m.shimi@dundee.ac.uk

patient, their surgical pathology and the proposed procedure, are made prior to undertaking surgery. Often, these assessments will require close liaison with the anaesthetic team who will care for the patient in the peri-operative period.

A number of Upper Gastrointestinal procedures carry notable risks, particularly Gastrectomy and Oesophagectomy, where the 30-day mortality has been estimated as high as 11% [1], despite advances in surgical technique and processes of care. This contrasts sharply with the much more favourable risk profile found in modern anti-reflux and weight management bariatric surgery, much of which now benefits from minimally invasive techniques, further reducing physiological disturbance.

In terms of surgical pathology, there is a huge spectrum between benign diseases, which have made little impact on the patients' physiology, and chronic or malignant conditions which have made a significant impact on the physiology and psyche of the patient. The debilitating effects of cancer and any pre-operative neo-adjuvant treatment cannot be over emphasised. Obesity, when "benign" impacts significantly on the cardio-respiratory and metabolic status of the patient and consequently elevates their risk profile.

Regardless of the condition of the patient, the proposed procedure or the surgical pathology, attention to individual patient selection, assessment and optimisation will need to be exercised to manage individual risk by taking all factors into consideration.

Anaesthetic Assessment

The majority if not all patients presenting for elective surgery will have been "pre-assessed" by an experienced anaesthetist prior to their elective admission. This often occurs at specific clinics that are supervised by anaesthetic medical staff, and are usually undertaken a period of weeks before the procedure is scheduled. This process provides an opportunity for the entire team responsible for patient care to ensure all necessary investigations are complete and comprehensive. It also provides an opportunity for patient optimisation when this is deemed necessary. With regard to Anaesthesia, this generally provides an opportunity to meet and assess the patient without the pressure of an immanent procedure. It also affords an opportunity to schedule cardiovascular fitness assessment tests as indicated, so that results can be fully analysed with the surgical team prior to admission.

Pre-assessment is an opportunity to meet not only the patient, but also their close family members, who will play an important role throughout the patient's journey through assessment, surgery and recovery. The importance of these "carers" throughout the process cannot be overestimated. They may be able to provide accurate and helpful observations, which will aid preoperative risk assessment; ask pertinent and important questions during the consent process and then act as a vital source of encouragement to the patient during preoperative exercise regimes, smoking cessation and any required dietary changes.

Engaging the patient's family/friends from an early point, and providing them with accurate and realistic information, as well as managing their expectation of events are of the utmost importance.

As with all surgery, a basic anaesthetic assessment should be undertaken. This should include a comprehensive history of the presenting problem, as well as their past medical, drug and social history. In addition, information should be collected on their nutritional history and status. It is particularly important to have access to previous anaesthetic history in the patient's medical charts, and the patients' recollection of the experience whilst making this assessment. Although most patients would not volunteer information on their airway history, careful probing should identify potential risks (Table **1**). The relevance of the accuracy of details should be made clear to patients and they should be sensitively encouraged to volunteer additional relevant information or anxieties, which may affect the anaesthesia or recovery. Anxieties around pain and analgesia should also be explored.

Specific Aspects of History Taking

Chemotherapy: Current advances in the treatment of oesophago-gastric cancer have strongly advocated the use of neo-adjuvant chemotherapy to try to minimise tumour bulk and spread prior to resection. This has significant relevance to the anaesthetist, in that chemotherapy predisposes the patient to infection. In addition, regimes including the use of epirubicin (in doses $>200\text{mgm}^{-2}$) are associated with impaired LV function [2]. Care must be taken to assess the timing of recent chemotherapy, and also its physiological effects, especially effects on White Blood Cell count, platelets and coagulation parameters.

Table 1. Important topics in basic anaesthetic assessment.

History Topic	Specifics
Past Medical History	History of significant cardiovascular, respiratory, gastrointestinal, renal and neurological disease. Symptoms of obstructive sleep apnoea (OSA).
Drug History	Current medication, recent neo-adjuvant chemotherapy (and the agents used), agents, which can influence coagulation mechanisms or platelet function.
Allergies	Medication, Latex, iodine/chlorhexidine allergies or intolerance.

(Table 1) contd.....

History Topic	Specifics
Social History (including substance misuse)	Available family support. Brief employment history and relevant occupational exposures. Cigarette smoking and alcohol consumption.
Nutritional History	Recent weight loss, and amount. Dietetic input and nutritional supplementation.
Previous Anaesthetic (personal or familial) history	Previous anaesthetic complications (personal or familial). Previous negative experiences around surgery (severe pain during recovery).
Airway History	Airway management history in previous anaesthetics. Airway Alert card. Sleep apnoea.

Examination

A thorough examination of the patient should be undertaken, with particular focus on the cardiac and respiratory systems, as these represent the areas, which can influence the decision to surgery. It is essential to detect any major abnormalities within both of these systems, and then investigate them appropriately.

Airway:

Virtually all UGI procedures under general anaesthesia require intubation of the trachea to facilitate surgical access and prevent aspiration of gastric contents.

Major UGI resection surgery for oesophageal and some gastric cancers will involve the placement of a Double-Lumen endo-tracheal tube. It is therefore, essential that a comprehensive assessment is made of the patient's airway. This will involve exploring their previous anaesthetic history, referring to previous anaesthetic documentation for any evidence of difficulties during attempted laryngoscopy, or more significantly ventilation. Examination of the patient is an integral part of the process. A commonly used system for predicting airway difficulties is the Mallampati grading system [3]. It is easily performed and standardised in reporting the findings. The patient is asked to protrude their tongue, with the head and neck in a neutral position. Based on the visible structures, 4 different scores may be awarded, a higher number denoting an increasing level of concern over a potentially difficult-to-manage airway (Fig. **1**).

Grade 1: Soft palate, uvula, fauces and pillars visible
Grade 2: Soft palate, uvula and fauces visible
Grade 3: Only soft palate visible
Grade 4: Soft palate not visible.

Should the preliminary assessment reveals features causing concern, a number of further investigations should be considered; including CT scanning of head and neck a

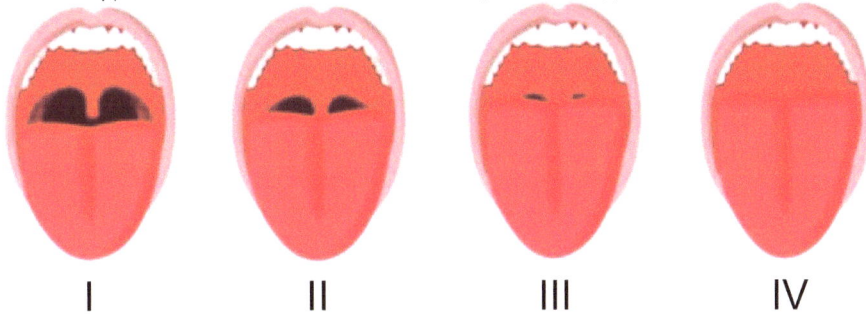

Fig. (1). Mallampati Grading Scale. The patient is asked to protrude their tongue, with the head and neck in a neutral position. Based on the visible structures, 4 different scores may be awarded, a higher number denoting an increasing level of concern over a potentially difficult-to-manage airway.

If there have been difficulties during previous attempts at airway management under anaesthesia, a patient may be issued with an "Airway Alert Card" (Fig. **2**). This acts as a prompt to future anaesthetists to firstly check the medical notes to determine the difficulties previously encountered or to seek notes from another institution, and secondly to be aware that the patient may pose a significant, ongoing airway challenge. Although the nature of this challenge may have changed from previous anaesthesia, the alert heightens awareness and enables appropriate planning of necessary expertise, alternative equipment and strategies.

Fig. (2). An airway alert card.

It is also prudent to assess patients presenting for weight management surgery for signs of Obstructive Sleep Apnoea (OSA), which may compromise post-operative airway care. As part of this assessment, both Body Mass Index (BMI) and neck circumference should be measured. A useful assessment tool is the STOP BANG system, detailed below:

1. S: Do you snore loudly (loud enough to be heard through closed doors)?
2. T: Do you often feel tired, fatigued or sleepy during the daytime?
3. O: Has anyone observed you stop breathing during your sleep?
4. P: Do you have/are you being treated for high blood pressure?
5. B: Is your BMI >35?
6. A: Are you aged >50 years?
7. N: Is your neck circumference >40 cm?
8. G: Is your gender Male?

A score of 3-4 positive answers indicates an intermediate risk of OSA, whereas a score >5 indicates a high risk of post-operative OSA.

Smoking History:

Many of the patients presenting for surgery may have smoked, some of them until very recently. With this reality comes a substantial burden of chronic cardiovascular and respiratory disease including ischaemic heart disease, peripheral vascular disease, chronic obstructive pulmonary disease and an increased likelihood of respiratory infection. Active smokers should be very strongly encouraged to stop smoking pre-operatively. Due to the addictive nature of the habit and inhaled nicotine, this can be very difficult. Active counselling support together with Nicotine replacement therapy can help.

Support in terms of nicotine replacement therapy (Fig. **3**) or engagement with self-help "Quit" groups may be of benefit.

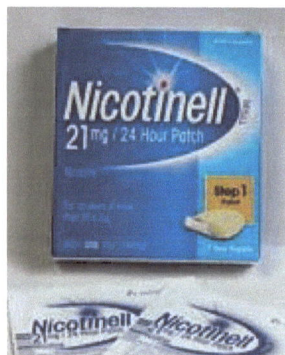

Fig. (3). Nicotine Replacement Patch Therapy

Nutritional Status:

Many of the patients presenting for UGI resection surgery and some with Achalasia requiring cardiomyotomy, will have a relatively compromised nutritional status. This is particularly true of cancer patients as their ability to ingest and absorb nutrients may have been substantially impaired for some time. Research has shown that patients presenting with the following criteria are at substantially increased perioperative risk of morbidity and mortality due to their poor physiological reserve.

• Body Mass Index (BMI) <18.5
• >20% total body weight loss
• Body weight <90% predicted
• Hypoalbuminaemia

At the other end of the nutritional spectrum, patients presenting for weight management surgery may also pose challenges. Whilst their body mass index is usually high, significant dietary restriction also leaves them at risk of micronutrient depletion. Care should also be taken with their nutritional assessment preoperatively, management of their liver reducing diet and management of blood sugars; especially in those patients on regular hypoglycaemic agents

Formal assessment of nutritional status, in the form of blood tests (see below) and measurements of BMI and fat reserves should be sought. If there is concern about a patient's nutritional status and reserve, the early involvement of the dietetic team should be considered. The surgical team should be alerted to institute measures, which could help improve the nutritional status. Timing of the definitive surgery may have to be reviewed until the patient's nutrition is improved sufficiently.

Psychology:

An often-neglected area of patient assessment is the psychology of patients facing major and often life-changing surgery and sometimes, prolonged recovery. The peri-operative period is a time of great anxiety and concern to both patients and their families. Early and realistic information concerning what to expect, both in terms of the operative period and also the recovery phase is essential. Some patients find the opportunity to meet and discuss issues with a patient who has gone through the same experiences useful.

It is also vital to be sensitive to the presence of depressive illness or anxiety states resulting from diagnosis of illness, particularly in the case of upper gastrointestinal cancer. There can be no doubt that the presence of depression acts as a risk for poor patient outcome and delayed or limited functional recovery. Therefore, aggressive, multi-disciplinary steps should be taken to alleviate this prior to surgery, insofar as this is possible.

Preoperative Investigations

The exact combination of investigations required for surgery will be dependent on a number of factors including the type of surgery, the patient's individual risk factors and their physiological ability to adapt to cardiovascular stress in the post-operative period.

Procedures such as invasive two or three stage oesophagectomy constitute some of the highest risk of all surgical procedures, and require careful planning. However, less than 1% of all mortality is directly due to intraoperative factors. Therefore, the majority of all mortality and morbidity result from patient-specific risk factors [4], which must be assessed and where possible, optimised pre-operatively.

All patients should have basic preoperative investigations performed. These include an electrocardiogram (ECG) and blood testing: including full blood count, renal and liver function. In addition, a sample for blood for transfusion cross matching should also be taken immediately prior to surgery.

These basic tests provide an important insight into the patient's current and chronic health, and can illuminate a number of conditions, such as chronic ischaemic heart disease, or chronic renal dysfunction. In patients with a history of cigarette smoking or respiratory disease, pulmonary function tests are also desirable to assess the degree of physiological function and estimate limitation.

Scoring Systems

Patients with a higher than average risk profile, or those having high-risk surgery, should have an advanced assessment of cardiovascular reserve. The objectives of this assessment are to provide an indication of the patients' fitness to withstand demanding surgery and their ability for subsequent recovery through measurement of oxygen consumption at the tissue level. A number of tests have been proposed [5]. These tests are collectively termed exercise ECG testing- the so-called "treadmill test". It has been hypothesised that despite their ready availability, these tests are less useful than anticipated, as they lack specificity for detecting problems and are unable to demonstrate a dynamic, cardiorespiratory response to physiological stress. As such, current practice has focussed on the use of exercise testing as a means of assessing cardiovascular "reserve". Echocardiography can be supplementary and is indicated in patients with valvular or ischaemic heart disease where additional information is required to ascertain ventricular function. A number of cardio-respiratory reserve tests have been proposed.

The ASA scoring system: The American Society of Anaesthesiologists' (ASA) classification is a subjective assessment of a patient's overall health, which is based on five classes (I to V).

I. Patient is a completely healthy fit patient.
II. Patient has mild systemic disease.
III. Patient has severe systemic disease that is not incapacitating.
IV. Patient has incapacitating disease that is a constant threat to life.
V. A moribund patient who is not expected to live 24 hour with or without surgery.

E Emergency Surgery, E is Placed After the Roman Numeral

This classification is used universally in the pre-operative assessment of all patients considered for surgery. Since inception it has been revised on several occasions and an 'E' suffix was included denoting an emergency case. Being simple and widely understood, ASA score also has been used in policy making, performance evaluation as an easy tool for audit, resource allocation, reimbursement of anaesthesia services and frequently is cited in clinical research as well.

Although the ASA classification of Physical Health is a widely used grading system for preoperative assessment of the surgical patients, multiple variations exist between individual anaesthetist's assessments when describing common clinical problems. In addition, it has been recognised not to be an accurate predictor of either risk or outcomes. Despite this valid criticism, it remains a widely applicable and useful system for individual patients as well as comparing groups of patients considered in research articles or policy and protocol standards. It is easy to apply and understand with little variation. It is easily adopted as a sole measure but often in conjunction with additional assessment measures of a patient's condition prior to surgery.

Duke Activity Status Index:

This scale seeks to quantify the patient's fitness based on the idea of Metabolic Equivalents (METS) (Table **2**).

It proposes that 1 MET equals an oxygen consumption of 3.5 mls/kg-1/min-1. Identifying a patient's ability to exercise and assessing METS accordingly should then produce an estimation of the maximal ability to deliver and consume oxygen. Though easy to perform at the bedside, this system is limited by patient over-estimation of their functional ability.

Table 2. MET Scoring Scale.

Physical Activity	METS
Light Intensity activities	<3
Sleeping	0.9
Watching television	1.0
Desk work, typing	1.5
Walking (2.7 km/h: very slow)	2.3
Walking (4 km/h: slow)	2.9
Moderate intensity activities	3 to 6
Bicycling (50 W stationary, very light effort)	3.0
Walking (4.8 km/h: moderate pace)	3.3
Home exercise, moderate effort	3.5
Walking (5.5 km/h: fast pace)	3.6
Bicycling (16 km/h)	4.0
Bicycling (1000 W, stationary, light effort)	5.5
Sexual activity	5.8
Vigorous intensity activities	>6
Jogging	7.0
Circuit training: vigorous effort	8.0
Running	8.0
Rope jumping	10

Exercise Testing

A number of schemes to test patient functional ability based on exercise tolerance have also been employed. The 6-minute walk test and the Incremental Shuttle Walk Test (ISWT) are both well published methodologies, and easily performed without specialist equipment. It has been identified that in the case of oesophagectomy, patients unable to complete greater than 350 m of the ISWT are at increased risk of morbidity and mortality [6]. Though perhaps more objective than a simple estimation of fitness, these tests are relatively crude and are subject to limitations in patient mobility, as distinct from their cardiovascular reserve (Fig. **4**). This is particularly true in those presenting for Bariatric malabsorptive procedures, where functional ability may appear far more depleted than expected, as patient body mass will limit weight-bearing exercise capacity, rather than cardiovascular limitations.

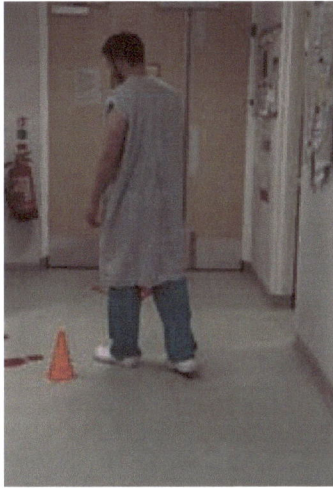

Fig. (4). Incremental Shuttle Walk Test (ISWT) Performed pre-operatively.

Cardio Pulmonary Exercise Testing (CPET): Formal CPET testing requires both specific technical equipment and the skills to interpret the data gathered. In recent times, it has seen considerable support as the gold standard to assess functional reserve. Usually performed on a cycle ergometer, CPET results are displayed as a "9-panel plot" (Fig. **5**).

Two values are of particular importance:

- Anaerobic Threshold (AT): the point at which metabolism becomes predominantly anaerobic due to lack of available oxygen in muscle tissue. Patients with an AT of <11 mls/kg^{-1} are at higher risk of morbidity and mortality.
- Maximum Oxygen Delivery (V_{O2} Max): the maximal amount of oxygen that the body is capable of delivering, a potent test of cardiorespiratory fitness. Patients with values <800 mls/min^{-1}/m^{-2} pose a high-risk proposition for major surgery.

Though a formal linear result between cardiovascular fitness and outcome has yet to be established, it is known that for high-risk surgeries such as thoracotomy, low AT and V_{O2}Max are associated with poor patient outcomes [7]. Currently CPET remains the most sensitive and specific test of cardiovascular fitness and where available, afford the anaesthetist early opportunity to identify the high-risk patient. It is difficult to use CPET in patients with who have arthritic problems in the lower limbs since it relies mainly on cycling with the use of the lower limb muscles for exercise.

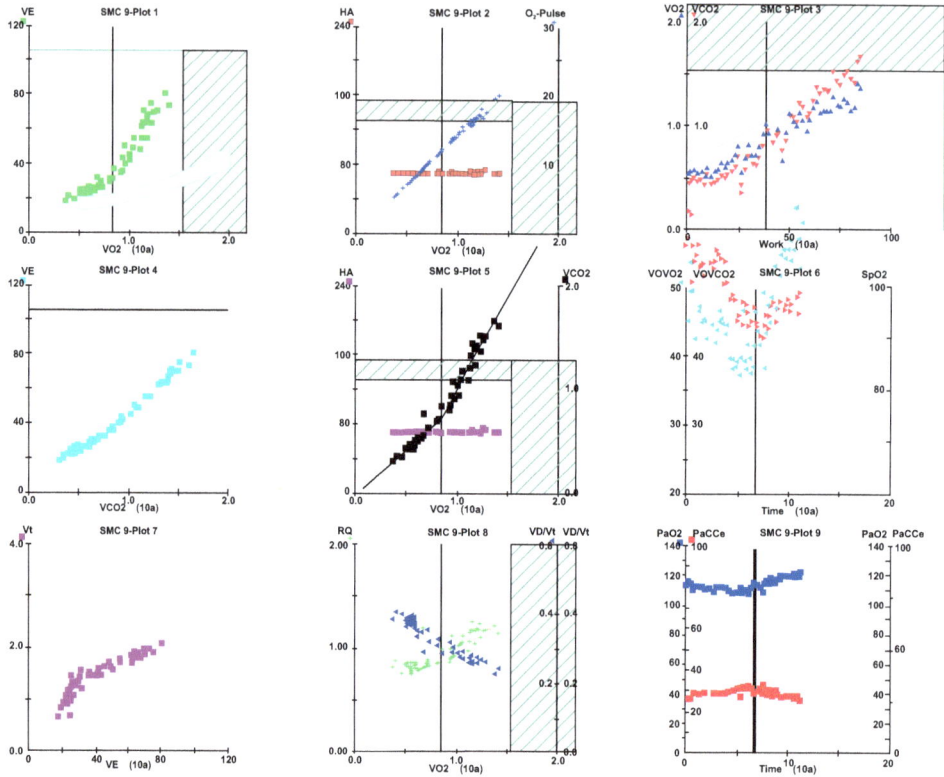

Measurement (peak)	Predicted	Measured	%Predicted	Plot #
VO2 (l/min)	1.854	1.412	76	1,3
Work Rate (Watts)	127	85	66	3
HR (bpm)	143	70	49	2
O2 Pulse (ml/beat)		20.2		5
Respiratory Quotient (RQ)	1.1-1.3	1.18		8
VE Max (l/min) BTPS	106.6	88.8	0	1,7
Breathing Reserve (%)	20-40	11		1,7
AT (l/min)	0.742	1.051		1,5,6,9
Slope Calculations			**(Normal Range)**	
VO2/Work (ml/min/watt)	10.3		8.7-11.9	3
HR/VO2kg (bpm/ml/kg)	3.8		3.0-4.0	2,5
VE/VO2 (L BTPS/L STPD)	27.5		23-26	1,6
VE/VCO2 (L BTPS/L STPD)	27.7		26-29	3

Version: IVS-0101-28-3b

Fig. (5). CPET Results showing 9-panel plot.

Pre-surgical Fitness Training

Even in patients with CPET-proven high cardiovascular risk, the effects of this risk can be ameliorated by undertaking prescribed and tailored pre-operative exercise programmes to improve cardiovascular fitness and conditioning. Such programmes coupled with dietary optimisation, adequate hydration and smoking cessation have been shown to be of benefit to patients, by improving their operative risk profile.

Exercise is similar to many drug interventions in terms of benefit in the secondary prevention of coronary heart disease and diabetes, rehabilitation after stroke and treatment of heart failure. Aerobic exercise is beneficial as it induces an improvement in major cardio-respiratory adaptations such as VO2 peak (max), cardiac output and heart rate. VO2 peak (max), being the best direct measurement of cardio-respiratory fitness, is an exceptional sign of health status. As such, it has been used as an independent predictor of mortality. Pre-operative oxygen uptake at anaerobic threshold of greater than 11 ml/min/kg was associated with decreased mortality after major surgery. After major surgery, post-operative complications have been attributed to deprived levels of global and local tissue oxygenation. This is attributed to insufficient cardio-respiratory fitness. It impacts on post-operative tissue healing particularly in anastomotic areas. Most peri-operative deaths in the elderly result from pre-existing cardiac or respiratory disease rather than surgical or anaesthetic complications. Major surgical procedures can increase oxygen demand of up to 50% above resting values. Exercise prior to surgery for individuals, who were not engaged in regular exercise, can result in reduced post-operative complications and hospitalisation time. A recent systematic review of pre-surgical exercise studies included eighteen studies on 966 participants with lung, colorectal and prostate cancers. Most studies showed preliminary positive changes in clinical outcomes with significant improvements in cardiorespiratory fitness, functional walking capacity and incontinence rate [8].

The pre-surgical fitness enhancement training should consist of three components:

a. *Aerobic training*: This mode of exercise should be pragmatic and dictated by patients' preference to include equivalent intensity of cycling, brisk walking, jogging or swimming or a combination.
b. Muscular Strength and Endurance (MSE) training (resistance training of upper, lower and trunk muscles). For this exercise, elastic bands with different levels of resistance and free weights (1, 1.5 and 2 kg) can be used to train arms, legs and trunk muscles. Repetitions of each exercise should be performed and increased progressively.
c. Inspiratory Muscle training (IMT) using an inspiratory threshold-loading device.

The three components should be performed five times per week initially for 1 hour, progressing to 1.5 hours. The objective is to increase the heart rate to 1.5 the resting value during training incrementally and for as long as possible.

On a practical level, fitness enhancement training (optimisation) should be encouraged for a number of weeks before surgery. Clearly this is not feasible for emergency surgery. However, for all elective surgery including cancer surgery such optimisation tilts the balance of risk in favour of the patient. For cancer surgery, the exercise programme could be undertaken during the period of neo-adjuvant chemo/radio therapy without delay to surgery.

CONDUCT OF ANAESTHESIA

Although anaesthetic techniques will vary depending on operative procedure, institutional experience, patient specific factors and individual preference; there is a high degree of commonality in anaesthetic techniques. In recent times, the advent of Enhanced Recovery Programs (ERPs) and Standardised Clinical Pathways (SCPs) are changing traditional techniques in an effort to enhance patient recovery times and improve outcomes. Despite this, there remains a strong evidence base for many areas of traditional anaesthetic techniques in UGI resection surgery.

The majority of patients presenting for benign UGI surgery are admitted on the day of surgery with a planned stay of 48 h or less. Patients with a high-risk profile including diabetics are usually admitted the day before surgery (or before) for optimization. In addition, patients scheduled to have high-risk surgery are admitted for optimization, acclimatization with ward structures and routines and for preparation for surgery.

Premedication

Sedatives: In all but the most anxious patients, sedative pre-medications are increasingly omitted. Concerns around dangers of gastric content aspiration, as well as the availability of potent, but short-acting anaesthetic agents have largely consigned the traditional "pre-medication" to history. This is particularly so in those presenting for anti-reflux surgery, in who obtunded airway refluxes due to sedation can have serious consequences in terms of aspiration risk. In very anxious patients, sedatives may still have a role in anxiolysis, but caution should be exercised to prevent over-sedation in the ward environment.

Gastric Prophylaxis: Regurgitation and aspiration of gastric contents at induction remains a serious complication, and is more commonly encountered in those with existing reflux disease or obstructive oesphago-gastric pathology. Premedication with H2-receptor antagonists or Proton Pump Inhibitor therapy is strongly advised to limit this danger.

Thromboembolism Prophylaxis: All patients undergoing major surgery remain at risk of thromboembolism, particularly those with active cancer and those with significantly raised Body Mass Index (BMI). A pre-operative dose of a low-molecular-weight heparin or similar agent is indicated. At least 12 hours should be allowed to elapse between the administration of this medication and attempts at thoracic epidural insertion.

Pre-operative carbohydrate drinks: Recent process advances in colorectal surgery have demonstrated the utility of pre-operative carbohydrate drinks in ensuring on-going normal bowel function and reduction of operative stress. Although this is an evolving field in UGI resection surgery, it is likely that pre-operative consumption of carbohydrate drinks will be of benefit to patients (Fig. **6**).

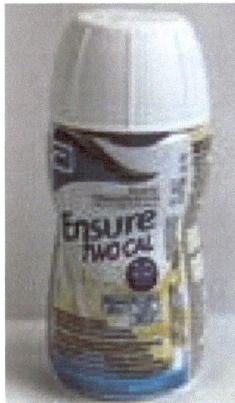

Fig. (6). Pre-operative Carbohydrate Drinks

Disinfectant mouthwashes are frequently helpful in reducing the bacterial flora of the obstructed upper gastro-intestinal tract. This is particularly important when the surgery involves anastomosis proximal to the obstruction where bacterial colonization may contaminate the operative site. Several studies have emphasized the importance and benefits of disinfectant mouthwashes for at least one week prior to surgery.

Monitoring

Routine monitoring (Oxygen saturation, non-invasive blood pressure, 3-lead ECG) is mandatory for all anaesthetic procedures; however, in the case of major upper gastrointestinal surgery is usually insufficient. The need for more invasive monitoring will be dictated by the patient's individual risks, and also the demands of the surgery being performed. In the case of oesophagectomy, a National Confidential Enquiry into Post-Operative Death (NCEPOD) report identified that measurement of direct invasive arterial blood pressure (94%), central venous pressure (88%), temperature (64%) and urine output (94%) were also commonly undertaken (Fig. **7**). This is in contrast to a minimally invasive anti-reflux procedure, where "routine" monitoring may be sufficient to ensure patient safety.

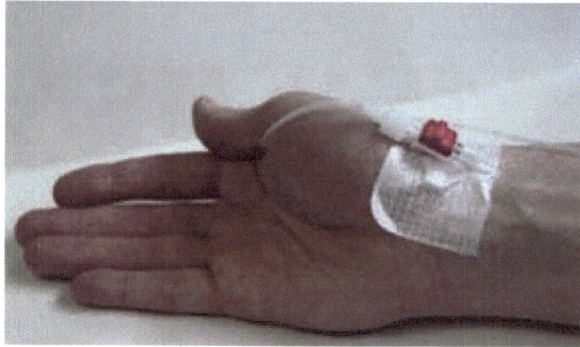

Fig. (7). Arterial line is for invasive blood pressure monitoring.

Capnography: This is considered mandatory throughout the procedure and increasingly into the recovery room/post-anaesthesia care unit, as it remains the only reliable way of detecting endotracheal tube misplacement or obstruction from an early point. Oxygen saturation monitoring is not sufficiently sensitive or specific to perform this function.

Cardiac Output Monitoring: It is increasingly recognised that optimal fluid administration is both challenging and essential to good patient outcome, particularly in the case of high-risk procedures involving an anastomosis. Though a number of studies have suggested that a restrictive strategy is associated with a better outcome, judging the individual requirements of a patient in a lengthy procedure can be a significant challenge.

Increasingly, cardiac output monitoring along with goal-directed fluid therapy are increasingly employed to address this problem. Though evidence of their absolute utility in upper GI surgery remains scant, there has been research to suggest an improvement in patient outcome in colorectal surgery. As such, it seems reasonable to advocate the use of cardiac output monitoring in major upper GI surgery, pending further evidence. It should be noted that the use of an oesophageal Doppler monitor is often impractical for UGI surgery; commonly used alternatives tend to rely on pulse-contour analysis. This uses data gathered from the patient's arterial line monitoring trace and makes a number of statistical assumptions about the patient to calculate cardiac output. It is a readily accessible monitor, though some experience is required to interpret the data in situations where cardiac output may be changing rapidly, such as in major haemorrhage.

Anaesthesia

Analgesia: Depending on whether the procedure is to be carried out open or using minimally invasive techniques, differing analgesic strategies may be appropriate. In major, open surgery with a high abdominal incision (particularly if a thoracotomy is anticipated), thoracic epidural analgesia (TEA) is thought to represent the optimal analgesic technique. The thoracotomy wound represents significant challenges in terms of postoperative respiratory function and recovery if analgesia is sub optimal The MASTER trial (Multi-centre Australian Study of Epidural Anaesthesia) showed that although Epidural use conferred no reduction in mortality or major morbidity compared to opiate based analgesia, it significantly improved pain scores and lowered rates of postoperative respiratory failure in high risk patients undergoing major upper GI surgery [9]. Multiple other studies have also demonstrated the utility of TEA, with one going so far as to suggest that TEA usage may actually reduce the risk of surgical complications such as anastomotic leakage [10]. As such, thoracic epidural analgesia remains the gold standard analgesia for UGI resection surgery.

If there are specific contraindications to TEA, the use of para-vertebral analgesic techniques can be considered, as they provide good quality analgesia, without a number of the cardiovascular effects of TEA. It should be noted that, in the case of oesophagectomy in particular, a paravertebral technique will only provide analgesia for the thoracotomy wound, and another analgesic technique for the laparotomy wound will be required. Recently, studies have observed considerable success in the use of rectus sheath catheters (either surgically or ultrasonographically placed) with a continuous infusion of local anaesthetics into the wound for up to 72 hours. This method of analgesia could be used in conjunction with a paravertebral block.

In less invasive surgery such as minimally invasive anti-reflux procedures and cardiomyotomy for acahlasia, a balanced analgesic regime comprising simple analgesics (*e.g.* regular paracetamol, opioids either enteral/parenteral) along with judicious use of local anaesthetic blocks (*e.g.* Tranvesus abdominis Plane blocks) is often adequate. An individual analysis of a patient's physiological reserve, particularly with regard to respiratory function is advisable before the analgesic strategy is finalised. In the case of minimally invasive bariatric surgery, it is often undesirable that patients receive large doses of long-acting opiate medications due to their effects on suppressing respiratory function. In these procedures, the use of local anaesthetics at laparoscopic port sites, coupled with simple oral analgesia should provide optimal, safe pain relief.

***Anaesthetic Technique*:** All major UGI surgery will require general anaesthesia, and therefore the main choice is between volatile or total intravenous techniques for maintenance of anaesthesia. Both have their advocates, though often individual or institutional experience will influence the final choice. What is essential is for the anaesthetist to become familiar with both but to have special knowledge and experience of a favoured method with all its pitfalls and how to overcome these. There will always be patients who would benefit from the application of one or other technique and the familiarity with both techniques is essential in those circumstances.

In the case of operative procedures requiring one-lung ventilation (OLV), there are theoretical benefits in the use of total intravenous techniques (Table **3**). However, no evidence exists to suggest that they result in an improved clinical outcome.

Table 3. Anaesthetic techniques, their advantages and disadvantages.

Technique	Advantages	Disadvantages
Volatile Anaesthesia	Familiarity. Volatile agents may have an immuno-modulatory effect on pulmonary inflammatory response after One-Lung Ventilation (OLV). Modern agents are short acting and quick in offset.	Environmental pollutants. Expensive agents and machinery to supply. May blunt hypoxic pulmonary vasoconstriction (HPV) during OLV, contributing to hypoxaemia.
Total Intravenous Anaesthesia	Protective of HPV during OLV. Short acting agents with predictable washout. Less atmospheric pollution caused by their use.	Require specific experience. Associated with increased risk of patient's awareness intra-operatively.

***Double Lumen Tube Insertion (DLT) for One Lung Ventilation (OLV)*:** In the case of two or three stage oesophagectomy when surgical access is via an open thoracotomy or occasionally in thoracoscopic surgery, it is often necessary to perform One Lung Ventilation (OLV). This facilitates collapse of the right lung to improve surgical access to the thoracic oesophagus. OLV can be achieved via a number of strategies, depending on unit experience and preference. They would include the use of a Double Lumen Tube (DLT) or the use of a single-lumen tube and a bronchial blocker.

A Double Lumen Tube (DLT) consists of a large endotracheal tube with a preformed bronchial extension (either left or right). This can be independently sealed by means of a bronchial lumen cuff, ensuring lung isolation and independent lung ventilation. By contrast, a bronchial blocker is a thin wire-like device with a balloon at the tip which may be passed down a standard single-lumen endotracheal tube, before being placed in the right or left main bronchus and inflated (often under fibre-optic guidance). This will result in the ability to perform One Lung Ventilation, though with less reliable lung isolation.

The commonest and most favoured method consists of the use of a single use DLT such as Bronchocath (Fig. **12**) for superior lung isolation and control of ventilation. Inserting a DLT is a complex process, and is summarized in the following images (Figs. **8**, **9** and **10**). There are a number of key points to consider:

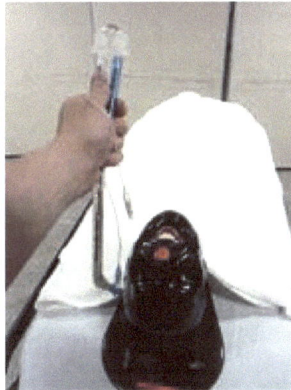

Fig. (8). Double lumen tube (DLT) orientation for tracheal intubation.

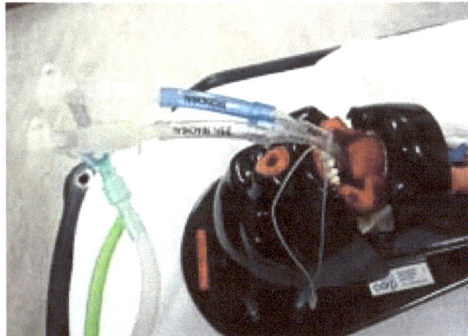

Fig. (9). DLT in situ, bronchial and tracheal lumens clearly marked.

- Size: selecting the correct size of DLT can be difficult. Convention suggests that either a 35 or 37 F DLT be selected for a female patient and a 39 or 41F for male patients. However, small-framed males may require smaller DLTs and large framed females may require larger DLTs.
- The exact selection of Right or Left DLTs remains a point of contention and research has not shown a difference in outcome dependent on this variable. The

choice is individual for the anaesthetist and is dictated by their custom and practice.

- The use of fibre-optic bronchoscopy to ensure optimal bronchial cuff placement both at the time of insertion and also after any patient movement (*e.g.* supine to lateral) is strongly advocated. Although this is an accurate method to ensure optimal cuff placement, manual one-sided occlusion and auscultation is also used.

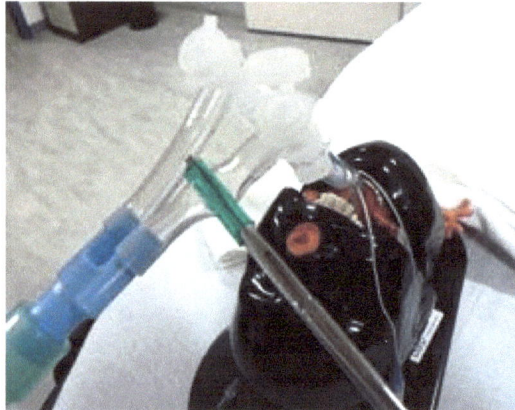

Fig. (10). Clamp position on tracheal lumen inlet, allowing air leak from bronchial tube to be detectable through tracheal lumen outlet.

Patient Preparation: The patient should be appropriately monitored and then anaesthesia induced. The lungs should be ventilated with 100% oxygen whilst neuro-muscular paralysis is instituted.

Inserting the Double Lumen Tube: Using a laryngoscope, a view of the glottis should be obtained. The DLT should be positioned at 90° to its intended final resting position, and the bronchial extension carefully passed into the glottis, followed by the rest of the DLT. Approximately half way down the trachea, the DLT should be axially rotated through 90° before being passed gently down until the black lines on the tube are within the glottis. Thereafter, the endotracheal balloon should be inflated until no gas leak is audible and endotracheal placement confirmed with capnography.

Checking Position of the ET Tube

Clinical Method: Observation to ensure both lungs are being ventilated (a combination of chest observation and auscultation) indicating the tracheal lumen is above the carina. A clamp is placed on the endotracheal lumen gas inlet and the port at the top of the endotracheal lumen is then opened. Ventilation should continue via the endobronchial lumen. Air is gently added to the bronchial cuff until no further air leak can be detected returning up the endotracheal lumen, through the open port. The total volume of air should not exceed 2.5 mls. Should more be required, it is likely that the bronchial lumen is misplaced (Fig. **11**).

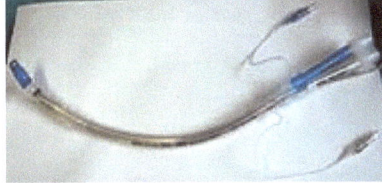

Fig. (11). Bronchocath: a commonly used type of Double Lumen Tube.

Fibre-optic Method: A fibre-optic bronchoscope (FOB) is passed down the endotracheal lumen port. Firstly, the tube is confirmed to be not abutting the carina, and that there is no accessory right upper lobe bronchus visible. Secondly, the position of the endobronchial lumen is observed, to ensure it is within the main bronchus. The cuff is gently inflated under direct vision, ensuring that the cuff does not herniate out with the bronchus and the FOB is used to check that the distal lumen is not obstructed.

If surgical techniques for minimally invasive thoracic access are used, then by positioning the patient semi prone on a wedge OLV may be avoided.

Ventilation Strategies

The topic of optimal ventilation during surgery has recently attracted renewed interest. In the case of major UGI surgery, and specifically oesophagectomy, it is well recognised that pulmonary complications independently predispose patients to increased morbidity and also mortality and are in fact the most common cause of death post oesophagectomy [4].

As such, careful selection and adjustment of ventilatory parameters during surgery is of the greatest importance, particularly during OLV, where the ventilated lung is at risk of iatrogenic injury.

A number of studies have proposed the use of both Pressure Controlled Ventilation (PCV) and Positive End Expiratory Pressure (PEEP), concluding that they offer superior ventilatory mechanics to other ventilation strategies. Suggested indices include:

- Tidal volumes of 5-6 mls kg^{-1} (lean body mass)
- Optimisation of PEEP by use of inflection point on volume-pressure curves
- Limiting plateau pressures <25 cm H_2O

- Limiting peak inspiratory pressures <35 cm H_2O
- Allowing Permissive hypercapnia

Whilst it would seem that PCV in particular reduces the risk of barotrauma by reducing Peak Airway Pressure (whilst PEEP reduces the risk of atelectasis trauma), it should be noted that this has not shown to correlate with an improvement in arterial oxygen tension. As such, strategies to manage hypoxaemia during OLV remain important, even with optimal ventilation parameters.

Management of Hypoxaemia during OLV

The locally developed and used algorithm describes the stepwise management of hypoxaemia during OLV. The initial step must always be to confirm that there has not been displacement or occlusion of the endobronchial lumen prior to other measures being instituted (Fig. **12**).

Thereafter, a number of other measures may improve either lung recruitment or oxygen carriage, as described below. It should be noted that in UGI surgery, the option of clamping the Pulmonary Artery of the collapsed lung, to limit a possible shunt mechanism, is not an option.

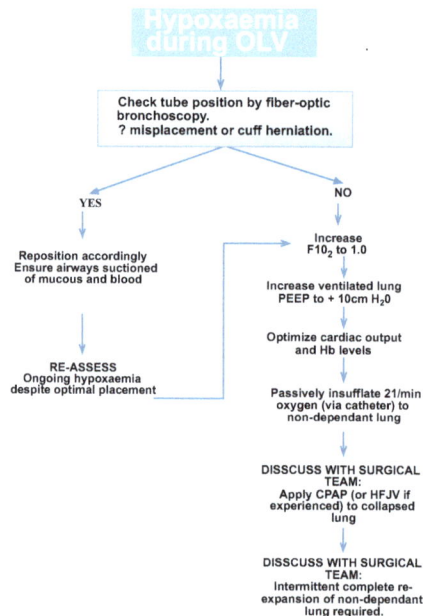

Fig. (12). Local algorithm for management of hypoxaemia during OLV

Development of hypoxaemia (*i.e.* arterial oxygenation <90%) during OLV may be explained by considering oxygen storage, dissociation of oxygen from haemoglobin, the relationship between ventilation and perfusion, and factors that reduce the effect of hypoxic pulmonary vasoconstriction.

There are two main strategies to manage hypoxaemia during OLV: prevention and treatment. Prevention of hypoxaemia may be achieved by ventilation of the patient's lungs with 100% oxygen with time for de-nitrogenation before OLV.

When profound hypoxaemia develops during OLV, it is necessary to treat the problem by increasing the inspired oxygen to 100% and, on some occasions, ventilating both lungs. Surgery may have to be discontinued whilst the problem is managed. The patient's lungs should be ventilated manually and checks should be performed. Strategies to manage hypoxaemia may be divided into three main categories: delivery of oxygen to the patient, treatment of causes associated with high airway pressure, and management of physiological hypoxaemia.

Positioning and Temperature Control

Major UGI resection surgery has the potential to be lengthy in nature, and therefore careful patient positioning with particular emphasis on pressure areas padding and care is essential to prevent iatrogenic injury. The use of gel-material padding to relieve pressure areas or of vacuum-mattress devices to ensure optimal position should be incorporated into practice

From the anaesthetic perspective, all positioning and pressure area care is important, but none more so than that of head and neck position monitoring ensuring the brachial plexus is not stretched when in the lateral position. Particular attention should be paid to the position and access to endotracheal tubes and lines, especially if the patient's position is altered during surgery.

Temperature control and prevention of hypothermia is also very important particularly for lengthy cases. During lengthy surgery, hypothermia can result in sub-optimal cardiovascular and respiratory parameters as well as worsening coagulopathy. Forced air warming blankets may be employed, but often their coverage is limited by the need for extensive surgical access. In such case, warming mattress devices should be considered. IV fluids should be warmed and the use of a circle system in the ventilator minimizes respiratory heat and moisture losses.

Temperature monitoring should be employed to prevent hyperthermia by over-warming.

Thromboembolism Prophylaxis

Whilst all patients should receive chemical thromboprophlaxis in the peri-operative period, mechanical means should also be employed during surgery. Usually, these will include the use of graduated elastic stockings and pneumatic leg compression devices, which can be engaged not only during surgery, but also into recovery and potentially beyond into critical care environments. These devices inflate and deflate at regular intervals to encourage the movement of peripheral venous blood to more central veins. In this way, they seek to artificially replicate the actions of the physiological muscle pump. Care to prevent thrombosis from poor positioning and venous stasis as well as dehydration should be undertaken.

Extubation

Extubation is a very important part of the anaesthesia process. It must be done gently and timed to coincide with the most appropriate time when patients have regained consciousness and are able to support their ventilation. The advent of enhanced recovery programs have shown that early extubation of patients is both safe and reduces morbidity and mortality, provided optimal analgesia and a satisfactory fluid status have been achieved [11]. In practice, most patients will be appropriate for extubation at the end of major UGI resection surgery, and with the use of short-acting general anaesthetic agents, this should be eminently possible.

The advent of the cyclo-dextrin "Sugamadex" is another major advance in ensuring all amino-steroid neuromuscular paralyzing agents are rendered ineffective at the end of a procedure, thus ensuring optimal return of respiratory muscle function. Though theoretically expensive, the use of this drug has a number of potential advantages in preventing post-operative respiratory insufficiency in the immediate post-extubation period. Some of the weight management bariatric patients require complete muscle paralysis to facilitate surgical access and the use of Sugamadex in this patient group allows safe extubation at the end of the procedure.

In rare cases, intraoperative complications or patient-specific factors may necessitate a period of ventilation in a critical care environment. Strenuous attempts to limit the duration of this further ventilation should be made by regular monitoring of the patient's respiratory status with appropriate adjustments to facilitate extubation.

When OLV has been performed, it is usually preferable to exchange the DLT for a single lumen tube prior to admission to critical care if post-operative ventilation is planned. Great care should be taken at this time as the patient remains at high risk of aspiration and attendant pulmonary complications due to their suppressed upper airway reflexes under anaesthesia. (Fig. **13**)

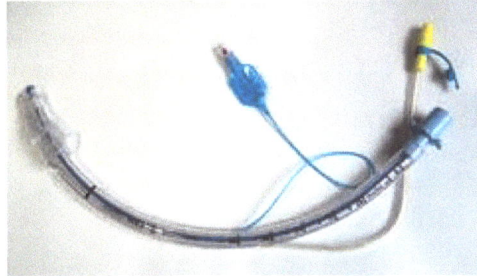

Fig. (13). Supra-glottic Suction Port tubes, commonly used in an ICU setting.The Immediate Post-Operative Period

Most patients will progress initially to an appropriate theatre recovery or a dedicated post-anaesthesia care unit. Full monitoring should be employed during this period, and X-rays to confirm central intravenous line placement and re-expansion of the lun g including chest drain placement should be obtained (Fig. **14**).

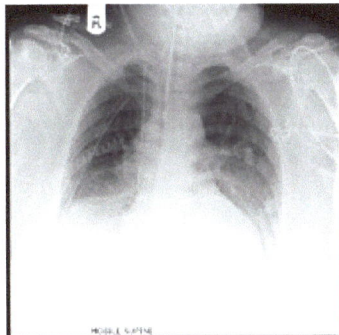

Fig. (14). Chest X-ray of patient in ICU, post oesophagectomy showing the endotracheal tube in situ with an expanded right lung after right thoracotomy. A naso-gastric tube is used to deflate the transposed gastric conduit.

Prior to return to a critical care environment, the patient should be thoroughly reviewed to ensure optimal analgesia and fluid management has been achieved. It is also helpful to set acceptable parameters and review fluid requirements, which need to be passed on to the receiving ward staff.

Patients who have undergone minimally invasive anti reflux procedures can safely be transferred to the ward from the recovery room. Bariatric surgery patients who have undergone weight management surgery present a greater challenge. Often a transfer device (Hover-mat) is used to aid transfer to and from the operating table and into bed. Hydraulic beds will allow the patient to be positioned in an optimal sitting position. If the patient uses a home CPAP machine this should accompany them to the recovery room and may be required along with some supplemental oxygen. Mobilisation in this group of patients is essential and should be started in the immediate post-operative period once they are awake and comfortable.

INFECTION AND ANTI-MICROBIAL THERAPY

Infective Complications

Many of the complications seen in the perioperative period involve infection. Of note, pulmonary infection and surgical site infections are of particular concern. After oesophagectomy, up to 40% of patients will experience significant pulmonary complications, predominantly infection, and up to 50% of those patients will die [12]. Anastomotic leakage, too, carries significant risks, occurring in up to 14% of patients, with mortality estimated at 5-35%. In particular, breakdown of a mediastinal anastomosis can be both difficult to identify and extremely injurious to the patient concerned, due to the intense inflammatory response and mediastinitis that may result.

A high index of suspicion, prompt recognition of complications including sepsis, along with rapid initiation of antimicrobial therapy is of paramount importance if these complications are suspected. Attempts to identify the pathogen in blood cultures, sputum samples and aspirates of pus from drains should be made, but they should not delay the initiation of broad-spectrum antibiotic therapy, as this intervention remains the single most important factor in the treatment of sepsis, with an increase in mortality of approximately 8% for every hour of delay in severely ill patients.

As well as antibiotic therapy, it is important to remember that the upper GI tract contains fungal and yeast species, which may also become pathogenic if continuity of that tract is breached. Early advice from specialist microbiology teams is strongly recommended; ensuring sufficiently broad antimicrobial and antifungal cover is instituted promptly (Fig. **15**).

In certain patients, antimicrobial therapy may prove insufficient, and more definitive, invasive measures are required. In the case of pulmonary infection; respiratory embarrassment and subsequent respiratory failure should provoke early consultation with Intensive Care services. Many of these patients are inappropriate for forms of non-invasive ventilation/mask CPAP due to the risks of distension of the gastric tube, anastomotic blood supply compromise and risk of aspiration, therefore early intubation and respiratory support may be required. Respiratory physiotherapy can assist in bronchial toilet in the un-intubated patient, but more definitive bronchoscopy and bronchial lavage is helpful in the intubated patient. This involves the direct removal of secretions from the respiratory tract, particularly those obstructing major bronchi. Washing with sterile saline can assist in this process.

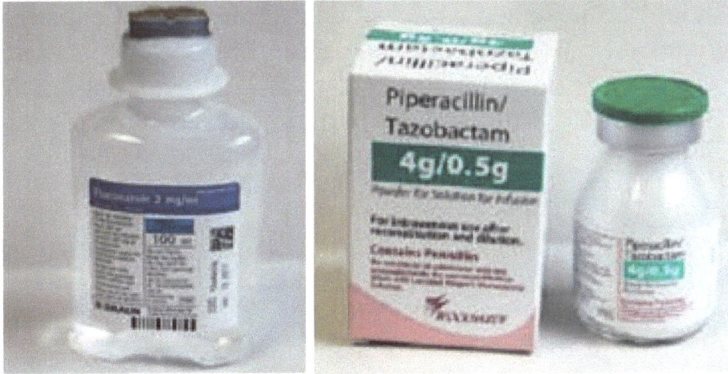

Fig. (15). Examples of Antibiotics and Antifungals used for the management of post-operative complications.

Due to the potential for inflammation after major surgery, there is a significant risk that many of these patients will go on to develop not only a pulmonary infection, but also a systemic inflammatory response, resulting in Adult Respiratory Distress Syndrome (ARDS). This requires prompt specialist intensive care management and carries a mortality risk in the region of 40%.

Small anastomotic leaks can often be managed with conservative measures (keeping the patient nil by mouth or placing a removable covered oesophageal stent) and antimicrobial therapy alone. In the case of larger leaks or abscess formation, additional surgical measures including thoracoscopic drainage may be required, necessitating further anaesthesia. Decisions for further surgery should not be taken lightly as these patients represent a considerable perioperative anaesthetic risk. Early consultation with critical care services is indicated to ensure adequate operative and post-operative support.

Routine Prophylaxis

The term surgical site infection (SSI) is used to encompass the surgical wound and infections involving the body cavities such as the peritoneal or thoracic cavity. SSI is one of the most common healthcare associated infections (HAI) and contributes to morbidity, mortality and delayed discharge from hospital. Risk factors which can increase the rate of surgical site infections include patient factors such as co-morbidities, poor nutritional status, obesity, smoking, and operation factors such as length of surgical procedure, multiple surgical sites, GI anastomosis and the use of foreign materials including drains.

Prophylactic administration of antibiotics inhibits growth of contaminating bacteria thus reducing the risk of infection. However, administration of antibiotics also increases the prevalence of antibiotic-resistant bacteria. Surgical antibiotic prophylaxis should be regarded as an adjunct rather than a substitute for, good surgical technique. Antibiotic prophylaxis should be regarded as one component of an overall, effective policy for the control of healthcare associated infection. The goals of prophylactic administration of antibiotics to surgical patients are to:

- Reduce the incidence of surgical site infection.
- Use antibiotics supported by evidence of effectiveness.
- Minimise the effect of antibiotics on normal bacterial flora.
- Minimise adverse effects.
- Cause minimal change to the patient's host defences.

Before surgery, patients scheduled to have resection should be adequately prepared by minimizing all risk factors such as cessation of smoking, and an increase in exercise levels. Oral decontamination with anti-septic mouthwashes should be commenced 5 days before surgery. Skin decontamination using aseptic baths should be done on the day of surgery. During major UGI resection surgery, all patients will require antibiotic prophylaxis due to the potential for leakage of gut organisms into the peritoneal or thoracic cavity. Exact agent selection will be governed by local guidance on antibiotic prophylaxis as well as known patient allergies. In general, selected agents should be active against a range of aerobic and anaerobic pathogens as well as anti-fungal agents where appropriate.

POST-OPERATIVE CARE AND MONITORING

The post-operative care and monitoring of patients after major UGI resection surgery can be more challenging than the operative course they have just undertaken. Given that few complications happen during the actual operative period, it stands to reason that most must occur post-operatively, making this period considerably more challenging than the one that preceded it. Good quality post-operative care is essential, requiring considerable multi-specialist input. However, recent advances in streamlining this process are showing promise, particularly in high-risk surgeries such as oesophagectomy and bariatric malabsorptive procedures.

Selection of Location

The nature of major surgery and the presence of invasive monitoring and thoracic epidural analgesia will often dictate the location of further patient care. Recent investigations into the role of Enhanced Recovery Protocols and Standardised Clinical Pathways for oesophagectomy have shown that it is both unnecessary and indeed undesirable to admit patients to the Intensive Care Unity (ICU), still ventilated, as a matter of routine. However, as the post-operative care of these patients is potentially complex, it is reasonable that they be admitted to critical care environments, and cared for by specialists experienced in critical care medicine, and the care of post-operative Upper GI surgery patients in particular (Fig. **16**).

In less invasive surgery, such as minimally invasive anti-reflux procedures, it is preferable that the patient's post-operative course be normalised as far as possible. Rather than critical care, emphasis should be placed on an early return to mobility and self-care in a ward environment, staffed by appropriately experienced clinicians and nurses familiar with the post-operative care of these patients.

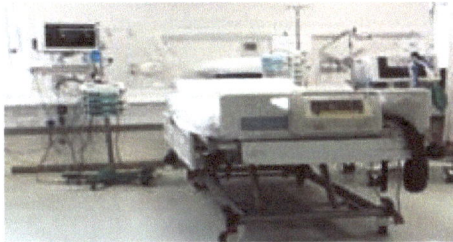

Fig. (16). A typical Critical Care Environment bed space.

Patients undergoing bariatric weight management surgery should be cared for in a ward area that is suitably equipped for their needs in terms of provision of suitable beds, seating *etc*. A culture that promotes early mobilisation and dietary support is essential.

Enhanced Recovery

A number of systems and processes to enable "Enhanced Recovery" after major UGI resection surgery have been described. Essentially, they seek to rapidly mobilise patients, ensuring early mobility to promote better respiratory outcomes. This relies on a wide range of other measures such as optimal analgesia and satisfactory fluid status to enable aggressive, early physiotherapy to take place. Efforts to ensure early nutrition, which can be with the aid of a feeding jejunostomy, are also essential, as patient nutritional status remains an important predictor of eventual recovery, particularly after cancer resection surgery. To this end, early specialist advice and access to high-calorie, nutritionally complete food supplementation is vital.

Though not present in all institutions, the use of Enhanced Recovery Protocols (ERBs) have been associated with a marked improvement in patient outcome (both morbidity and mortality) as well as shorter stays in hospital and reduced costs. Indeed, a recent Cochrane review strongly endorsed their use in improving outcome after oesophagectomy, with some centres claiming to have reduced mortality to as little as 1% after the adoption of ERBs [13].

Goal Directed Fluid Therapy in First 24 Hours

A continuing point of controversy is optimal fluid therapy after major surgery. There is much conflicting evidence in other areas of surgery, particularly after colorectal resection, but relatively little after major upper GI surgery. Restrictive fluid administration strategies have been shown to have potential benefits. This is likely due to less pulmonary oedema and anastomotic oedema resulting from excessive fluid administration.

Certainly, it would seem reasonable that careful monitoring and optimisation through the use of a cardiac output monitor (such as a Pulse Contour Analysis Monitor: see above) represents a sensible intervention to monitor and limit fluid administration. In this way fluid challenges can be given and their effects quantified quickly in terms of effect on Cardiac Output. However, use of these monitors relies on the availability of such equipment out with the operating theatre environment, and also in the presence of skilled staff familiar with their use.

Vasopressor Use

Traditionally, there has been great resistance to the use of vasopressor therapy in the post-operative period, with concerns around arterial vasoconstriction resulting in ischaemia and necrosis of anastomoses. However, more recent work has suggested that this may not be the case, with no association shown between short-acting vasopressor use and anastomotic leak. Indeed, preventing excessive fluid administration whilst maintaining mean arterial pressure in the presence of Thoracic Epidural Analgesia may well necessitate the use of vasopressor/inotropic support. The administration of these agents should be undertaken by those experienced and familiar with their use., Specialist care should ensure that low blood pressure is not caused by other factors, such as sepsis.

Respiratory Sufficiency and Role of Physiotherapy

Respiratory complications remain both one of the most common and also the most serious adverse events after major UGI resection surgery. Indeed, they are the most common cause of death after major surgery. Multiple factors must be controlled to prevent respiratory complications from occurring, ranging from prevention of aspiration by 30-degree head-up tilt on the patient's bed, to cautious fluid therapy as discussed above.

The importance of the physiotherapy team in post-operative management cannot be over-emphasised. Judicious chest physiotherapy as well as the use of techniques such as incentive spirometry is vital in ensuring optimal respiratory outcomes, often in patients with substantial smoking histories and pre-existing pulmonary pathology (Fig. **17**). An incentive spirometer is a device where a predetermined amount of respiratory effort is required to lift three plastic balls up in plastic tubes. In this way, patients are required to take tidal volume breaths and generate greater levels of positive end expiratory pressure, leading to greater lung recruitment.

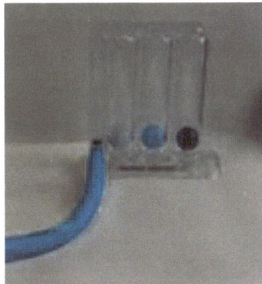

Fig. (17). Incentive Spirometer for use either before surgery or in the post-operative period.

The safe use of non-invasive ventilatory techniques resulting in either continuous or intermittent positive airways pressure remains an unanswered question with concerns around anastomotic breakdown potentially limiting their use. Early discussions between surgical, anaesthetic/intensive care and physiotherapy teams should be undertaken if a patient has been identified as potentially requiring such therapy (Fig. **18**).

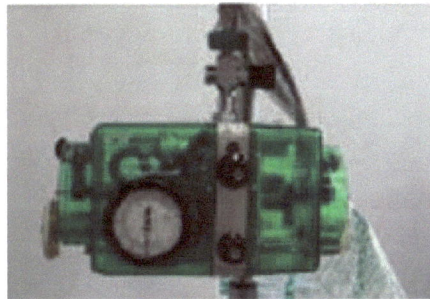

Fig. (18). Device for positive pressure recruitment manoeuvres ("The Bird").

Recognising and Managing Early Complications/Problems

A number of complications are common after major upper GI surgery, several of which (pulmonary infection/inflammation and anastomotic leakage) have already been discussed. Further complications can include the following:

Cardiac Arrhythmia: perhaps the most common complication, particularly after oesophagectomy where it is thought to occur in up to 60% of patients. Atrial Fibrillation (AF) remains the most common arrhythmia, though ventricular tachyarrhythmias have also been reported. AF is independently associated with a number of other complications, including pulmonary infection, anastomotic leakage and surgical sepsis. Unfortunately, it remains difficult to control; with studies suggesting neither beta-blockade nor prophylactic digitalisation have any beneficial effect. There is currently much interest in the role of statins in preventing perioperative AF, though the mechanism of this action remains unclear. In practice, the management of AF is two-fold; the first step is to try to identify a treatable cause, for example electrolyte abnormalities such as hypokalaemia or low magnesium, which can be treated by intravenous supplementation. Other causes of AF such as infection require treatment of the underlying precipitant cause. The second part is to determine of AF is compromising cardiac output. If AF is compromising cardiac output, blood pressure or organ perfusion then steps should be taken to either control the heart rate with drugs such as Beta-blockers or to restore sinus rhythm either pharmacologically with amiodarone or electrically using DC cardioversion. It can be difficult to restore and maintain sinus rhythm if the underlying driving cause is not treated.

Venous Thromboembolism (VTE): Cancer patients in particular remain at high risk of VTE post operatively, with rates of up to 20% observed. It is unsurprising that this carries a substantial risk of morbidity and mortality. This effect is likely worsened by adjuvant chemotherapy, which may result in endothelial damage, predisposing VTE (particularly regimes including cisplatin and 5-fluorouracil). Prophylaxis remains the mainstay of therapy, with chemical and mechanical means as well as early mobilisation providing the best reduction in risk (Fig. **19**).

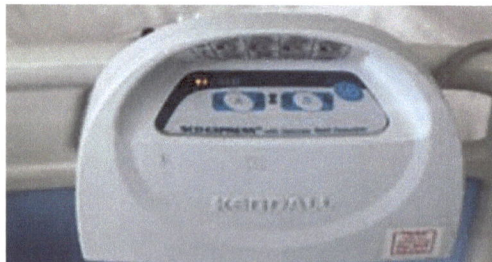

Fig. (19). Flowtron Compression Device pump.

Chylothorax: This is a relatively uncommon complication after oesophagectomy. It usually presents with an on-going cloudy milky-white output from the thoracic drain. It is thought to occur in less than 4% of patients and is due to damage to the thoracic duct during thoractomy. Conservative measures such as elimination of fat from the diet are usually sufficient, but invasive therapy such as thoracic duct ligation via a repeat thoracotomy is definitive but associated with an increase in mortality.

CONSENT FOR PUBLICATION

Not applicable.

CONFLICT OF INTEREST

The authors declare no conflict of interest, financial or otherwise.

ACKNOWLEDGEMENT

Declare none.

REFERENCES

[1]   Chang AC, Ji H, Birkmeyer NJ, Orringer MB, Birkmeyer JD. Outcomes after transhiatal and transthoracic esophagectomy for cancer. Ann Thorac Surg 2008; 85(2): 424-9.
[http://dx.doi.org/10.1016/j.athoracsur.2007.10.007] [PMID: 18222237]

[2]   Mercuro G, Cadeddu C, Piras A, *et al.* Early epirubicin-induced myocardial dysfunction revealed by serial tissue Doppler echocardiography: correlation with inflammatory and oxidative stress markers. Oncologist 2007; 12(9): 1124-33.
[http://dx.doi.org/10.1634/theoncologist.12-9-1124] [PMID: 17914082]

[3]   Mallampati SR, Gatt SP, Gugino LD, *et al.* A clinical sign to predict difficult tracheal intubation: a prospective study. Can Anaesth Soc J 1985; 32(4): 429-34.
[http://dx.doi.org/10.1007/BF03011357] [PMID: 4027773]

[4]   Ferguson MK, Martin TR, Reeder LB, Olak J. Mortality after esophagectomy: risk factor analysis. World J Surg 1997; 21(6): 599-603.
[http://dx.doi.org/10.1007/s002689900279] [PMID: 9230656]

[5]   Ridgway ZA, Howell SJ. Cardiopulmonary exercise testing: a review of methods and applications in surgical patients. Eur J Anaesthesiol 2010; 27(10): 858-65.
[http://dx.doi.org/10.1097/EJA.0b013e32833c5b05] [PMID: 20689441]

[6]   Murray P, Whiting P, Hutchinson SP, Ackroyd R, Stoddard CJ, Billings C. Preoperative shuttle walking testing and outcome after oesophagogastrectomy. Br J Anaesth 2007; 99(6): 809-11.
[http://dx.doi.org/10.1093/bja/aem305] [PMID: 17959592]

[7]   Win T, Jackson A, Sharples L, *et al.* Cardiopulmonary exercise tests and lung cancer surgical outcome. Chest 2005; 127(4): 1159-65.
[PMID: 15821190]

[8]   Singh F, Newton RU, Galvão DA, Spry N, Baker MK. A systematic review of pre-surgical exercise
        intervention studies with cancer patients. Surg Oncol 2013; 22(2): 92-104.
        [http://dx.doi.org/10.1016/j.suronc.2013.01.004] [PMID: 23434347]

[9]   Rigg JR, Jamrozik K, Myles PS, *et al.* Epidural anaesthesia and analgesia and outcome of major
        surgery: a randomised trial. Lancet 2002; 359(9314): 1276-82.
        [http://dx.doi.org/10.1016/S0140-6736(02)08266-1] [PMID: 11965272]

[10]   Michelet P, D'Journo XB, Roch A, *et al.* Perioperative risk factors for anastomotic leakage after
        esophagectomy: influence of thoracic epidural analgesia. Chest 2005; 128(5): 3461-6.
        [http://dx.doi.org/10.1378/chest.128.5.3461] [PMID: 16304300]

[11]   Lanuti M, de Delva PE, Maher A, *et al.* Feasibility and outcomes of an early extubation policy after
        esophagectomy. Ann Thorac Surg 2006; 82(6): 2037-41.
        [http://dx.doi.org/10.1016/j.athoracsur.2006.07.024] [PMID: 17126107]

[12]   McKevith JM, Pennefather SH. Respiratory complications after oesophageal surgery. Curr Opin
        Anaesthesiol 2010; 23(1): 34-40.
        [http://dx.doi.org/10.1097/ACO.0b013e328333b09b] [PMID: 19858717]

[13]   Rotter T, Kinsman L, James E, *et al.* Clinical pathways: effects on professional practice, patient
        outcomes, length of stay and hospital costs. Cochrane Database Syst Rev 2010; Mar 17: CD006632.
        [http://dx.doi.org/10.1002/14651858.CD006632.pub2]

CHAPTER 2

Peri-Operative Care After Oesophago-gastric Surgery

Amy Sadler and **Shaun McLeod**[*]

Department of Anaesthesia, Ninewells Hospital and Medical School, Dundee, Scotland, UK

Abstract: Adult critical care is an important, high profile and high-cost area of modern healthcare provision. Postoperative management after elective oesophago-gastric surgery for cancer has a huge bearing on mortality and morbidity. Assessment of the impact of surgery requires reliable tools that assess the morbidity and mortality risks, including the severity of the surgical insult. These tools have evolved over the last century but are not patient specific. In general, intensive care provides level 3 care to patients requiring mechanical ventilation where as a high dependency unit (level 2 care), has a vital role in patients requiring support for a single failing organ system. Post-operative monitoring, analgesia and nutrition are the main tenets of critical care.

Tissue injury secondary to surgical trauma produces profound changes to all body systems and triggers the stress response. Although considerable effort has gone into defining the stress response over the past century, very little advance has been made to negate or modify the stress response or its effects on the surgical patient. The surgical insult also produces inherent changes to ventilatory mechanics. The combination triggers single or multi-organ failure. The main systems affected in this cascade are the respiratory, cardiovascular and renal systems. Hepatic and coagulation systems failure tend to be late and multi-factorial. Critical care units have evolved in the multifaceted management of these failing systems.

Keywords: Anaesthesia, Analgesia, Discharge criteria, Post-operative care, Critical care, Scoring systems, Post-operative monitoring, Nutrition, The stress response, System support, Modes of ventilation.

POST-OPERATIVE CARE

Patients undergoing major upper gastrointestinal (GI) surgery may require post-operative critical care for a number of reasons. A significant number of these patients have significant co-existing medical problems and are of advanced age.

[*] **Corresponding author Shaun McLeod:** Department of Anaesthesia, Ninewells Hospital and Medical School, Dundee DD1 9SY, Scotland, UK; Tel: +44 1382 660111; E-mail: shaun.mcleod@nhs.net

In addition, by nature of the diseases affecting the oesophagus and stomach, patients tend to be malnourished. The surgical procedures tend to be complex, of long duration, with significant blood loss and fluid and electrolyte shifts. The site of the access wound(s) and extent of dissection can cause severe post-operative pain. The procedures are associated with high physiological stress response and can lead to profound physiological upset including respiratory failure. Profound cardiovascular adaptations occur in the post-operative period, which can have significant impact on tissue perfusion. Finally, the majority of patients who have had a resection will have a critical anastomosis, which requires adequate perfusion of oxygenated blood to heal.

Postoperative management after elective oesophago-gastric surgery for cancer has a huge bearing on mortality and morbidity. Thoracic-abdominal incision with associated pain, extended operative time with consequent extracellular fluid shifts, single lung ventilation, and potential for prolonged postoperative mechanical ventilation and comorbidities in patients with cancer, all contribute to high perioperative risk. Respiratory problems remain the major cause of both mortality and morbidity after oesophago-gastric surgery for cancer. A specific pulmonary disorder, acute respiratory distress syndrome (ARDS) occurs in 10-20% of patients after oesophagectomy. ARDS mortality exceeds 50%. Atrial fibrillation, that complicates recovery in 20 to 25% of patients after oesophagectomy, contributes to make the outcome worse. Anesthesiologists have adopted advanced clinical strategies known to optimize patient outcome. Decreased postoperative mortality and morbidity have been associated with epidural analgesia, bronchoscopy to clear persistent bronchial secretions, intraoperative fluid restriction and early extubation. It has been shown that setting up early respiratory physiotherapy and mobilisation may improve functional recovery.

Adult critical care is an important, high profile and high-cost area of modern healthcare provision [1]. Critical care services are atypical in the wide heterogeneity of their patients. This is in part a reflection of the way in which these services have evolved. The need for intensive care is related to the severity of the patient's clinical condition and the need for invasive monitoring and treatment. The development of intensive care units (ICUs) and high dependency care units (HDUs) has followed on from the realisation that severely ill patients benefit from a higher intensity of medical and nursing care than is usually available at a normal ward level.

Scoring Systems

Over the last decade, postoperative mortality after oesophago-gastric surgery has declined, in part due to specialisation and better patient selection. Nevertheless, the impact of the quality of surgery and postoperative care in patients who undergo gastro-oesophageal resection, in particular for cancer, remains unclear due to variations in case. It has long been recognised that a risk prediction model that could determine an individual patient's risk for a specific surgical operation would be very useful in pre-operative assessment, patient selection, the consent process and will serve as a good guide in post-operative management including a determination of the level of critical care required.

Assessment of the impact of surgery requires reliable tools that assess the morbidity and mortality risks, including the severity of the surgical insult. The POSSUM (Physiological and Operative Severity Score for the enUmeration of Mortality and Morbidity) model was developed for predicting post-operative mortality using cohorts of general surgical patients [2]. This was subsequently revised to P-POSSUM using the same set of variables as POSSUM but with a different logistic regression equation. Both POSSUM and P-POSSUM scoring systems use a 12-factor physiological score and a 6-factor operative severity score. POSSUM has been reported to be superior, compared with the Acute Physiology And Chronic Health Evaluation (APACHE) II tool, in predicting postoperative death in patients who undergo major surgery in a high-dependency unit. Attempts have been made to modify the POSSUM scoring system for specific surgical procedures such as oesophago-gastric surgery. This model has been adapted into a specialised model for the prediction of risk-adjusted post-operative mortality in oesophageal and gastric surgery (O-POSSUM). O-POSSUM appears to be good at predicting mortality following gastric cancer surgery but not as good after oesophageal resections. By contrast, P-POSSUM appears to be the most useful risk prediction model for oesophageal resections but substantially over predicted the risk in gastric resections. Attempts have been made to modify the POSSUM scoring system for predicting morbidity for upper gastrointestinal surgery. However, a deficiency of the current POSSUM models is that they are not based on a good understanding of the pathophysiological process that results in morbidity and mortality following cancer surgery. In addition, all severity-scoring systems have with the caveat that they have been derived from the statistical analysis of large cohorts of patients and are not for a specific individual.

Levels of Post-Operative Care

The definition and nomenclature for different levels of critical care are different in different parts of the world. The distinction between a patient requiring ICU and a patient requiring HDU may be complex and reflect local unit set-up and policies. In the UK, the Department of Health has recommended 4 levels of care from the normal ward environment to the high-end intensive care unit (Table 1).

Table 1. Levels of critical (intensive) care.

Level	Appropriate Patients
Level 0	Patients whose needs can be met in a general ward. Examples include intravenous therapy and observations required less frequently than 4 hourly.
Level 1	Patients at risk of deterioration whose needs can be met on a ward with additional support and advice if needed. This includes patients recently discharged from a higher level of care.
Level 2	Patients requiring detailed observation and/or intervention. This includes single organ support, pre-operative optimisation, specific or extended post-operative care and recent discharge from a higher level of care. In addition, patients receiving basic respiratory support, basic or advanced cardiovascular support and patients receiving renal support.
Level 3	Patients requiring advanced respiratory support or basic respiratory support with further support for 2 or more organ systems.

As such, critical care within this continuum is provided in levels 2 and 3 units. Although there is wide variation between individual units, an ICU will provide level 3 care to patients requiring mechanical ventilation or support for 2 or 3 failing organ systems. An HDU, on the other hand, has a vital role in patients requiring support for a single failing organ system (excluding advanced respiratory support) and those who will benefit from more detailed observation and care than can be provided on a normal ward.

Post-Operative Monitoring

Acute deterioration in critical ill and post-surgical patients is often preceded by changes in physiological parameters, such as pulse, blood pressure, temperature oxygen saturation (SpO2) and respiratory rate. In addition, urinary output provides a functional monitor of a complex interplay between intra-vascular volume and kidney perfusion. With more acutely ill patients, central venous pressure monitoring is also essential. These are the basic parameters, which require monitoring in any critical care environment. If relevant changes in the patient's vital parameters are recognized early, excess mortality and serious adverse events (SAEs) such as cardiac arrest may be prevented. Sufficient monitoring and care is of paramount importance for the safe outcome of patients in the post-operative period. However, adequate interpretation of changes in physiological parameters and an appropriate action / response must follow. Early accurate recognition and initiation of treatment of the critically unwell patient avoids progression to higher levels of morbidity, excessive utilization of costly resources, such as escalation of care to ICU, and shorter inpatient stay, a pressing issue in a climate of intense financial constraint.

Over the last decade, the clinical value of continuous monitoring of arterial blood pressure and arterial pulse pressure variation (PPV) to guide fluid management (goal-directed therapy) has been demonstrated. This has led to the adoption of continuous monitoring in critical care units. The choice between invasive and non-invasive monitoring will depend to a large extent on personal preference, training, available facilities and the level of nursing and medical input. Recognising the risks associated with invasive monitoring and the evolution of and accuracy of non-invasive monitoring equipment, translated to most critical care units adopting non-invasive monitoring whenever practical. However, invasive monitoring remains necessary in the acutely ill patients. In these patients, the need for invasive monitoring should be evaluated regularly, the risks anticipated and mitigated as appropriate.

The use of the pulmonary artery catheter for monitoring cardiac output (CO) has declined. Several techniques have emerged to estimate CO. Arterial pressure waveform analysis computes cardiac output from the arterial pressure curve. The method of estimating cardiac output for these devices may need to be calibrated by an independent measure of cardiac output. Some newer devices can estimate cardiac output from an arterial curve obtained noninvasively with photoplethysmography, allowing a noninvasive beat-by-beat estimation of cardiac output [3]. The main advantage of pulse contour analysis is to provide a real-time estimate of cardiac output. The calibrated devices provide a reliable estimate of cardiac output but are invasive and require frequent calibrations. However, the uncalibrated devices have a low reliability when vascular resistance changes to a larger extent.

CRITICAL CARE MANAGEMENT

The general medical and nursing care needs of all critical care patients can be extrapolated to those patients post major upper GI surgery [1]. This consists of general preventive and active measures (Table **2**).

Table 2. Aspects and constituents of management considered in critical care units (all levels).

Aspect of Care	Constituents of Care
Prophylaxis of deep vein thrombosis	Anti-thromboembolic stockings Prophylactic low molecular weight heparin Early mobilisation
Prophylaxis of stress ulcers	Use of proton pump inhibitor or H_2 receptor antagonist Establish enteral feed as early as possible
Nursing care	Personal and oral hygiene Care and limitation of pressure areas Head-up tilt to the bed

(Table 2) contd.....

Aspect of Care	Constituents of Care
Physiotherapy	Respiratory system Musculoskeletal system
Psychosocial aspects	Support and information for both patient and family

The multi-disciplinary critical care team has a major role for all patients within critical care. Daily input from medical and nursing staff as well as dietetics and physiotherapy facilitates a holistic approach to patient management. Input from infection control, biochemistry, renal and haematology physicians become increasingly important in patients with comorbidity and after complex surgery.

Post-Operative Analgesia

Pain can be significant after upper abdominal and thoracic surgery. It is a potent stimulator of the stress response and has a detrimental effect on respiratory and cardiovascular function. Pain can originate from both wound and visceral elements. The method of analgesia chosen will depend on the undertaken surgical procedure, patient characteristics and preferences, local expertise and available facilities. Most commonly in major upper GI surgery this involves epidural analgesia, other regional local anaesthetic techniques and systemic patient-controlled analgesia (PCA).

Epidural Analgesia: Thoracic epidural analgesia has traditionally been regarded as the gold standard of analgesia for major oesophago-gastric surgery with evidence that it is associated with decreased respiratory complications and reduced anastomotic leakage [4]. However, thoracic epidural is not necessarily a panacea as there are risks associated with insertion and removal, have a reasonable failure rate, and an association with hypotension reflecting reduced systemic vascular resistance. Depending on local guidelines, the presence of an epidural catheter for analgesia may necessitate nursing in a specific area such as a high dependency unit.

Other Regional Analgesia Techniques: Paravertebral blockade is practiced in patients undergoing thoracotomy at some hospitals, particularly in oesophagectomy patients. Compared to thoracic epidural analgesia, complications may be reduced but further clinical trials are required to directly compare the two modalities.

Systemic Patient-Controlled Analgesia (PCA): Although an analgesic alternative, use of systemic opiate PCAs have largely been superseded by regional techniques in appropriate patients. Opiates given in this manner are associated with potentially inferior analgesia and increased systemic side effects such as nausea and vomiting, pruritus and sedation. However, they do remain an option. They may be invaluable for patients in whom regional anaesthesia is contra-indicated and may also be used as second-line management in case of regional anaesthesia failure. They are often used as a step-down option after a period of epidural analgesia.

Multi-Modal Analgesia: In addition to the above, the importance of multi-modal analgesia should not be overlooked. Unless contra-indicated, patients should also be prescribed paracetamol and consideration given to non-steroidal anti-inflammatory drugs where appropriate. Other systemic agents that may be of additional benefit in refractory pain are usually introduced with specialist guidance and include clonidine, lignocaine and ketamine.

Post-Operative Nutrition

Patients undergoing upper GI surgery may have a poor background nutritional status and/or may have required a period of nutritional optimisation prior to surgery. Consideration needs to be given to their on- going nutritional management in the post-operative period. Depending on the undertaken surgical procedure, a feeding jejunostomy or gastrostomy tube may have been inserted during surgery. Enteral feeding *via* the gastric or jejunal route can commence soon after surgery. This will provide essential nutrition for these patients and prevent further weight loss as a result of the catabolic stare. However, in some cases a prolonged period of fasting with inability to feed orally or enterally may be encountered in some critical care patients. If this is predicted to be of more than a few days' duration, then parenteral nutrition should be instituted early.

Discharge from Critical Care

The step-down of a patient from ICU to HDU and then to the ward is a critical process. In this process, there will be reduced levels of nursing care, monitoring and certain specific treatments. However, specialist input remains available to all patients albeit at a reduced rate. It is essential that a discharge summary and suggested on going management plan, accompany the patient in the transfer process. The importance of clear communication and organisation in the process of transfer cannot be overemphasised. In addition, there must be clear guidelines as to the action to be taken if the patient were to deteriorate on the ward. This should include the suitability or otherwise of re-admission to critical care. This is a dynamic situation and subject to re-evaluation and assessment if and when the situation arises. The overall guiding principle has to be determined by a risk assessment and assessment of the probability of a positive outcome.

PATHO-PHYSIOLOGY OF SURGERY

The Stress Response

Tissue injury secondary to surgical trauma produces profound changes in endocrine-metabolic function and defense mechanisms (inflammatory, immunological) in the surgical patient, leading to an increase in catabolism, immunosuppression and postoperative morbidity. Major upper GI surgery by virtue of its complexity stimulates a significant physiological stress response. The stress response has the net effect of releasing endogenous energy stores. In evolutionary principles, this stress response confers a survival advantage to the injured organism by availing all stored energy to healing the effects of injury. It increases an injured animal's chance of survival. However, in the context of modern surgery particularly in elderly patients with significant co-morbidity, the stress response can be detrimental.

The response is characterised by activation of the sympathetic nervous system and the hypothalamic-pituitary axis. Resulting systemic changes include cardiovascular stimulation with tachycardia and potential arrhythmias, intense protein catabolism with inhibition of glucose utilisation, and release of inflammatory cytokines [5].

During a significant physiological insult, oxygen delivery mechanisms may be unable to meet demand and anaerobic metabolism ensues. This leads to an oxygen debt, which needs to be "paid off" and necessitates a period of increased oxygen consumption that continues after the initial stimulus has ceased. This is the cornerstone to postoperative management within a critical care environment where oxygen delivery can be improved with the manipulation of cardiovascular and respiratory parameters.

In addition to the systemic physiological stress response, there will be additional local factors, which depend on the impact of surgical trauma on specific organs at the site of surgery *e.g.* acute lung injury, pneumothorax, chylothorax and ileus.

Post-Operative Respiratory Changes

After surgery, alterations in ventilatory mechanics are characterised by a reduction in functional residual capacity (FRC) and vital capacity (VC). As the FRC reduces, it approaches the lung closing volume leading to airway closure during tidal ventilation with resultant atelectasis and hypoxia. Contributory factors include prolonged recumbency, poorly controlled pain, decreased thoracic compliance and pleural collections. In the immediate postoperative period, a rise in oxygen consumption can further exacerbate a mismatch in oxygen supply versus demand. The whole cascade results in respiratory failure.

Respiratory failure is a syndrome of inadequate gas exchange due to dysfunction of one or more essential components of the respiratory system. This includes the chest wall (including the diaphragm), airways, the alveolar-capillary unit, pulmonary circulation and the controlling nervous system particularly the brain stem. In *Type I* respiratory failure, hypoxaemia is the main feature with PaO2 less than 60 mmHg. It reflects a failure of oxygen exchange due to alveolar flooding and is refractory to supplemental oxygen. This is due to a ventilation/ perfusion (V/Q) mismatch or shunting of blood such as in pulmonary embolism. The main causes of this type of respiratory failure include pneumonia, pulmonary oedema (cardiogenic and non-cardiogenic), atelectasis, and pulmonary embolism. In *Type II* respiratory failure, hypercapnia (PaCO2 > 45 mmHg) is the main feature but hypoxaemia is secondary. It reflects a failure to exchange or remove carbon dioxide as a result of decreased alveolar minute ventilation (V_A). Although it is accompanied by hypoxaemia, this tends to correct with supplemental oxygen. It results from decreased minute ventilation (MV) relative to demand and from increased dead space ventilation. The main causes of this type of respiratory failure include chronic obstructive airways disease, asthma, obesity and neuromuscular and chest wall disorders. *Type III* respiratory failure is a sub-category of type I and type II. It represents peri-operative respiratory failure. It is due to abnormal abdominal or chest wall mechanical excursions as a result of surgery or post-operative pain. Obese individuals and previous smokers are at an increased risk of this type of respiratory failure after surgery. It results in low functional residual capacity (FRC) leading to atelectasis. It can result in type I or II respiratory failure with a mixed picture being common. It can be ameliorated by adequate analgesia, posture, incentive spirometry and a lower intra-abdominal pressure. In certain parts of the literature, *type IV* respiratory failure is described. It describes patients who are intubated and ventilated as part of their resuscitation for shock. The aetiology of shock can be septic, cardiogenic or hypovolemic. The goal of ventilation in these patients is to improve gas exchange and to decrease the load on respiratory muscles, which in effect lowers their oxygen consumption.

In order to discern the type of respiratory failure, arterial blood gasses (ABGs) quantify the magnitude of gas exchange abnormality and can help to identify the type and chronicity of respiratory failure. Additional tests in the post-surgical patient should be guided by the clinical picture and include a blood count, cardiac serological markers, microbiology of secretions and drain output, chest radiography, electrocardiography and less frequently, echocardiography. To help ascertain the aetiology for the deterioration in respiratory function in a surgical patient, a contrast enhanced CT of at least the operation field is mandatory.

The general management includes ensuring an adequate airway, supplemental oxygenation or ventilation, together with circulatory support as necessary. This should be followed by treatment of the cause of deterioration. Specific post-operative respiratory issues include pneumonia, pneumothorax, pulmonary oedema, acute lung injury (ALI) and pulmonary embolus. Post-operative measures for minimising respiratory dysfunction should be advocated and involve provision of adequate analgesia, nursing in a semi-erect position, use of humidified oxygen, early mobilisation and pulmonary physiotherapy.

BODY SYSTEM SUPPORT

Respiratory Support

Although all post-operative and deteriorating patients should be considered for supplemental oxygen, the clinical scenario would dictate the subsequent respiratory support required and the urgency of this [6]. In general, respiratory support can be subdivided into non-invasive and invasive ventilatory support [7].

Non-Invasive Ventilation

This includes high flow oxygen administration, Continuous Positive Airway Pressure (CPAP) and Bi-level Positive Airway Pressure (BIPAP). Non-invasive ventilation should be considered in patients with exacerbations of COPD, cardiogenic pulmonary oedema, obesity with hypoventilation syndrome.

High flow oxygen can be administered *via* face mask or nasal prongs. Humidified high flow nasal oxygen can provide comfortable therapy with reduced FiO_2 dilution and a degree of CPAP. Continuous Positive Airway Pressure (CPAP) should be considered in Type 1 respiratory failure. It requires a co-operative patient to wear a tightly fitting face mask or high flow nasal cannulae. It maintains a set airway pressure through the patient's own respiratory cycle. In addition, it can increase FRC, aid alveolar recruitment and decrease pulmonary shunts.

Bi-level Positive Airway Pressure (BIPAP) should be considered in Type 2 respiratory failure and respiratory acidosis. It also requires a co-operative patient to wear a tightly fitting mask. It delivers a higher pressure during inspiration and a lower one in expiration. The tidal volume delivered is determined by lung compliance and the set driving pressure. It can decrease work of breathing and improve diaphragmatic function.

Invasive Ventilation

This is also termed "mechanical ventilation". This is usually delivered in Level 3 intensive care units (ICU). There is sufficient evidence that most patients will benefit from early extubation after surgery, provided adequate analgesia is maintained [4]. However, a subgroup of patients will remain intubated and ventilated after their initial surgical procedure. This is usually indicated when a period of post-operative optimisation is required. A further group of patients may require intubation and ventilation as a result of intra-operative or early post-operative complications. In other patients, the indications for mechanical ventilation include cardiac or respiratory arrest, tachypnoea with respiratory fatigue, respiratory acidosis, refractory hypoxaemia, and inability to protect the airways as a result of decreased level of consciousness. In addition, mechanical ventilation should be considered in patients with shock associated with excessive respiratory work.

The goals of mechanical ventilation include correction of hypoxaemia and hypercapnia and improvement of cardiac function by decreasing preload, afterload and metabolic demand.

There are numerous invasive ventilatory modes used in ICU, which aim to balance optimal gas exchange with prevention of complications associated with mechanical ventilation [8]. Names for different modes vary but the more commonly found modes set the time, pressure, volume or both. Other modes are triggered by or synchronise with the patients breathing efforts (Table **3**).

Table 3. Modes of ventilation and their features.

Mode of Ventilation	Features
Pressure Control Ventilation	Each breath is delivered to a set pressure. Fluctuations in tidal volume can result.
Volume Control Ventilation	Each breath is delivered to a set volume. Fluctuations in airway pressure can result.
Synchronised Intermittent Mandatory Ventilation (SIMV)	Ventilator will deliver set breaths at set tidal volume or inspiratory pressure. If the patient makes additional inspiratory effort, the machine will detect this and augment the breath.
Pressure Regulated Volume Control (PRVC)	Set tidal volume is delivered to give the lowest inspiratory pressure.
Pressure Support Ventilation (PSV), also known as Assisted Spontaneous Breathing (ASB)	Ventilator senses patient inspiratory effort and then increases pressure to a set level, which is then maintained until expiration is triggered.
Airway Pressure Release Ventilation	Time in inspiration is longer than in expiration. Aim is to maximise alveolar recruitment.

Another important concept within ICU ventilation is Positive End Expiratory Pressure (PEEP). PEEP is a set level of pressure maintained during expiration, which helps to prevent alveolar collapse and promote compliance.

Mechanical ventilation can lead to 'volutrauma' (alveolar over distension) and barotrauma (excessive pressure), and ventilation strategies are selected to minimise these complications. The aim is to achieve satisfactory arterial blood gasses (ABGs) rather than normal ABGs.

Weaning from Mechanical Ventilation

Weaning is attempted if the original cause of respiratory failure has been addressed, respiratory parameters indicate improvement, and sedation, pain, nutritional status and electrolytes are all optimised. The various modes of ventilation can be used to gradually reduce ventilator support. In a few patients, a tracheostomy may be considered to aid on going ventilatory support (by reducing dead volume) and eventual weaning.

Cardiovascular Support

Peri-operative cardiovascular complications confer significant morbidity and mortality. A combination of pathophysiological and cardiovascular changes can occur. Sepsis, pain, major blood loss, fluid shifts or electrolyte disturbances are examples. In addition, there may be underlying cardiovascular co-morbidity *e.g.* pre-existing ischaemic heart disease. Often, it is the combined sum of all these factors operating on the individual patient. In the majority of cases corrective measures and support are mainly pharmaceutical. Exact timing and dose selection and frequency can be challenging. Frequently, titrating the supportive measures is preferable to applying quoted doses.

Tissue oxygenation depends upon arterial oxygen content and tissue perfusion determined by Cardiac output (CO). CO is a function of heart rate and stroke volume, which in turn, is determined by preload (ventricular end-diastolic volume or pressure), contractility and afterload (the pressure the heart needs to inject against). This inter-relationship means that cardiovascular disturbance may reflect increased or reduced circulating volume, primary "pumping" issues and increased or reduced afterload. These factors can potentially be monitored and modified within the critical care environment. A commonly seen manifestation of cardiovascular disturbance after upper GI surgery is arrhythmia, particularly atrial fibrillation that has many causes (Table **4**). Other common cardiovascular manifestations include cardiac ischaemia, which may be silent, and development of pulmonary oedema. Cardiovascular therapy in critical care aims to optimise tissue perfusion and thereby reduce tissue hypoxia.

Table 4. Causes of postoperative atrial fibrillation after upper GI surgery.

- Sepsis
- Increased age
- Pre-existing cardiac disease
- Blood loss and fluid shifts derangement
- Extensive intra-thoracic dissection
- Chest drain position
- Anastomotic leak

In addition to clinical examination, further indicative parameters that can be monitored include urine output (indicating renal perfusion), lactate (indicative of tissue perfusion), blood pressure, central venous pressure (CVP) and cardiac output (Table **5**).

Table 5. Methods of Cardiac Output Monitoring and their features.

Method of Monitoring	Features
Pulse contour analysis	• Contour of arterial line waveform used to estimate cardiac output and other haemodynamic measurements
Aortic doppler measurement	• Usually *via* trans-oesophageal echocardiography • May be inappropriate depending on surgical site
Thermo dilution	• Requires pulmonary artery catheter • Distal thermistor measures temperature change following saline injection
Transthoracic bio-impedance	• Non-invasive • Correlates rate of change of thoracic electrical resistance to cardiac output

Monitoring CVP can give an early indication of under filling or overdistention of the venous collecting system. Normally, increased venous return results in an augmented cardiac output without significant changes in CVP. Poor right ventricular function or a challenged pulmonary circulation can raise the right atrial pressure and CVP. Hypovolaemia or vasodilatation in most circumstances result in reduced venous return and a fall in right atrial pressure and CVP.

Fluid status needs to be monitored carefully in post-operative upper GI surgery patients with both hypovolaemia and hypervolemia avoided. Regular clinical review of these patients is a necessity and cannot be over-emphasised. Hypovolaemia can lead to hypotension and decreased tissue perfusion. Hyperperfusion can also put a strain on the heart and potentially reduce cardiac contractility and ultimately tissue perfusion. Both scenarios will at best delay tissue healing, which may impact on anastomotic healing. Peri-operative hypotension with evidence of hypovolaemia and reduced organ perfusion will need careful monitored fluid challenges. If tissue perfusion and cardiac output remain poor once hypovolaemia has been corrected, then consideration should be given to vasoactive drug use within a critical care environment (Table **6**).

Table 6. Examples of vasoactive drugs.

Drug	Main Receptor Targets	Effect	Use
Metaraminol	α1-adrenoceptors	Arteriolar vasoconstriction	Low SVR states
Noradrenaline	α-adrenoceptors	Arteriolar vasoconstriction	Low SVR states *e.g.* sepsis
Adrenaline	α- and β- adrenoceptors (mainly β1 at low dose)	Positive inotropy and chronotropy	Low cardiac output states
Dobutamine	α- and β- adrenoceptors, dopamine receptors	Reduces SVR and increases cardiac output	Cardiogenic shock

SVR = systemic vascular resistance.

Renal Support

Acute kidney injury (AKI) is a clinical syndrome characterised by a rapid reduction in renal excretory function underpinned by a variety of causes. Acute kidney injury is classically divided into pre-renal, renal (intrinsic) and post-renal.

Acute kidney injury has now replaced the term acute renal failure and a universal definition and staging system have been proposed to allow earlier detection and management of AKI [9]. Acute kidney injury has been demonstrated to be an independent risk factor for mortality mainly due to bleeding and sepsis. AKI is defined when one of the following criteria is met:

• Serum creatinine rises by ≥ 26 µmol/L within 48 hours <u>or</u>
• Serum creatinine rises ≥ 1.5 fold from the reference value, which is known <u>or</u>
• Presumed to have occurred within one week <u>or</u>
• Urine output is < 0.5 ml/kg/hour for >6 consecutive hours

The reference serum creatinine should be the lowest creatinine value recorded within 3 months of the event. If a reference serum creatinine value is not available within 3 months and AKI is suspected.

Acute kidney injury staging (1 – 3) can be performed using serum creatinine or urine output criteria. It has been demonstrated that as the stage of AKI increases so does the risk of mortality. Up to 30% of cases with AKI may be preventable, with a further significant percentage potentially remediable through simple interventions such as volume repletion, discontinuing and/or avoiding certain potentially nephrotoxic agents and earlier recognition of conditions causing rapid progression of AKI. Avoidance of pre- and peri-operative hypovolaemia is an essential component of patient management.

Following surgery, the body's physiological response is to retain sodium and water. The selection of the type of fluid to be prescribed is important as excessive peri-operative fluid therapy with 0.9% sodium chloride can potentially lead to hyperchloremic acidosis, sodium, chloride and water overload which contributes to postoperative morbidity and mortality whereas excessive peri-operative fluid replacement with 5% dextrose will increase the risk of developing hyponatremia. Fluid replacement prescriptions should be tailored to the needs of the patient. Potassium containing solutions (Hartmann's and Ringer's Lactate) should be used cautiously in patients who develop progressive AKI, due to the potential risk of exacerbating hyperkalaemia.

When a diagnosis of AKI is made, general supportive measures include optimisation of haemodynamic status by appropriate fluid therapy, administration of vasopressors and/or inotropes and treatment of any underlying sepsis. Nephrotoxic medications should be stopped. Nephrotoxic contrast agents should only be used when it is absolutely necessary and in consultation with renal physicians.

It is important to monitor the patient's volume status throughout the episode of AKI. This remains an essential part of patient management in the recovery phase. Patients may develop a polyuric phase during which they are at an increased risk of developing a negative fluid balance and electrolyte disturbance including hypernatraemia and hypokalaemia. There will need to be careful consideration about when to reintroduce medications such as antihypertensive medication and diuretics.

In general, there is no specific pharmacological therapy proven to effectively treat AKI secondary to hypoperfusion injury and/or sepsis. Loop diuretics have been used to convert patients with oliguric AKI to non- oliguric AKI, to facilitate the management of fluid and electrolyte disturbances and reduce the requirement for renal replacement therapy (RRT). However, the use of loop diuretics is associated with an increased risk of failure to recover renal function and mortality, possibly related to the resultant delay in commencing RRT timeously. Dopamine is a non-selective dopamine receptor agonist which at low-dose (0.5-3.0 µg/kg/min) induces a dose-dependent increase in renal blood flow, natriuresis and diuresis in healthy humans. However, there is no good evidence to support any important clinical benefits from dopamine to patients with or at risk of AKI. Fenoldopam is a selective dopamine A-1 receptor agonist that decreases systemic vascular resistance whilst increasing renal blood flow to both the cortex and medullary regions in the kidney. There is good evidence that fenoldopam reduces the need for renal replacement therapy and mortality in patients with AKI [10]. However, additional studies are necessary to confirm this effect.

In patients with severe or continuing AKI there may be no other option than to commence renal replacement therapy (RRT) [11]. RRT using pumped veno-venous methods *via* dedicated venous catheters should be initiated once AKI is established and unavoidable but before overt complications have developed.

The choice of renal replacement therapy modality should be guided by the individual patient's clinical status, medical and nursing expertise, and availability of modality. The currently available therapies include intermittent haemodialysis (IHD), various forms of continuous renal replacement therapy (CRRT) including continuous haemofiltration and haemodialysis/filtration and newer "hybrid" therapies such as extended duration dialysis (EDD), sustained low-efficiency dialysis (SLED) and the Genius® system. Most clinicians chose intermittent haemodialysis/haemofiltration for cardiovascularly stable patients, and continuous or hybrid therapies for those with cardiovascular compromise and multi-organ failure [12].

CONSENT FOR PUBLICATION

Not applicable.

CONFLICT OF INTEREST

The authors declare no conflict of interest, financial or otherwise.

ACKNOWLEDGEMENT

Declare none.

REFERENCES

[1]   Short MN, Ho V, Aloia TA. Impact of processes of care aimed at complication reduction on the cost of complex cancer surgery. J Surg Oncol 2015; 112(6): 610-5.
[http://dx.doi.org/10.1002/jso.24053] [PMID: 26391328]

[2]   Dutta S, Horgan PG, McMillan DC. POSSUM and its related models as predictors of postoperative mortality and morbidity in patients undergoing surgery for gastro-oesophageal cancer: a systematic review. World J Surg 2010; 34(9): 2076-82.
[http://dx.doi.org/10.1007/s00268-010-0685-z] [PMID: 20556607]

[3]   Monnet X, Teboul JL. Minimally invasive monitoring. Crit Care Clin 2015; 31(1): 25-42.
[http://dx.doi.org/10.1016/j.ccc.2014.08.002] [PMID: 25435477]

[4]   Chandrashekar MV, Irving M, Wayman J, Raimes SA, Linsley A. Immediate extubation and epidural analgesia allow safe management in a high-dependency unit after two-stage oesophagectomy. Results of eight years of experience in a specialized upper gastrointestinal unit in a district general hospital. Br J Anaesth 2003; 90(4): 474-9.
[http://dx.doi.org/10.1093/bja/aeg091] [PMID: 12644420]

[5]   Finnerty CC, Mabvuure NT, Ali A, Kozar RA, Herndon DN. The surgically induced stress response. JPEN J Parenter Enteral Nutr 2013; 37(5) (Suppl.): 21S-9S.
[http://dx.doi.org/10.1177/0148607113496117] [PMID: 24009246]

[6]   Chiumello D, Brioni M. Severe hypoxemia: which strategy to choose. Crit Care 2016; 20(1): 132.
[http://dx.doi.org/10.1186/s13054-016-1304-7] [PMID: 27255913]

[7]   Shekar K, Davies AR, Mullany DV, Tiruvoipati R, Fraser JF. To ventilate, oscillate, or cannulate? J Crit Care 2013; 28(5): 655-62.
[http://dx.doi.org/10.1016/j.jcrc.2013.04.009] [PMID: 23827735]

[8]   Goligher EC, Ferguson ND, Brochard LJ. Clinical challenges in mechanical ventilation. Lancet 2016; 387(10030): 1856-66.
[http://dx.doi.org/10.1016/S0140-6736(16)30176-3] [PMID: 27203509]

[9]   Thakar CV, Christianson A, Freyberg R, Almenoff P, Render ML. Incidence and outcomes of acute kidney injury in intensive care units: a Veterans Administration study. Crit Care Med 2009; 37(9): 2552-8.
[http://dx.doi.org/10.1097/CCM.0b013e3181a5906f] [PMID: 19602973]

[10]   Landoni G, Biondi-Zoccai GG, Tumlin JA, *et al.* Beneficial impact of fenoldopam in critically ill patients with or at risk for acute renal failure: a meta-analysis of randomized clinical trials. Am J Kidney Dis 2007; 49(1): 56-68.
[http://dx.doi.org/10.1053/j.ajkd.2006.10.013] [PMID: 17185146]

[11]   Kanagasundaram NS. Renal replacement therapy in acute kidney injury: an overview. Br J Hosp Med (Lond) 2007; 68(6): 292-7.
[http://dx.doi.org/10.12968/hmed.2007.68.6.23567] [PMID: 17639824]

[12]   Palevsky PM, Zhang JH, O'Connor TZ, *et al.* Intensity of renal support in critically ill patients with acute kidney injury. N Engl J Med 2008; 359(1): 7-20.
[http://dx.doi.org/10.1056/NEJMoa0802639] [PMID: 18492867]

CHAPTER 3

Nutrition for Oesophago-gastric Disorders

Joanne Thomson[1] and **Sami M. Shimi**[2,*]

[1] *Department of Nutrition and Dietetics, Ninewells Hospital and Medical School, Dundee, Scotland, UK*

[2] *Department of Surgery, Ninewells Hospital and Medical School, Dundee, Scotland, UK*

Abstract: Oesophageal disorders can impact locally on food delivery to the stomach while gastric disorders can interfere with reservoir function and chemical digestion. These restrictive disorders prevent anabolism and contribute to catabolism in order to maintain function. However, many oesophago-gastric disorders can impact on the energy balance through their systemic effects such as sepsis or cancer cachexia as two notable examples. These are catabolic disorders and despite adequate intake malnutrition is the end result. Malnutrition is prevalent in most patients with oesophago-gastric disorders particularly in patients with cancers of the oesophagus or stomach. In addition, the effects of therapeutic modalities delivered to the oesophagus or stomach such as surgery, chemo and radiotherapy can also influence a catabolic state either directly or indirectly. The local, systemic and therapeutic effects on energy balance have to be addressed by a thorough screening, assessment, appropriate therapy and continuous monitoring of nutritional status.

All patients with reduced oral intake and / or weight loss as a result of mechanical or functional obstruction in the oesophagus or stomach should be screened and referred for dietetic assessment and management if appropriate. The overall goal of dietetic therapy in oesophago-gastric disorders is to address the energy imbalance, restore the energy requirements and improve symptoms in order to maintain function and survival.

Keywords: Cancer cachexia, Dumping syndrome, Energy balance, Enteric nutrition, Nutrition, Malnutrition, Risk assessment, Nutritional requirements, Oral nutrition supplements, Parenteral nutrition.

NUTRITION AND MALNUTRITION

Apart from their other functions, the oesophagus and stomach are the natural gateways for the entry of fluid and nutrients entry into the digestive tract. As such, this places them in a central position to deliver the required hydration and nutritious material for the continuing survival and function of the individual.

* **Corresponding author Sami M. Shimi:** Department of Surgery, Ninewells Hospital and Medical School, Dundee DD1 9SY, Scotland, UK; Tel: +44 1382 660111; E-mail: s.m.shimi@dundee.ac.uk

It also places these organs at risk as a result of their early contact with contaminated or injurious material before it is decontaminated or diluted further down the digestive tract. Regular adequate hydration is essential for the function of all body systems. Without adequate hydration, multiple body systems will cease to function. Ingestion of tasty nutritious material is important for delivering the required energy for the individual but is also a pleasurable part of social functioning. Inability to ingest adequate nutritious food, results in an imbalance between energy supply and demand which unless addressed results in detriment of the individual.

Oesophageal disorders can impact locally on food delivery to the stomach while gastric disorders can interfere with reservoir function and chemical digestion. However, many oesophago-gastric disorders can impact on the energy balance through their systemic effects such as sepsis or cancer cachexia as two notable examples. In addition, the effects of therapeutic modalities delivered to the oesophagus or stomach such as surgery, chemo and radiotherapy can also influence a catabolic state either directly or indirectly. The local, systemic and therapeutic effects on energy balance have to be addressed by a thorough screening, assessment, appropriate therapy and continuous monitoring of nutritional status.

The overall goal of dietetic therapy in oesophago-gastric disorders is to address the energy imbalance, restore the energy requirement and improve symptoms in order to maintain function and survival (in conjunction with other treatment modalities). In this context, dietetics therapy is one of the cornerstones of the overall treatment strategy for the individual with these disorders. For some disorders such as gastro-oesophageal reflux disease or peptic ulceration, the goal of dietetic treatment is to alter the type of food intake to reduce gastric acidity and if the patient is overweight, to reduce the amount or proportion of nutrients intake to lose weight. For disorders, which functionally impair transit in the oesophagus (achalasia) or stomach (gastroparesis), the goal of dietetic therapy is to improve food tolerance by altering the texture of food and promoting low texture foods. For disorders which mechanically interfere with the passage of food in the oesophagus or stomach (cancer or benign strictures) the aim of dietetic treatment is to select fortified foods at the appropriate consistency which can pass through stenotic areas more easily. Patients, who are malnourished who cannot maintain adequate oral food intake, may benefit from oral supplements. Patients who are unable to have adequate oral intake but have a functioning GI tract may benefit from additional enteric feeding. The parenteral route can be used, to provide adequate nutrition if dietary requirements cannot be met by the oral or enteric routes, (post-operative states, sepsis, trauma).

Malnutrition

Malnutrition is defined as a state of nutrition in which a deficiency or excess (or imbalance) of energy, protein and other nutrients causes measurable adverse effects on tissue/body form (body shape, size and composition) and function, and clinical outcome. In practical terms, the criteria for diagnosis of malnutrition are dependent on the measured Body Mass Index (BMI), quantification of recent (over 3 – 6 months) weight loss and current / recent dietary intake. A diagnosis of malnutrition is made if the BMI is less than 18.5 kg/m^2 or there has been weight loss of 10% (or more) in the past 3-6 months. Using the same criteria, an individual could be considered being at risk of malnutrition if the BMI is less than 20 kg/m^2 or there has been weight loss of 5-10% in the past 3-6 months.

Malnutrition is prevalent in most patients with oesophago-gastric disorders particularly in patients with cancers of the oesophagus or stomach. Approximately 80% of patients with oesophago-gastric cancer are thought to have or are at risk of malnutrition at the time of diagnosis. Malnutrition and weight loss impacts negatively upon treatment response, post-operative recovery and are also associated with morbidity, mortality and reduced quality of life [1]. Expert dietetic advice is an essential part of a cancer patients care from the point of diagnosis. The cause of malnutrition will ultimately determine the best dietetic treatment and goal. Every patient has to be considered on an individual basis. However, regardless of the cause of malnutrition, it imparts poorer overall clinical outcomes for the patient.

Many oesophago-gastric conditions particularly cancer are insidious and remain sub-clinical in the early stages of the disease process. Even at presentation, patients often present with minimal or vague symptoms. Indeed, a common presentation is with unexplained weight loss. At the time of diagnosis, after symptoms are noticed, oesophago-gastric cancer is often at an advanced stage in more than 60% of individuals.

The development of malnutrition, resulting from an imbalance between energy input and output, is often multi-factorial. Reasons for increased energy expenditure include metabolic alterations such as cachexia, post-operative recovery, infection and wound healing. A reduced dietary intake due to a reduced appetite is often exacerbated by other symptoms, from the disorder or side effects from treatment including nausea, vomiting, pain, low mood, taste changes and constipation. This exacerbates the existing nutritional deficit. The reduced dietary intake may also be due to mechanical swallowing difficulties. Dietetic modifications cannot alter the energy expenditure part of the balance equation. However, changes to dietary intake (energy input) may address the balance.

Cancer and cancer treatments impact negatively on the nutritional status of the majority of cancer patients (90%) thus malnutrition is a common problem in this patient group. Up to 20% of cancer patients die from the effects of malnutrition or the effects of treatment rather than from cancer itself. Nutritionally, oesophageal and gastric cancers affect food intake in different ways. Oesophageal cancer and strictures mechanically affect food delivery into the stomach. Gastric disorders including cancer can also affect food transit through the stomach as a result of mechanical or functional obstruction. However, gastric distension in the presence of mechanical obstruction can also contribute to early satiety, reduced stomach capacity for food and fluid, loss of appetite associated with painful distension and impaired digestion.

Causes of Malnutrition in Patients with Oesophago-gastric Cancer

Localized Effects of Tumour: Tumours of the oesophagus and stomach mechanically interfere in the consumption of nutrients. The resultant malnutrition depends on tumour extent. Dysphagia tends to occur relatively late in the presentation of these tumours as the oesophagus distends to accommodate the ingestion of food or liquid to pass the tumour. Most cancers involve at least a 4-cm length of the oesophagus before diagnosis and the average patient will have had 3- to 6 months of dysphagia and some weight loss. Other patients will report reflux type symptoms, odynophagia, coughing or choking on food, which makes them afraid or reluctant to eat. This places them at high risk for malnutrition from the time of diagnosis.

Systemic Effects of Tumour: Many patients with oesophageal or gastric cancer develop cancer cachexia as the disease progresses. This consists of weight loss, debilitation, and anorexia. The aetiology of cancer cachexia is poorly understood but it is thought to be related to paracrine tumour secretions such as cytokines. Patients with cancer cachexia experience increased catabolism despite a decrease in energy intake causing an increase in nutritional needs and further nutritional depletion [2].

Treatment Effects: The side effects of treatment are major contributing factors to the malnutrition and wasting syndrome commonly observed in patients with oesophago-gastric cancer. The surgery can have profound effects on the patient's ability to consume adequate nutrition. Changes in the anatomy and reservoir size result in early satiety, reflux, nausea, vomiting, and vitamin and mineral deficiencies. In cases where a vagotomy is performed, gastric stasis may occur. Colonic or jejunal interposition, anastomotic leaks, anastomotic strictures substantially delay resumption of oral intake, which leads to inadequate oral intake in patients postoperatively. Chemotherapy and radiation therapy can also reduce the size of the tumour and thus relieve dysphagia, but these treatments can have profound gastrointestinal toxicity. Nausea, vomiting, diarrhoea, and stomatitis occur with cisplatin and 5-fluorouracil therapy, while the most predominant symptoms of mediastinal radiation are esophagitis with dysphagia, odynophagia, reflux, and oesophageal strictures. Nutritional side effects of chemotherapy usually resolve following treatment; however, the first symptoms of radiation damage from mucosal injury begin within two to three weeks after the start of therapy. Most cancer programs now advocate combined- modality therapy, resulting in more toxicities and little time for nutritional repletion.

NUTRITIONAL ASSESSMENT

All patients with reduced oral intake and / or weight loss as a result of mechanical or functional obstruction in the oesophagus or stomach should be screened and referred for dietetic assessment if appropriate. In particular, patients with oesophageal or gastric cancer should be referred for dietetic assessment once the diagnosis is made. Hospital-based clinicians, disease specific specialist nurses or primary care practitioners, usually make the referral. Patients with a cancer diagnosis can also be referred from oesophago-gastric multi-disciplinary team meetings. After referral, patients can be seen and assessed by hospital-based dieticians, community dieticians or independent dietetic practitioners [3].

The initial part of the dietetic care process involves identification of patients who are malnourished and require dietetic input or patients who may be at risk of developing malnutrition. Following identification of those requiring dietetic input a comprehensive dietetic assessment following a diet focused clinical assessment to gather relevant information is carried out. This is then interpreted to inform a dietetic care plan in conjunction with the patient.

Screening

Screening for malnutrition should be carried out using a validated tool. In the U.K. screening in adults for malnutrition is commonly carried out using the 'Malnutrition Universal Screening Tool' (MUST) [4]. Alternative tools including Patient Generated Subjective Global Assessment can also be used and may be more relevant to the Oncology patient group. MUST is a five-step guide which identifies patients with malnutrition or who are at risk of developing malnutrition based on an assessment of their BMI, any unplanned weight loss over the past 3-6 months and any acute disease state or likelihood of no oral intake over 5 days. The BMI score (0 – 2) is combined with the weight loss score (0 – 2) and the acute illness score (0 or 2) to produce an overall risk of malnutrition. A cumulative score of 0 is assigned a "low" risk status, 1 is assigned a "medium" risk status and a cumulative score of 2 or more is assigned a "high" risk status for malnutrition. The over all risk score is then used to follow the appropriate dietetic management guideline to be adopted.

Current management guidelines indicate that a patient who is found to be at low risk of developing malnutrition, with a MUST score of 0, does not require immediate referral to the dietitian but that they should continue to be MUST screened for malnutrition at appropriate intervals. Those identified to be at moderate risk of developing malnutrition, with a MUST score of 1, are monitored for 3 days and managed using the food-first approach by setting goals to increase oral intake with additional monitoring. In practical terms, immediate care staff are expected to offer and encourage full-cream milk and additional snacks with regular monitoring of compliance. If a patient is found to be at high risk of malnutrition, with a MUST score of 2 or above, an immediate referral to the dietetic department for assessment by a dietitian should be initiated.

Referrals can enter the dietetic service from nursing staff in inpatient settings, General Practitioners in the outpatient setting or other healthcare providers based on the score of the MUST screening tool. Patients should be screened at regular intervals as determined by their care setting. Patients attending for outpatient appointments should be screened for malnutrition on their first visit.

In addition to the MUST referral criteria, patients can enter the dietetic service *via* the Upper Gastro-Intestinal Cancer Pathway. This is a process, which aims to optimise outcomes for patients who are diagnosed with oesophageal or gastric malignancy. Pathways are usually developed by the Upper Gastro-intestinal multi-disciplinary team and are institution/site specific but include input from the dietitian at all stages. Patients can also be referred to the dietitian *via* the oesophago-gastric Clinical Nurse Specialist often prior to a diagnosis. It is the role of the Specialist Upper GI dietitian to identify the patients at risk of malnutrition and the necessary dietetic input by using relevant information including; BMI, weight history and eating habits. The dietician can then attach a score using the MUST principles. This amounts to a risk assessment, which defines the intervention priority. Subsequently, patients can be seen in a clinic setting, within an agreed time frame, for completion of a more thorough assessment.

Due to the nature of oesophago-gastric malignancy, many patients are likely to need some dietary advice at presentation. This may include advice on dietary modification for dysphagia or advice to improve nutritional intake depending on the patient's symptoms. Some may need additional nutritional support.

Dietetic Assessment

Anthropometry: Accurate weight and height should be obtained and used to calculate a body mass index (BMI). If this is not possible there are alternative measurements that can be used to estimate body mass index but they tend to be less accurate. BMI is a weight to height ratio and is used as an indicator of nutritional risk to stratify patients in to underweight, desirable, overweight or obese categories (Table **1**). The following calculation eq. (1) is used to derive the BMI;

$$BMI = Weight\ (kg)\ /\ Height\ (m^2) \tag{1}$$

Table 1. WHO Classification of BMI ranges.

BMI Range (kg/m^2)	Weight Category
<18.5	Underweight
18.5 - 24.9	Desirable
25 - 29.9	Overweight
≥ 30	Obese

BMI can be used to estimate and monitor chronic changes in protein energy status and this can be used to estimate the risk of malnutrition. Another indicator of a patient's risk of malnutrition is percentage weight change (Table **2**). This is used to determine a patient's acute change in protein energy status over the past 3-6 months. This is calculated by eq. (2):

$$Percentage\ Weight\ Loss = [Usual\ Weight\ (kg) - Current\ weight\ (kg)]\ /\ Usual\ Weight\ (kg)\ x\ 100 \tag{2}$$

Table 2. Use of percentage body weight loss to estimate risk of malnutrition. Adapted from BAPEN [4].

Percentage Body Weight Reduction	Significance
<5	'Normal' Variation
5-10	Greater than normal variation and early indicator of increased risk of malnutrition
> 10	Clinically Significant

Special consideration must be applied for those who have additional fluid on board such as patients with edema or ascites as this can inflate a patient's true body weight. A dry weight should be estimated in this instance and used as an alternative to calculate weight change and BMI.

Determining weight change can be challenging if a patient is unable to recall their weight history. Often information relating to practical changes can prove vital in the assessment of a patient's nutritional status. For example, the presence of weakness, loose skin, loose fitting jewelry or clothing or a recent change in belt buckle hole.

Biochemical Markers/Biochemistry: These have a limited value in identifying nutritional status as many of these factors are affected by the disease state. They can however be useful in indicating hydration status *e.g.* Urea, sodium and potassium. However, these must be considered in relation to the overall clinical situation as many factors can affect these results. C-Reactive Protein and White Cell Count are often used as part of a dietetic assessment as an indication of current inflammation or infection suggesting a metabolic stress response, which alters energy expenditure.

Clinical Assessment: Clinical factors include; current diagnosis, past medical history, details of clinical tests/results and medications or proposed treatment. Taken together with other assessments, clinical factors are important in signifying the acute disease effects and proposed treatment, which can alter the overall malnutrition score and necessitate additional dietetic nutritional input.

Dietary Assessment: Details of dietary intake can be gathered using a range of methods including a dietary 24 hours recall from the patient or a diet history of 'usual' dietary intake. Details of dietary intake are analysed and compared to the patients estimated nutritional requirements. Other factors that are likely to be explored include recent changes in dietary habits and the possible reasons for this, the presence of symptoms limiting food intake and any difficulty with swallowing.

Environmental Assessment: In addition to analysis of anthropometric data, biochemistry, dietary intake assessment and details about a patients' clinical condition it is important to consider the psychosocial aspects of a patient in their natural environment (home or supported accommodation) as these can influence dietary intake. Important factors such as meal provision, ability and access to resources to shop and prepare meals and snacks for themselves and mood, which can also have an effect on nutritional intake, should all be explored.

Calculation of Nutritional Requirements

Nutritional requirements of a patient are essential in determining the extent to which nutritional support is required. Using an equation, the dietitian can calculate a patient's estimated nutritional requirements, which is based on an estimation of their energy expenditure. This will be used as a baseline figure (starting point) for basing their assessment on. This should be reviewed at regular intervals and adjusted accordingly, taking in to account changes in clinical condition i.e. improving CRP and WCC as an indication of a reduction in metabolic stress and energy output. Clinical judgment should be used and a rationale provided for all observed changes.

Measuring basal metabolic rate (BMR) is difficult in practice and requires advanced techniques. As a result, the majority of dietitians' estimate BMR in order to calculate total energy expenditure (TEE). There are many reported methods, which can be used to estimate a patient's basal metabolic rate. There are advantages and disadvantages to each method and dieticians should use a convenient method, which is familiar to them recognizing its pitfalls. The equations produce estimates of nutritional requirements, which are roughly similar with minor variations. All equations estimate the Basal Metabolic rate (BMR) and add a correction factor for diet induced thermogenesis (DIT), physical activity (Table 3) and stress to indicate total energy expenditure (TEE).

Stress factors corrections are provided by professional specialty organisations such as the Parenteral and Enteral Nutrition Group (PENG), which relate to a range of clinical conditions. For patients with cancer, a 0-20% correction could be applied. The lower end of the range should be used in the first instance and on-reassessment, adjusted accordingly. Cancer can inflict a hypometabolic or hypermetabolic state although oesophageal and gastric cancers are likely to induce a hypermetabolic state. As a general principle, the stress factor should be assumed at 0% unless there are factors to suggest otherwise such as; presence of infection, recent surgery, raised temperature, raised WCC or CRP indicating an inflammatory response.

Table 3. Correction factor for activity. Adapted from Elia [5].

Activity	Correction Factor (%)
Bed Bound Immobile	10
Bed Bound Mobile/Sitting	15-20
Mobile on the ward	25

For those considered to have an activity level or function to that of a healthy individual a physical activity level (PAL) correction factor should be applied. In order to balance input and output, nutritional requirements must at least balance total energy expenditure (TEE). Protein requirements are usually calculated first and the balance of the energy requirements divided between carbohydrates and fats. Nitrogen Requirements are used to calculate protein requirements by multiplying by 6.25 to give total estimated protein requirements (Table 4).

Table 4. Estimated Nitrogen and protein requirements in different metabolic states. Adapted from Elia [5].

Status	Nitrogen Requirements (Range) in gms/Kg/day	Protein Requirement (Range) in gms/Kg/day
Normal	0.17 (0.14 - 0.20)	1.06 (0.87 – 1.25)
Hyper metabolic 5-25%	0.2 (0.17 - 0.25)	1.25 (1.06 – 1.56)
Hyper metabolic 25-50%	0.25 (0.20 - 0.30)	1.56 (1.25 – 1.87)
Hyper metabolic >50%	0.3 (0.25 - 0.35)	1.87 (1.56 – 2.18)
Depleted	0.3 (0.20 - 0.40)	1.87 (1.25 – 2.5)

Carbohydrates should comprise 30 – 70% of total energy requirements and fats should provide approximately 30 – 35% of total energy requirements. Standardised feeds should also provide electrolytes, micronutrients, vitamins and trace elements in appropriate measures. Reference tables, produced by professional specialty organisations, usually provide these proportions. Fluid requirements are calculated on the basis of age and body weight. For those who are less than 60 years old, 35 ml/kg body weight and for those who are 60 years old or older, 30 ml/kg body weight.

Once the nutritional requirements are calculated, dietetic input may include, food first advice, dietary counseling, oral nutritional supplementation (ONS), enteral nutrition (EN) or Total parenteral nutrition (TPN). The exact input will depend on the patient's ability to meet the requirements. Comparison of dietary intake to nutritional requirements will be calculated and an estimated nutritional deficit figure calculated for both energy and protein. Dietetic intervention will aim to negotiate manageable patient-centered goals with the patient to overcome barriers to adequate nutritional intake. Dietetic advice will be influenced by dietary impairment (reduced oral intake), presence and severity of symptoms, which affect oral intake and nutritional deficit.

Dietetic Goals

Examples of goals of dietetic treatment throughout the patient journey include:

- Prevention of further weight loss
- Maximisation of oral intake
- Improvement of nutritional status to promote treatment response
- Improve nutritional status prior to surgery
- Aid weight gain to improve reserves for surgery
- Minimise nutritional deficit or losses

A holistic approach should be adopted and consideration of patients' abilities in relation to shopping for food, meal preparation, social circumstances, psychological mood and environmental barriers should be made.

Refeeding Syndrome

This is a metabolic complication that can occur with the initiation of nutrition following a period of reduced dietary intake. The re-introduction/presence of carbohydrate forces the body to change from the fasted to the fed state or a catabolic to anabolic state. Insulin secretion is increased in response to the presence of carbohydrate. This initiates uptake of potassium, phosphate and magnesium in to the cells reducing plasma levels of these electrolytes and increasing the likelihood of associated complications [6]. Steps can be taken to minimise the risks of developing related complications with the gradual re-introduction of nutrition in those who are at increased risk in accordance with re-feeding guidelines set out by the British Association of Parenteral and Enteral Nutrition [7].

Cancer Cachexia

This is a complex metabolic process that accelerates the breakdown of fat and protein, reduces protein synthesis and increases resting energy expenditure resulting in weight loss [2]. Anorexia, fatigue and low mood are also symptoms of the condition, which contribute to malnutrition. Cancer cachexia can result in progressive weight loss regardless of nutritional intake. Without radical treatment of the underlying cancer, the condition is often irreversible despite dietary changes and nutritional support.

NUTRITIONAL MANAGEMENT

Dietitians should be involved at the earliest point following a patient's presentation after screening. Patients with a diagnosis of cancer should be referred early due to the high incidence of malnutrition in patients with OG cancer. At the time of diagnosis 80% of those with upper gastrointestinal cancers have already lost weight [8]. Identifying and treating malnutrition early in those with a cancer diagnosis is associated with better treatment outcomes and may help to improve patient's prognosis.

Multi-disciplinary team approach including a dietician should be adopted. Patients are individually discussed at a regular Multi-disciplinary team meeting with consideration given to their diagnosis, current fitness, any co-morbidities, stage of cancer and nutritional status, all of which help to inform a thorough treatment plan. Dietetic intervention following a diagnosis of oesophago-gastric malignancy should take a patient-centered approach but is often influenced by the planned clinical treatment, patient's symptoms, patients' nutritional needs as well as patients' wishes. Although the overall treatment goals do not necessarily focus on addressing weight loss primarily, they are taken into consideration as one of the factors, which influence treatment outcome and managed appropriately.

Symptom Management

Often dietary intake can be improved with medical management of associated symptoms such as; nausea, vomiting, pain, constipation, by using anti-emetics, adequate analgesia, laxatives or prokinetic agents as required. Dietary management can accompany this. If nausea and vomiting is a problem, patients should be encouraged to eat small portions of food or light meals and at regular intervals, every 2-3 hours if possible. High calorie fluids should also be encouraged, as these are often easier to manage. Ginger containing foods and drinks can sometimes help to settle symptoms of nausea. Dry foods such as crackers, biscuits, cold foods may be easier to manage than stews. Other symptoms, include regurgitation of foodstuffs due to partial obstruction, early satiety due to tumor bulk or tumor associated gastroparesis, reduced appetite due to low mood or the disease state itself.

Dietetic management should focus on the patient's ability to eat and texture modification. If weight loss and reduced overall nutritional intake are a problem, dietary advice may include food fortification to increase the energy content of foods, the use of high energy high protein dietary intake, or the use of energy dense foods. Texture modification to soft or liquid diet is recommended to treat dysphagia due to oesophageal obstruction or to treat recurrent vomiting due to gastric outlet obstruction.

The stage of disease and its impact on functional ability of the individual patient should be considered carefully. Some patients may not have the ability to purchase or prepare meals and a meal delivery service may need to be put in place. Alternatively, the dietician may recommend tinned, packet, ready-meal foods to ease the pressure on meal preparation. A holistic approach should be adopted when trying to implement such change with patients. Social and environmental factors may contribute as barriers to adequate nutritional intake. These should be managed sensitively.

Nutritional support in the form of Oral Nutritional Support, Enteral Nutrition (EN), parenteral nutrition (PN) may need to be considered if dietary intake alone is not enough to meet the patient's nutritional needs. The oral route may however be unsuitable due to an obstructing lesion.

Curative Approach

Patients with a lower stage of cancer who are sufficiently fit for a radical approach are managed with a curative intent. The range of treatments offered with a curative intent include, surgery after neo-adjuvant chemotherapy, radio or chemotherapy. In order to withstand the radical approach and to improve treatment outcomes, it is important that these patients maintain an adequate nutritional intake. Patients with an adequate oral intake may benefit from texture modification, food fortification, the use of energy dense foods or oral supplementation. If adequate oral intake could not be maintained (*e.g.* due to dysphagia), patients should be considered for placement of a self-expanding stent. Some patients will require additional enteral nutrition and a few will benefit from total parenteral nutrition depending on the extent of weight loss and ability to maintain oral intake.

Palliative Approach

A palliative treatment option for those with oesophageal cancer, which is deemed incurable, is the placement of an oesophageal stent. Self-expanding metal stents can achieve immediate palliation of dysphagia. They are placed endoscopically and place minimal burden on the debilitated patient. The focus of dietary advice for these patients is on texture modification to minimise the risk of the stent blockage (Fig. **1**).

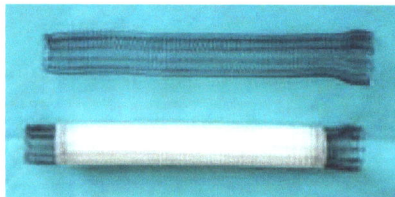

Fig. (1). A self-expanding metallic stent for the treatment of oesophageal or pyloric obstruction. An uncovered and a covered stents are shown.

Once the stent has been placed, 20% of patient may experience pain necessitating opiates analgesia until the stent is fully expanded. Patients should start taking a fluid only diet including water, tea, coffee, fruit juice, milk, milkshakes, clear soups, bovril, stock. Gradually, patients are able to tolerate semisolid and then moist food over a few days. Once taking foods, patients should be advised to take frequent sips of fluids in between mouthfuls to encourage any debris from foodstuffs to pass through the stent in to the stomach. Patients should be advised to take energy dense foods with or without oral supplements. Reflux is a common symptom following stent placement and antacid medications are often prescribed to minimise these symptoms. This will help patients to progress from taking fluids to a diet containing soft, moist foods.

Although the aim of the stent placement is to enable to patient to maintain a near-normal dietary intake, there are certain foods that are more likely to result in the stent blocking. Patients should be advised to avoid such foods. These include bread and rolls which often form a bolus when they mix with digestive juices (saliva), fruit or vegetables that have a tough skin such as apples, pears, tomatoes, peppers, orange piths, stringy vegetables such as celery and salad and tough, dry and grizzly meats.

Patients should be advised to avoid skins of fruit and vegetables. They should also be advised to peel and cook fruits or vegetable to moisten and soften their consistency. Vegetables can be added to sauces or soups and fruits can be stewed and eaten as part of a snack or a pudding. Patients should be encouraged to add plenty of sauces and gravy with meals to moisten the consistency of food.

Recommended dietary changes include taking small mouthfuls of food, chewing food well, taking time over eating, taking sips of fluids following mouthfuls of food and Sitting upright whilst eating and for 30-60 minutes following consumption of food to aid transit through the oesophagus. These dietary changes take time to establish and patients need to be reminded of them on a regular basis. Issuing them with a reminder card often helps.

If the stent does become blocked, patients should be advised not to panic and to stop eating when they feel a choking episode. Standing up and walking for a short distance, sometimes helps. Taking sips of fluids such as luke warm water or fizzy drinks sometimes helps to dislodge the obstructing bolus in either direction. If patients perceive no improvement over 2 hours, they are advised to contact their general practitioner or to visit the emergency department.

The aims of dietetic treatment in this patient group are focused on offering dietary advice to minimise dysphagia and increase confidence with eating. Due to the negative impact of dysphagia patients tend to lose confidence in eating a diet containing 'normal' textures. It can therefore take varying time frames for patient to progress their eating habits to more solid food. If a nutritional deficit is evident which is often the case, patients should be advised to maximise the overall nutritional intake to improve energy levels. This may include food fortification, high protein high calorie food choices but also in the form of oral nutritional supplements to supplement oral intake from diet. In patients with advanced cancer, dietetic input is less of a priority. Other symptom management is often a higher priority. This however should not exclude basic dietary advice as appropriate.

Oral Nutritional Support

The preferred method of providing nutritional support for a patient who has been identified as being malnourished or is at risk malnutrition is *via* the oral route. Dietary advice should focus on optimising the patient's nutritional intake by a combination of texture modification, meal pattern and content changes including snacks and food fortification. If the 'food-first' approach is not adequate to meet a patient's nutritional needs, dietary advice may need to include Oral Nutritional Supplements.

Food Fortification

In patients who have a reduced appetite due to the disease or symptoms of the disease, it is important that the food they do consume counts significantly towards their overall requirements. Patient compliance with treatment goals is increased if the focus is on modifying foods already taken as part of their usual diet and includes their favorite foods. The aim here is to increase the energy density of foods rather than the volume of food. Food fortification advice is always patient specific but may include general advice such as adding in full-cream milk or butter to mashed potatoes, adding crème fraiche, yoghurt or cream to soups, grating cheese over main meals, adding creamy sauces or gravy to main meals, topping porridge or cereals with dried fruit, honey or jam (Fig. **2**).

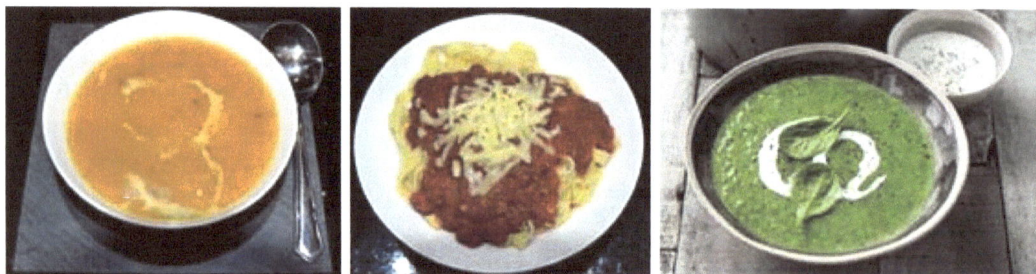

Fig. (2). Examples of fortified food in soups and main meals.

Meal Pattern and Content

Patients with a reduced appetite will usually eat less because they do not feel hungry. It doesn't mean that because they don't feel hungry that their body doesn't need the energy. It is important encourage patients to try to maintain a normal meal pattern consisting of breakfast, lunch and dinner as much as possible. It is difficult to re-introduce this routine once it is lost. Patients may find it easier to take smaller meal portions at usual times or to take multiple 'mini-meals'. Eating more frequently can help to optimise calorie and protein intake.

Introducing snacks and modifying them to include a high calorific and protein content can be just as nutritious as nutritional supplement drinks. Snack ideas can include adding butter and cheese to plain biscuits or crackers, eating breadsticks or crisps with dip and snacking on malt loaf with spread (Fig. **3**). Patients should be encouraged to include high calorie nourishing drinks and fluids such as milk, milkshakes, smoothies with yoghurt, milk or ice cream, hot chocolate or fruit juices. Fizzy juices can also be taken but with care if reflux is an issue as fizzy juices may exacerbate reflux symptoms.

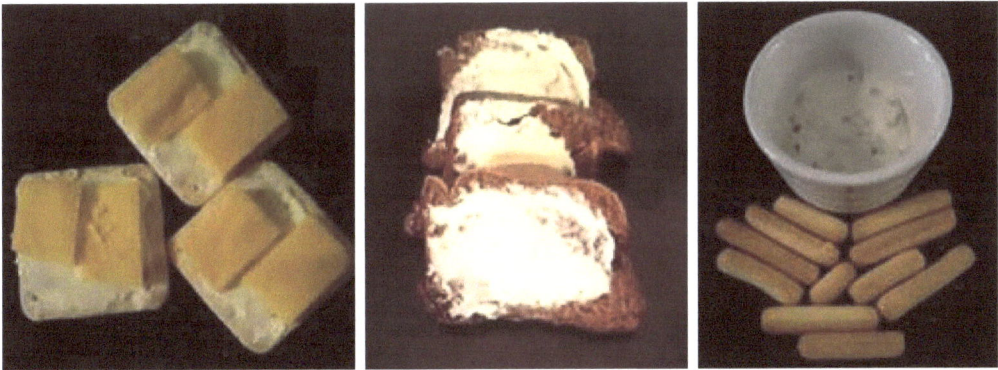

Fig. (3). Examples of "food first" snack ideas with energy and protein content which is comparable to oral nutritional supplements.

Texture Modification

This is based on a soft or liquidized diet. Patients with dysphagia may require texture-modified diet to meet their needs if they cannot tolerate solid textures in a normal diet. Dietary modification should be patient centered and advice should be given to suit the individual's tolerance. Most patients know their own tolerance and the advice should be focused on methods of texture modification rather than on extent. The advice may include pulverising or liquidising meals or adding extra sauces and gravy to moisten the consistency of foods. Cooking pastas and vegetables well, should also be encouraged. Patients should be encouraged to eat smaller pieces of meat in small mouthfuls with adequate chewing to ease swallowing.

High calorie fluids, "little and often" approach to eating and food fortification is incorporated in to texture modification advice for patients to maximise oral intake. In patients who are unable to take an adequate oral intake to meet their nutritional needs oral nutritional supplements should be considered.

Oral Nutritional Supplementation

This is non-invasive and less expensive than other methods of nutritional support. It can also help patients to maintain their independence with regards to their nutritional intake. They allow patients to be creative and to take ownership of their nutrition and approach to their illness. Oral nutritional supplements contain energy in varying quantities of carbohydrates, fat and protein and they also include vitamins and minerals. Some also contain fiber. Typical energy content ranges from 1.5 - 2.4 kcal/ml and they contain 10 – 20 g of protein. The general expectation would be to consume between 1-3 per unit day however a patient with dysphagia whose oral intake may be restricted to a liquid texture only, may require more than 3 units to meet their estimated nutritional requirements. They are usually offered as a supplement to dietary intake to take between meals. However, they can be offered as a sole source of nutrition for those with limited ability to take oral diet but can manage liquids.

There are many different types of oral nutritional supplements (ONS), which are marketed and can be prescribed in accordance with the Advisory Committee on Borderline substances (ACBS), prescribing criteria, and these include ONS such as milkshake drinks, juice drinks, yoghurt-based drinks, savory Soups, liquid Shots, puddings, jellies, ready-mixed or powdered preparations. These should be used in addition to food intake if the patient is able to take food and not used as a meal replacement.

Each of the products is available in various flavors. The type and flavor of supplements prescribed are largely based on patient's preference. The more concentrated supplements in a smaller volume can be offered to patients who prefer smaller volumes due to taste or who have a depressed appetite. Patients who have higher nutritional requirements would be recommended a higher energy and protein supplement. The palatability of supplements can be improved by mixing them in milkshakes, ice cream floats, milky puddings or smoothies. They could also be mixed with water to make diluting juice or jelly, freezing them as ice-lollies or ice cubes or using them as warmed drinks (Fig. **4**). Patients who are expected to take these supplements on a longer-term basis will need creative ideas to help with the compliance. Recipe ideas can be provided from dietitians.

The supplements are usually well tolerated however it should be mentioned that the juice based supplement drinks tend to have a higher carbohydrates content than the milk-based alternative. Patients with diabetes may experience fluctuations in their blood glucose levels on using this type of supplement. Close monitoring of their blood sugar levels are therefore encouraged and the GP or Diabetic Specialist Nurse can alter the diabetic medication accordingly to ensure that blood glucose levels are stable. Nutritional supplement products are available on prescription. Similar products such as powdered varieties are available to buy in supermarkets and pharmacies.

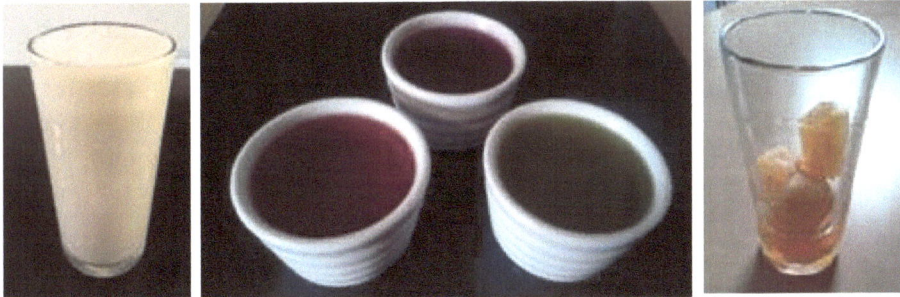

Fig. (4). Oral nutritional supplements can be consumed directly as a drink, made into jelly or frozen and used as ice cubes.

Oral Nutritional Support may not provide every patient's nutritional needs. If a patient is unable to consume adequate oral intake, artificial nutritional support including enteral nutrition and parenteral nutrition, may need to be considered.

Enteral Nutrition

Enteral tube feeding refers to the provision of a nutritionally complete feed directly in to the digestive tract *via* a tube. It can be used as a sole source of nutrition to meet all nutritional requirements or as a supplement to oral intake or parenteral nutrition to provide part of a patient's nutritional requirements [9]. Artificial nutrition support is indicated when oral intake is absent or likely to be absent for a period >5–7 days. Earlier instigation may be needed in malnourished patients. Support may also be needed in patients with inadequate oral intake (less than 60% of their estimated nutritional requirements) for 10 days or longer periods [10]. Enteral feeding can be used in unconscious patients and those with swallowing disorders. There is good evidence to suggest that early post pyloric enteral feeding is generally safe and effective in postoperative patients, even if there is apparent ileus. In addition, the evidence suggests that early enteral feeding after major gastrointestinal surgery reduces infections and shortens length of stay.

It may be necessary to bypass an oesophageal or gastric obstruction (mechanical or functional) preventing nutritional intake *via* the oral route. Another indication may be that a patient is unable to eat and drink due to symptoms of cancer such as dysphagia or reduced appetite enabling adequate oral intake, side effects of cancer treatments such as mucositis or due to unsafe oral intake (risk of choking). Enteral nutrition is also beneficial in providing nutrition pre-operatively and post-operatively until oral intake can be re-established.

Routes of Feeding

There are several different enteral routes of feeding and some of the most common methods of enteral nutrition are described below.

Naso-enteric Feeding: This includes naso-gastric and naso-jejunal feeding. A feeding tube is inserted into one of the nostrils of the patient and the end tip of the tube is positioned in the stomach (nasogastric) or proximal jejunum (naso-jejunal). Fine bore silk feeding tubes tend to be the most comfortable for nasogastric feeding and longer naso-jejunal tubes for naso-jejunal feeding (Fig. 5). The tube is used to deliver nutrition in a liquid form directly in to the stomach or jejunum. The feeding can be provided continuously *via* a feeding pump or boluses (in naso-gastric feeding) can be administered several times throughout the day.

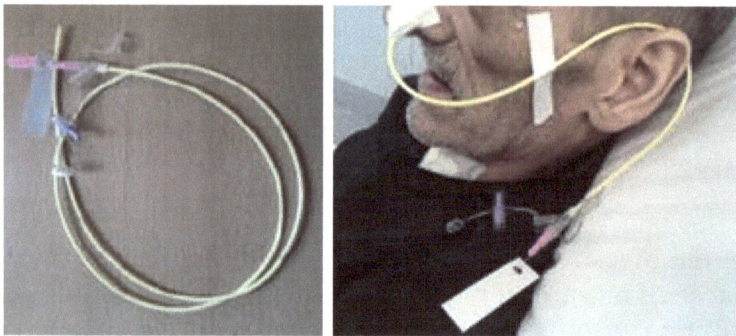

Fig. (5). Fine bore silk nasogastric feeding tube in use to feed a malnourished patient.

Nasogastric tubes can be placed on the ward but naso-jejunal tubes require endoscopic insertion. Prior to commencing feeding or administering water flushes or medication the position of the nasogastric tube must be checked preferably radiologically. Prior to each use following confirmed placement, a syringe is used to draw up a small amount of fluid from the stomach. The normal environment of the stomach is acidic and the acidity of the fluid drawn up is checked using a PH indicator strip. If the reading is less than 5 it is safe to feed. If the level is above this, this could indicate that the position of the tube is in not in the stomach. The position of the tube will need to be checked each time it is to be used for feed, medications or fluid flushes using the above method.

Nasogastric or naso-jejunal feeding is a short-term method of enteral feeding and is generally used for periods of 4-6 weeks. If it is to be used for longer periods, the tube will need to be replaced regularly and more permanent route of feeding should be considered such as; Percutaneous Endoscopic Gastrostomy (PEG), Percutaneous Endoscopic Gastrostomy with a jejunal extension (PEJ) or a surgically placed Jejunostomy tube (Fig. **6**). Nasogastric feeding can be problematic in patients who have recurrent vomiting. This increases the risk of tube dislodgement and in-turn can put the patient at increased risk of aspiration of feed in to the lungs, which can be serious. For these patients jejunal feeding would be indicated. Some patients may not tolerate the nasogastric tube. If a patient pulls on the tube it may dislodge or displace. A bridle can be used to secure the tube and reduce the risk of displacement. Bridles are expensive and are not suitable for all patients.

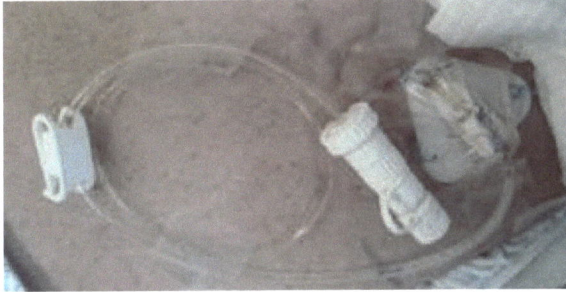

Fig. (6). Freka® feeding jejunostomy tube in situ.

Nasogastric feeding tends to be less well tolerated in patients with gastric cancer. There are many reasons that may contribute to this intolerance. The stomach capacity may be affected by the tumor bulk. Additionally, the tumor may involve the stomach wall or nerves and prevent gastric distension. Patients perceive a feeling of fullness or early satiety, which can lead to nausea and vomiting which reduce their tolerance to higher rates of feed. This can make it difficult to meet their nutritional needs. The use of medications such as PPIs, prokinetic agents and anti-emetics may help. Naso-jejunal tubes tend to be thin and are more susceptible to blocking. Regular water flushes before and after feeding and medications are essential to minimise this risk.

Gastrostomy Feeding: A gastrostomy is a tract formed between the stomach and the skin overlying the stomach to deliver feed directly into the stomach. A gastrostomy is usually used as a method of feeding in patients requiring longer term feeding. For patients, gastrostomy feeding is more cosmetically accepted than naso-gastric feeding. This method is also indicated for patients with oral mucositis, which can often result from chemotherapy treatment. As with naso-gastric feeding, this tube can also be used to deliver water flushes and medications. There are various types of gastrostomy tubes, which differ in the method of placement and the site of feeding.

Percutaneous Endoscopic Gastrostomy (PEG) tubes are placed endoscopically (Fig. 7). The tubes can remain in-situ for several years prior to being replaced.

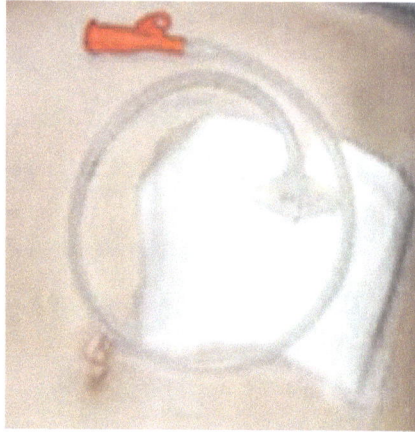

Fig. (7). Percutaneous Endoscopic Gastrostomy (PEG) tube in a malnourished patient with achalasia for pre-operative feeding.

Radiologically Inserted Gastrostomy (RIG) tubes are placed radiologically. The tube is usually held in place with an internal balloon and a bumper on the outer part of the skin. The balloon volume will usually be filled to a maximum of 4 ml. This will be routinely checked and adjusted by the dietitian, district nurse or other healthcare professional. Post-Pyloric Feeding site is chosen if a patient has an increased risk of aspiration with gastric feeding due to vomiting or regurgitation. Patients with obtunded consciousness who are at risk of aspiration will benefit from this site of feeding.

In Percutaneous Endoscopic Jejunostomy (PEJ) the jejunal tube is placed *via* the gastrostomy tract and guided endoscopically or radiologically in to the jejunum.

Surgical Jejunostomy Tube Feeding: A feeding tube is usually placed at the time of surgery, directly into the jejunum. The feeding tube is held in position by a sutured fixator onto the skin. The tube can remain in place for several months before needing replaced. These tubes are suitable for long-term feeding. The tubes can however inadvertently fall out and intermittently block with dried up food debris. Regular water flushes will minimize blocking. Regular inspection of the sutured skin fixator and site of insertion will insure the absence of infection and prevent the tubes falling out.

Types of Feed

The choice of feed to be given is influenced by a patient's nutritional requirements, any abnormality of gastrointestinal absorption, motility, or diarrhoea loss, and the presence of other system abnormality, such as renal or liver failure. Most commercial feeds contain 1.0 kcal/ml, with higher energy versions containing 2 kcal/ml. They are generally available in fiber free and fiber enriched forms. They are nutritionally complete but expert dietetic advice should be sought. Three types of feeds are generally available.

Polymeric Feeds: contain nitrogen as whole protein. The carbohydrate source is partially hydrolysed starch and the fat contains long chain triglycerides. Their content of fiber is variable and although most authorities recommend that fiber should be included.

Predigested Feeds: contain nitrogen as either short peptides or, in the case of elemental diets, as free amino acids. Carbohydrate provides much of the energy content with the content variable in both quantity and the proportion provided as LCTs and medium chain triglycerides (MCTs). The aim of "predigested diets" is to improve nutrient absorption in the presence of significant malabsorption. Their importance is probably greater in mal-digestive rather than malabsorptive states, and in patients with a short gut and no colon their high osmolality can cause excess movement of water into the gut and hence higher stomal losses.

Disease Specific and Pharmaco-nutrient Feeds: are specifically formulated for patients with organ failure or feeds containing large quantities of nutrients with potential pharmacological activity. Patients with respiratory failure are often given feeds with a low carbohydrate to fat ratio in order to minimise carbon dioxide production, but it should be recognised that this type of feed requires higher oxygen availability, and avoidance of overfeeding is probably the more important in limiting respiratory demands. Renal patients will often require modified protein, electrolyte, and volume feeds while liver patients may need low sodium low volume feeds. Sodium supplemented enteral or sip feeds are not available commercially but can be very useful in the management of patients with high output stomas who tend to become salt depleted. Low residue or no residue types of feed are recommended for patients with entero-cutaneous fistulae while waiting for these to heal.

Feeding Regimen

This is formulated to meet the patient's individual requirements and is usually developed by an experienced dietitian. However, emergency regimes for out-o--hours use may also be available in some institutions. These tend to be used in the short-term which prevents delay in introducing enteral nutrition before a dietitian is available to undertake a full nutritional assessment of a patient. If the patient has been following a near to normal diet prior to commencing enteral feeding, a standard whole protein feed (1 kcal/ml) containing fiber will be used initially. Once a patient is established on enteral feeding a more concentrated feed (typically 1.2-2.0 kcal/ml) can be introduced. This will allow the volume of the feed to be reduced and the timescale for feeding to be reduced without compromising calorie and protein intake. A slow transition between different types of feed is necessary to minimise any unwanted side effects.

Tolerance/GI Complications

Hypertonic or concentrated feeds delivered to the stomach can result in nausea, vomiting and distension as they slow gastric emptying. Hypertonic or concentrated feeds delivered to the jejunum may result in cramping and loose stools as they result in an osmotic gradient with a net absorption of fluid in to the intestine. Slow transition to a more concentrated feed can allow the body to adjust to the change in feed and improve tolerance. If loose stools/ diarrhoea is an issue it is important to rule out the possibility of infection so a stool sample should be sent for testing. Medications should also be reviewed by the pharmacist and modified if required. If neither of these resolve symptoms, the fiber content can be adjusted and tolerance may be found with a lower osmolality feed or one without fiber. If malabsorption is thought to be the causative factor a semi-elemental or elemental feed can be offered. Pancreatic Enzyme Replacement Therapy may also be beneficial in this instance. If constipation is an issue and the patient is on a fiber-free feed, a slow transition to a fiber containing feed should help to ease constipation. Laxatives may also be prescribed. Assessment of the patient's fluid intake will also be completed as lack of adequate fluid intake can also lead to constipation.

Tube Blockages

There is a higher risk of the enteral feeding tube blockage with administration of medication *via* the tube. This is particularly common with naso-jejunal tubes as they tend to be smaller in diameter. Regular water flushes before and after administration of feed or medication is essential. Blocked tubes can often be cleared with a flush of warm water (or cool boiled/sterile water if the route of entry is *via* the jejunum). If this is unsuccessful the tube will have to be replaced.

Methods of Administering Feed

Feed is usually administered *via* a feeding pump but drip-feeding can also be used if pumps are not available. The feed could be infused continuously (over 24 hours) or over a shorter period of time. Shorter feeding regimens can be more convenient for some patients but may not be tolerated by all. Feeding over shorter periods tend to require the feed to be administered at an increased rate, which can cause distension, abdominal cramps or diarrhea. Feeding regimens should be tailored to the tolerance of individual patients. Overnight feeding is convenient for patients who are mobile during the day provided that they can tolerate the short period feeding. In addition, overnight feeding will allow patients to indulge in the pleasure of eating small amounts during the day to supplement the feeding requirements. Some patients with gastric feeding may bolus enteral feed or nutritional supplement drinks down their feeding tubes at routine intervals through the day. These are usually administered *via* a syringe. This is not appropriate in jejunal feeding as there is no stomach reservoir to hold the contents and this could lead to abdominal cramps and bloating. As the feed is usually alkaline, this can neutralise gastric acidity and increase the risk of infection. Gastric feeding must allow for a minimum of four-hour break periods to enable the gastric pH to return to normal.

Enteral Feeding and Drug Interactions

The absorption and efficacy of certain medications can be altered by the feed if the route of administration is also *via* the enteral route. Adjustments can be made to patients' enteral feeding regimes to allow for a break period. In order to promote absorption of medications, a short break period in feeding both before and after administration of certain medications will enable medications to work effectively.

Parenteral Nutrition

Parenteral nutrition (PN) is the delivery of nutrients directly in to the bloodstream *via* the intravenous route. It can be used in isolation as the sole source of nutrition or in conjunction with nutrition *via* the oral or enteral route [11]. To ensure patients receive all the necessary nutrients, total parenteral nutrition (TPN) should provide fluid, energy source from carbohydrates (glucose), fatty acids, and protein (as amino acids), electrolytes, fat and water-soluble vitamins and trace elements. PN can be adjusted to suit individual needs *e.g.* removal or addition of certain electrolytes, addition of extra fluid etc. The type of PN bag prescribed for a patient can be altered in view of a patient's clinical condition. Electrolyte containing bags can have further electrolytes added to them if required. Alternatively, electrolyte-free or electrolyte selective bags can be administered. Bags containing different types of fat are also available as well as fat-free bags, which are often used in those with liver dysfunction [12].

A thorough dietetic assessment should be carried out prior to commencing TPN including assessment of baseline biochemistry and hydration status. As with ONS and EN methods of feeding, consideration must be taken of patients at risk of re-feeding syndrome and a detailed assessment of recent nutritional intake and nutritional status will help to determine this. Feeding should be commenced according to local guidelines. Dietetic assessment of a patient for parenteral nutrition should include the indications for parenteral feeding, appropriate venous access, current biochemistry including blood glucose levels and hydration status.

Indications

The primary indication for the use of TPN is an inaccessible or non-functioning gastro-intestinal tract. This may be due to an obstruction not passable *via* the enteral route, a post-operative ileus or inadequate nutrition *via* the enteral route due to severe malabsorption or a severe catabolic state.

Access and Associated Issues

The preferred access for parenteral nutrition is delivery directly in to a central vein, but peripheral venous nutrition (PVN) *via* a peripheral vein can be used for a short period (less than 2 weeks) (Fig. **8**).

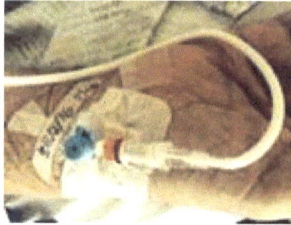

Fig. (**8**). Peripheral venous nutrition *via* a peripheral venous catheter

The use of a central vein can reduce the incidence of thrombotic phenomena associated with the indwelling catheter and constituents of the feed. Central venous feeding can be *via* a central venous catheter (CVC) or dedicated Hickman line, or a peripherally inserted central catheter (PICC) (Fig. **9**).

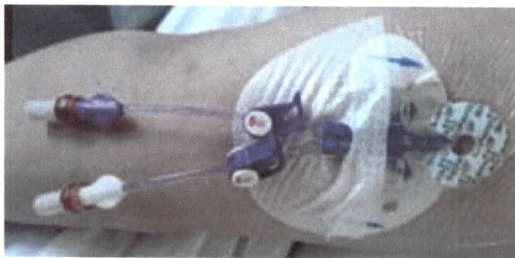

Fig. (**9**). Double lumen PICC® line used for intravenous nutrition.

Peripheral parenteral nutrition involves daily re-siting of a peripheral cannula to alternate areas. It is not suitable for patients with poor venous access. There is a risk of bruising, phlebitis and general discomfort at the access site. The feed used in parenteral nutrition can be a skin irritant but preparations with a low osmolarity and neutral PH are better tolerated. PVN does restrict the rate of infusion and limit the types of feed, which can be administered. Infusion line infection can occur with all types of access catheters. This is a particular problem with lines which are peripheral, not dedicated to feeding, remain in situ for long (more than 2 weeks) and if used by inexperienced staff.

Feeding Regimen

The goal of parenteral nutrition in dietetic treatment is to provide all elements of nutrition including fluids, electrolytes, micronutrients, trace elements, vitamins and minerals whilst the oral or enteral routes are unavailable for ingestion and/ or digestion. In patients where the oral or enteral routes are partially used, parenteral nutrition may be used to supplement the intake. A suitable regimen attempts to meet the nutritional needs of the individual. The anabolic Nitrogen (protein) requirements are met and the balance is supplied as lipids and carbohydrates. Additives of electrolytes etc., supplement the feed and are informed by the patient's biochemistry. The feed is supplied in bags to run over 24 hours delivering the fluid requirements of the individual. The bags should be protected from sunlight and must be used within a short period of supply. The feed should be infused with a calibrated pump.

The nutritional needs of patients receiving TPN should be routinely monitored. Routine monitoring of anthropometry, biochemistry, blood glucose levels, fluid balance, bowel function, liver function and weight should also be monitored routinely. A repeat assessment of nutritional requirements should be undertaken so that complications can be minimised. Overfeeding a severely malnourished or catabolic patient should be discouraged. This can add metabolic stress onto already challenged systems due to the effects of excess glucose and lipid. A gradual increase in the rate of feeding is more tolerable with high fat or glucose feeds. The patient's physical and psychological tolerance of the feeding regimen should be closely monitored and changes introduced to address intolerance. When TPN is no longer required a gradual reduction in infusion rate (over a few days) is preferable to a sharp stop. During the period of gradual rate reduction oral nutritional supplements could be introduced to avoid nutritional deficit.

In those feeding for longer than two weeks cyclical feeding should be considered to avoid unnecessary stress on the liver and to avoid restricting the mobility of the patient. Patients who may require TPN on a longer-term basis should be considered for home parenteral nutrition (HPN) by the Nutrition Support team. This team provides comprehensive assessment for suitability, appropriate training and support for suitable candidates.

Assessment and Monitoring

Biochemistry: Baseline biochemistry should be checked prior to commencing TPN. To minimise the risk re-feeding syndrome, correction of phosphate, potassium and magnesium levels should be done rapidly.

Blood Glucose Levels: Optimal blood glucose range in patients receiving TPN is between 4 – 12 mmol/l. If levels regularly exceed this range, a sliding scale insulin regimen should be commenced as per institution's local protocols. The continuous infusion of glucose *via* TPN over a 24-hour period rather than cyclically can help keep blood glucose levels more stable by reducing insulin resistance.

Fluid Balance: TPN can provide a significant volume of fluid (2 – 3 liters). Monitoring of fluid input and output is essential. Patients receiving TPN can be at risk of fluid overload. Significant volumes of fluid may also come from additional IV preparations including antibiotics, medications, oral consumption or enteral nutrition. Risk of dehydration should also be monitored particularly in excessive fluid output states *e.g.* high drain and fistula output, renal failure etc.

Liver Dysfunction: Liver dysfunction can occur with extended use of PN. Clinicians should initially focus on early detection and prevention. Serial biochemical monitoring of liver enzymes is essential. However, deranged liver function tests are more indicative of the patient's general clinical condition rather than TPN induced dysfunction. If there is a clinical suspicion that liver dysfunction may be induced by TPN, break periods of 8 or more hours per day can reduce insulin levels and stabilise liver enzymes [13].

NUTRITION OF THE SURGICAL PATIENT

Pre-operative Nutrition

All patients should be screened for malnutrition and if indicated referred for a dietetic assessment prior to surgery. Optimisation of nutritional status helps to reduce post-operative infection risk and promote wound healing. There is evidence to suggest benefits from pre-operative nutrition for 7-14 days in those who are severely malnourished to reduce surgical stress and promote recovery. Shorter periods of feeding do not show significant benefit. Recent guidelines suggest that pre-operative nutrition should be considered in those who are severely malnourished and that elective surgery should be postponed to allow a period of pre-operative nutrition [14]. Pre-operative nutrition should be provided *via* the enteral route as opposed to PN.

Immunonutrition

This has been a controversial issue for a long time [15]. The potential to modulate the activity of the immune system by interventions with specific nutrients is termed immunonutrition. Major surgery is followed by a period of immunosuppression that increases the risk of morbidity and mortality due to infection. Improving immune function during this period may reduce complications due to infection. Three potential targets exist for immunonutrition: mucosal barrier function, cellular defense, and local or systemic inflammation. The nutrients most often studied for immunonutrition are arginine, glutamine, branched chain amino acids, n-3 fatty acids, and nucleotides. Combinations of some or all of these nutrients are present in commercially available enteral feeds. Parenteral formulas containing glutamine or n-3 fatty acids are also available. Trials of immunonutrients indicate several beneficial clinical effects, particularly in surgical patients. However, doubts remain about the efficacy of this approach in critically ill patients, with contradictory findings among trials [16].

Post-operative Nutrition

Surgery induces catabolic changes due to the activation of stress hormones and an inflammatory response. This catabolic state increases the body's energy requirements. Current practice encourages re-introduction of nutrition as soon as possible after surgery to promote recovery and reduce complications [17]. In practice, this is difficult to achieve after major abdominal surgery due to ileus, anastomosis or sedation / analgesia regimens. Ironically, these are the patients who will have additional energy requirements. In these patients, many surgical units insert feeding jejunostomy tubes at the time of the index surgery to be used prophylactically after surgery. Others rely on naso-jejunal feeding tubes inserted after surgery. Other units introduce nutritional supplements such as high energy, high protein drinks routinely after surgery as soon as oral intake is tolerated.

Enteral Feeding

Feeding *via* a surgically placed feeding jejunostomy or *via* a naso-jejunal / nasogastric tube can commence as early as 24 hours after major abdominal surgery. Sterile water flushes should be administered every 6 hours following placement of the feeding tube. Feeding can start 24 hours after surgery. A standard polymeric feed (1 kcal/ml) is preferable in the first instance. The feed should commence at a low rate (10 mls per hour) and increased over days as tolerated. Once tolerance is established, the feed may be changed to an alternative more concentrated feed (1.5 kcal/ml) to provide more nutrition within a smaller volume. Oral intake should also commence when tolerated, subject to the overall clinical condition of the patient. At this point it is appropriate to aim for overnight top up feeding to give scope for oral intake to improve during the day. The guiding principle should be to meet the nutritional requirement of the post-operative patient. Prior to discharge, patients and carers should receive training on enteral feeding *via* the feeding pump. Institutions will have their local protocols for feeding and training. If patients have pancreatic insufficiency or malabsorption, a semi-elemental feed or peptide-based feed should be used to promote absorption. At home, patients can continue to have overnight top up feeds until their pre-operative weight is restored. This is usually between 6 weeks and three months after surgery. When the community dietician is satisfied with the nutritional status of the patient, the feeding tube could be removed.

Dietetic Advice After Discharge

Patients should be advised to select a low fiber diet since a high fiber diet will make patients feel distended for a longer period. Whenever possible, patients should focus on high protein and high calorie (energy dense) calorific foods. Patients should be advised to eat slowly and chew food well to minimise digestion efforts. They should remain upright during and 30-60 minutes after meals. They should limit fluid intake with meals to avoid filling up on fluid, which can limit calorific intake at meals. Patients should be advised to eat small frequent meals and snacks i.e. 6-8 times daily. Patients should keep snacks readily available particularly if leaving the house or are going out for extended periods. Patients should choose high calorific drinks within their tolerance limits. Advice may also include tips to overcome specific symptoms such as nausea.

Nutritional Consequences of Surgery

Weight loss: Failure to gain weight or even weight loss is common after major abdominal surgery particularly after gastric surgery. Significant weight loss can be encountered in patients who have had post-operative complications. The resulting diminished calorie intake is the major factor but malabsorption of fat and Nitrogen and decreased small bowel transit time may be responsible in some patients. Although mild steatorhoea is not uncommon, severe fat malabsorption is rare unless there is a coexisting small bowel disease (*e.g.* Gluten enteropathy), bacterial overgrowth or pancreatic disease.

Anaemia: Iron-deficiency anaemia manifesting with microcytosis and hypochromia of red cells is common after gastrectomy. The incidence of this complication is high and increases with time after gastrectomy. The exact reasons for the anaemia are not clear but lack of acidic pH and gastric juices are probably responsible for the decreased absorption of iron in foods. Prophylactic treatment with oral iron is recommended for all patients after gastrectomy. By increasing the supply of iron in the small bowel, sufficient absorption can take place to restore or keep iron levels in the normal range.

Macrocytic anaemia can also develop as a result of Vitamin B12 deficiency. The loss of intrinsic factor after gastrectomy significantly impairs Vitamin B12 absorption. In addition, the lack of acid environment, which normally facilitates the release of Vitamin B12 in ingested food, can be responsible. Fortunately, the healthy liver stores large amounts of Vitamin B12 and megaloblastic anaemia is rare. Patients usually have an abnormal Schilling test. Treatment is with three monthly injections of cyanocobalamine. Folate deficiency is rare and is only encountered after total gastrectomy. It results from poor dietary intake. Supplementary oral folate is recommended in these patients.

Bone Disease: The duodenum is the major site of calcium absorption. Several years after gastric resections with duodenal exclusion patients can develop osteoporosis (loss of bone substance) or osteomalacia (bone demineralization). Patients are usually females and present with bone pains, weakness and stress fractures. Their biochemistry shows a raised alkaline phosphatase (bone specific) and serum calcium. Radiology shows evidence of bone rarefication. Treatment is with oral calcium and Vitamin D supplements or with bi-phosphonates.

Dumping Syndrome: A common side effect after oesophageal or gastric surgery is dumping syndrome. The syndrome consists of post-prandial vaso-motor (systemic) and gastrointestinal symptoms. The vaso-motor symptoms (palpitations, vasodilatation, hypotension and fainting) occur within minutes of eating and are due to hypovolaemia accompanied by diminished cardiac output and peripheral resistance. The attacks are typically precipitated by high carbohydrate meals. This is due to the rapid transit of hyperosmolar food into the jejunum. Fluid shifts into the small bowel cause bloating, pain and diarrhoea. The fluid shift decreases intravascular volume cause hypervolemia, which manifest as hypotension and tachycardia. Inappropriate release of GLP-1 activates sympathetic outflow causing vasomotor symptoms. Early dumping syndrome generally occurs within 30 mins after eating however it may present up to 2 hours later depending on the food consumed. Symptoms include flushing or sweating, a feeling of weakness or tiredness, dizziness, urgency to defecate with loose bowels or diarrhea. Patients should be advised to eat small, dry meals rich in protein and fat but low in carbohydrates. Patients should avoid drinking fluids with meals. Fluids could be consumed at least 30 minutes after meals. Additives, (fiber or pectin), which slow gastric emptying can be beneficial. In late dumping, or reactive hypoglycaemia, glucose is rapidly absorbed from carbohydrates triggering inappropriate insulin release resulting in late hypoglycaemia with sweating, tremor, dizziness, poor concentration and occasionally fainting. This tends to occur 2 – 3 hours after eating. The diagnosis could be confirmed by an extended glucose tolerance test, which demonstrates an initial hyperglycaemia followed by hypoglycaemia. This tends to respond to dietary measures including low-carbohydrate, high protein meals. In addition, patients should be advised to carry glucose tablets with them to ingest if they experience reactive hypoglycaemia [18].

CONTINUOUS MONITORING OF NUTRITION

Continuous Management of the Surgical Patient

Routine dietetic follow-up is important following oesophageal and gastric surgery as many dietetic issues can arise which have a detrimental effect on the patients well-being and possibly survival. These include weight loss, reduced appetite, early satiety, reflux and dumping syndrome. The altered anatomy following oesophagectomy or gastrectomy, necessitate immediate adjustments in diet and nutrition. The reduced stomach capacity, absence or altered position, necessitate adjustments to meal sizes and frequency. In addition, patients may have persistent psychological effects resulting from a cancer diagnosis. The combination can result in difficulty to maintain an adequate nutritional status or achieve weight gain after surgery. Many patients develop fear of eating certain foods, which stem from unpleasant past experiences before surgery such as dysphagia for solids. Others may become socially isolated fearing meals out with the privacy of their home, which they perceive may expose dietary modifications or anti-social symptoms after meals. Caring family members may inadvertently pressure patients to increase their portion sizes. These family members often feel guilty when the patient develops untoward symptoms as a result. Continuing dietetic support in the short term can alleviate some of the patient's anxieties and enable them to adjust to their ne anatomy and eating habits. In addition, the dietetic involvement monitors the patient's nutritional status, which in itself is reassuring to patients and relatives.

Dietary advice should be practical and focus on adjustments to meal frequency and nutrient density. If necessary, patients could be advised on how to fortify foods to increase the energy density or they could be supplied with samples of different oral nutritional supplements. Practical advice could be given on reducing fluid consumption around meal times. Advice can also be provided on "problem foods" which produce untoward symptoms. Despite all efforts, some patients are not able to meet their nutritional requirements. The dietician is well placed to flag up these patients for further investigations and to recommend artificial nutritional support. The dietician should regularly assess progress, measure treatment outcomes and adjust nutritional goals.

Continuous Management of the Oncology Patient

It is important for patients to receive dietetic input before and throughout their oncological treatment to prevent further weight loss. Maintaining a desirable nutritional status can also enhance the response to treatment. The Focus of dietary input is usually on dietary changes to overcome barriers to oral intake associated with the side effects of chemotherapy treatment. These include reduced appetite, nausea, vomiting and taste changes. Advice will include a "little and often" approach to eating, choosing favorite foods, high calorie fluids and energy dense foods. Dry foods should be encouraged if nausea and vomiting are persistent. If reduced appetite or taste changes are reported, dietary intake can be improved by trying different foods, marinating meats or adding herbs, sauces and flavorings can often help. Fortunately, most of these symptoms are short lasting and disappear after treatment. Foods found to cause symptoms during treatment may become desired after treatment.

Radiotherapy can initiate different symptoms, which impair nutrition such as sore mouth, poor appetite and diarrhoea. Reducing the fiber content can help the diarrhoea. Adequate fluids should be encouraged to replace the losses. Soft moist foods should be encouraged in patients with oesophagitis or a sore mouth.

Continuous Management of Patients with Palliative Intent

In terminal stages of the disease, symptoms such as dysphagia often worsen. Dietary management usually focuses on texture modification coupled with energy dense foods and high calorie fluids. The role of dietetic management in these patients is to support the patient to maximise their nutritional intake to maintain a level of functionality for as long as possible together with general symptoms control.

Ethical Issues in Nutritional Management

The decision to use enteral tube feedings or parenteral nutrition for patients with advanced incurable disease requires careful consideration of the aims of such treatment. It is difficult to justify expensive and often invasive methods of nutritional support in patients who are not expected to have a worthwhile survival. This is particularly so, if patients' quality of life is compromised by the disease (cancer) or its symptoms. Conditions for which "artificial" feeding (such as enteral or parenteral nutrition) should be considered carefully include end-stage disease, advanced dementia, and a persistent vegetative state. Indeed, some patients express a desire to have no support whatsoever, even in the form of intravenous hydration. The decision to deliver basic support should be discussed with the family in terms of prognosis, anticipated consequences of not receiving hydration or nutrition, risks involved in administering support, and cost. In many patients, the provision of enteral support *via* tube feeding can provide a better quality of life by restoring some degree of strength and energy and allowing patients to eat for enjoyment rather than feeling pressured to maintain energy or weight. Ultimately, the choice for nutritional support in the end-stage cancer patient must lie between the treating clinician and the patient together with the family and carers. The choice options and consequences must be informed by advice from an experienced health care team.

CONSENT FOR PUBLICATION

Not applicable.

CONFLICT OF INTEREST

The authors declare no conflict of interest, financial or otherwise.

ACKNOWLEDGEMENT

Declare none.

REFERENCES

[1]   Choi WJ, Kim J. Nutritional care of gastric cancer patients with clinical outcomes and complications: A Review. Clin Nutr Res 2016; 5(2): 65-78.
        [http://dx.doi.org/10.7762/cnr.2016.5.2.65] [PMID: 27152296]

[2]   Anandavadivelan P, Lagergren P. Cachexia in patients with oesophageal cancer. Nat Rev Clin Oncol 2016; 13(3): 185-98.
        [http://dx.doi.org/10.1038/nrclinonc.2015.200] [PMID: 26573424]

[3]   Russell MK. Functional assessment of nutrition status. Nutr Clin Pract 2015; 30(2): 211-8.
        [http://dx.doi.org/10.1177/0884533615570094] [PMID: 25681483]

[4]   BAPEN. The 'MUST' explanatory booklet A guide to the 'Malnutrition Universal Screening Tool' ('MUST') for adults 2003.

[5]   Elia M. Quantitative biology and nutritional support. Clin Nutr 2003; 22 (Suppl. 2): S33-5.
        [http://dx.doi.org/10.1016/S0261-5614(03)00155-9] [PMID: 14512050]

[6]   Walmsley RS. Refeeding syndrome: screening, incidence, and treatment during parenteral nutrition. J Gastroenterol Hepatol 2013; 28 (Suppl. 4): 113-7.
        [http://dx.doi.org/10.1111/jgh.12345] [PMID: 24251716]

[7]   BAPEN (2012, 1st April) Refeeding syndrome: Identification of those at Risk

[8]   Bruera E. ABC of palliative care. Anorexia, cachexia, and nutrition. BMJ 1997; 315(7117): 1219-22.
        [http://dx.doi.org/10.1136/bmj.315.7117.1219] [PMID: 9393230]

[9]   Scott R, Bowling TE. Enteral tube feeding in adults. J R Coll Physicians Edinb 2015; 45(1): 49-54.
        [http://dx.doi.org/10.4997/JRCPE.2015.112] [PMID: 25874832]

[10]   Weimann A, Braga M, Harsanyi L, *et al.* ESPEN Guidelines on Enteral Nutrition: Surgery including organ transplantation. Clin Nutr 2006; 25(2): 224-44.
        [http://dx.doi.org/10.1016/j.clnu.2006.01.015] [PMID: 16698152]

[11]   Inayet N, Neild P. Parenteral nutrition. J R Coll Physicians Edinb 2015; 45(1): 45-8.
       [http://dx.doi.org/10.4997/JRCPE.2015.111] [PMID: 25874831]

[12]   Braga M, Ljungqvist O, Soeters P, Fearon K, Weimann A, Bozzetti F. ESPEN Guidelines on
       Parenteral Nutrition: surgery. Clin Nutr 2009; 28(4): 378-86.
       [http://dx.doi.org/10.1016/j.clnu.2009.04.002] [PMID: 19464088]

[13]   Hwang TL, Lue MC, Chen LL. Early use of cyclic TPN prevents further deterioration of liver
       functions for the TPN patients with impaired liver function. Hepatogastroenterology 2000; 47(35):
       1347-50.
       [PMID: 11100349]

[14]   Allum WH, Blazeby JM, Griffin SM, Cunningham D, Jankowski JA, Wong R. Guidelines for the
       management of oesophageal and gastric cancer. Gut 2011; 60(11): 1449-72.
       [http://dx.doi.org/10.1136/gut.2010.228254] [PMID: 21705456]

[15]   Calder PC. Immunonutrition. BMJ 2003; 327(7407): 117-8.
       [http://dx.doi.org/10.1136/bmj.327.7407.117] [PMID: 12869428]

[16]   Wong CS, Aly EH. The effects of enteral immunonutrition in upper gastrointestinal surgery: A
       systematic review and meta-analysis. Int J Surg 2016; 29: 137-50.
       [http://dx.doi.org/10.1016/j.ijsu.2016.03.043] [PMID: 27020765]

[17]   Wheble GA, Benson RA, Khan OA. Is routine postoperative enteral feeding after oesophagectomy
       worthwhile? Interact Cardiovasc Thorac Surg 2012; 15(4): 709-12.
       [http://dx.doi.org/10.1093/icvts/ivs221] [PMID: 22753430]

[18]   Berg P, McCallum R. Dumping Syndrome: A review of the current concepts of pathophysiology,
       diagnosis, and treatment. Dig Dis Sci 2016; 61(1): 11-8.
       [http://dx.doi.org/10.1007/s10620-015-3839-x] [PMID: 26396002]

CHAPTER 4

Pathology of the Oesophagus and Stomach

Shaun Walsh[*]

Department of Pathology, Ninewells Hospital and Medical School, Dundee, Scotland, UK

Abstract: The oesophagus and stomach present a wide spectrum of benign and neoplastic conditions. Understanding the pathology of these conditions has always been important to the surgical management of these diseases. The advent of modern molecular pathological techniques has greatly expanded our knowledge of the underlying pathogenesis of these conditions and now directly affects practice. The integration of this new knowledge with standard histopathological techniques presents new challenges to the pathologists and surgeon alike. This chapter discusses benign and malignant pathology of the oesophagus and stomach, with repeated emphasis on new knowledge where these influence practice.

By far, the commonest conditions affecting the oesophagus and stomach are benign. However, these conditions can impact heavily on affected individuals. Although relatively rare, cancers carry a huge burden on the individual and society. Specific management and prognosis for these conditions are dependent on accurate diagnosis, which is the realm of pathology. In this regard, the patient presentation, clinical and diagnostic findings together with chemical pathology (Biochemistry), where appropriate, are essential in guiding the pathologist to apply sophisticated pathological essays that clinch the diagnosis. In some circumstances, pathology is also important in identifying the aetiology, pathophysiology and malignant potential of some conditions.

Keywords: Adenocarcinoma, Carcinogenesis, Gastritis, Oesophagitis, Squamous cell cancer, Pathogenesis, Risk factors, Molecular pathology, Stromal tumours, Lymphoid tumours.

PATHOLOGY OF BENIGN CONDITIONS

Oesophagitis

Oesophagitis is defined as inflammation of any cause within the oesophageal wall. The commonest cause of oesophagitis is chemical injury induced by refluxed acid (and bile) from the stomach. While acid reflux per se is a normal physiological process, excessive acid reflux induces symptoms and with the full-

[*] **Corresponding author Shaun Walsh:** Department of Pathology, Ninewells Hospital and Medical School, Dundee DD1 9SY, Scotland, UK; Tel: +44 1382 660111; E-mail: shaun.walsh@nhs.net

Sami M. Shimi (Ed.)

ness of time, causes the inflammatory changes. Infective oesophagitis tends to be caused by specific bacterial, viral and fungal organisms. While the majority of people exposed to these infective agents do not succumb to their virulent processes, these organisms can rapidly invade immunologically compromised people. The oesophagus is a proximal port of entry of ingested foodstuff and other materials. As such, it is susceptible to direct contact injury of noxious materials causing corrosive oesophagitis but also susceptible to contact inflammation of allergens in primed individuals. Medication induced injury is a common but often unrecognised cause of oesophagitis. Radiation induced oesophagitis is well recognised in patients receiving radiotherapy where the oesophagus is within the treatment contours. In addition, a number of specific disorders are associated with oesophagitis including bullous dermatoses, Bechets's syndrome, Crohn's disease and aphthous oesophagitis.

Reflux Oesophagitis

The commonest cause of oesophagitis worldwide is reflux oesophagitis in which gastric contents including acid and digestive juices are refluxed into the squamous lined oesophagus from the stomach. Predisposing conditions include all causes of raised intra-abdominal pressure, of which the single most important is obesity. However, not all patients with reflux oesophagitis are obese and abnormal gastro-oesophageal sphincter function plays an important role. Reflux oesophagitis is a chronic condition and is associated with characteristic pathological features. These include epithelial basal cell hyperplasia, elongation of the lamina propria papillae together with influx of inflammatory cells including eosinophils and neutrophils [1, 2]. This constellation of biopsy features usually allows the pathologist to arrive at a diagnosis of oesophagitis most likely due to reflux. Reflux oesophagitis, when severe, may be associated with ulceration. Biopsies in such cases are likely to reveal fibrino-purulent exudate and elements of granulation tissue, which are non-specific responses to the loss of the protective surface epithelium. Rarely, elements of fibrotic scar tissue may be present which may correlate with stricture formation in severe cases. In chronic cases, the repeated exposure to acid and bile influences the basement membrane cells to undergo protective changes to survive in such a hostile unfamiliar environment. A clone of cells changes cell type, which is better adapted to the enteric milieu. Such supervening metaplasia may occur with replacement of the native squamous epithelium by an admixture of columnar epithelial cells of gastric and sometimes intestinal phenotype. This metaplastic response is most commonly termed as Barrett's oesophagus based on the original description by Norman Barrett, a thoracic surgeon in the 1950s [3, 4].

Infective Oesophagitis

Rarely oesophageal inflammation may be due to infective organism. Infective oesophagitis is best classified according to the offending organism and the commonest organisms include herpes virus, cytomegalovirus and the fungal infection caused by *candida albicans*. As might be expected these conditions are more commonly found in immuno-compromised patients. It is important for endoscopists to provide sufficient clinical information to the pathologist dealing with the biopsy including an indication when a suspicion of such predisposition exists. Although these organisms are often recognisable on routine histopathological stains, special histochemical and immunohistochemical studies may be required to establish the diagnosis in difficult cases. There are other rare causes of infective oesophagitis but these are beyond the scope of this discussion.

Eosinophilic (Allergic) Oesophagitis

Over the past two decades' clinicians and pathologists have identified a further subtype of chronic oesophagitis, which has an allergic aetiology. This condition is most commonly termed as eosinophilic oesophagitis [5]. This condition is associated with an allergic response to a variety of possible dietary components or allergens including wheat, dairy and nuts. Endoscopically, the condition is often characterised by concentric rings or so called trachealization of the oesophagus. On biopsy, a massive number of intraepithelial eosinophils are most often identified (Fig. **1**). These eosinophils often form micro-abscesses and are present throughout the mucosal layer. While there is no absolute number of intraepithelial eosinophils, which may be used to distinguish eosinophilic oesophagitis from reflux oesophagitis most pathologists would accept a count of greater than 15 eosinophils per high power microscopic field as being diagnostic. Recognition of this condition is important as anti-allergy type treatment rather than anti-reflux type treatment is necessary.

Gastritis

Gastritis is defined as gastric mucosal inflammation of any cause. It is most commonly classified clinically and pathologically as acute or chronic. Acute gastritis is often associated with systemic injury including sepsis, shock or burns and also head injury. It may also be associated with ingestion of corrosive substances. Pathological changes include mucosal erosions with surface inflammatory exudates, congestion, haemorrhage and active inflammation. In contrast, chronic gastritis is a more clinically burdensome problem, which effects large numbers of patients and is classifiable on aetiological grounds or morphological grounds. Of these, the former is most clinically useful. The three main types are autoimmune gastritis, bacterial *Helicobacter Pylori* driven gastritis and chemical gastritis.

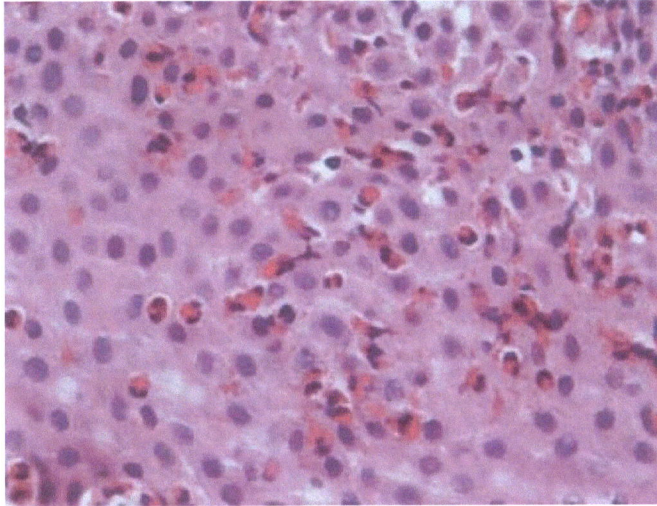

Fig. (1). Eosinophilic oesophagitis is characterised by a massive infiltrate of intraepithelial eosinophils.

Autoimmune Gastritis

Autoimmune gastritis is an immunological disorder associated with autoantibody production to parietal cells and/or intrinsic factor [6]. This condition is characterised by progressive loss of the specialised acid secreting epithelium of the gastric corpus mucosa and may be associated therefore with inability to absorb vitamin B12 in the small bowel (due to a lack of complex factor normally produced by the gastric mucosa) giving rise to the condition termed pernicious anaemia. Histopathologically, the normal oxyntic lining of the corpus mucosa is progressively lost and replaced by severe chronic inflammation associated with intestinal metaplasia and generalised mucosal atrophy. It may also be associated with neuroendocrine cell hyperplasia. Surface bacterial organisms are usually not present. Importantly, it may be complicated by epithelial dysplasia, either low or high grade, highlighting its pre-malignant potential (Fig. **2**).

Bacterial Chronic Gastritis

This type of gastritis is probably the most common type globally and is caused by infection with the non-invasive Gram-negative bacillus *Helicobacter pylori* [7]. Rarely, other Helicobacter species such as *Helicobacter heilmannii* may also produce a similar picture. Here, the surface Helicobacter organisms do not invade the epithelium or deeper tissues but instead incite a chronic active inflammatory reaction, which produces associated epithelial injury leading to erosions and ulceration. *Helicobacter pylori*-type organisms are recognisable on routine

Haematoxylin and Eosin staining but many centres also employ special stains such as a modified Giemsa stain in order to highlight the organisms (Fig. **3**). *Helicobacter pylori* gastritis is associated with peptic ulcer disease within both the duodenum and stomach. It is also critical to the development of low grade gastric lymphomas derived from the so-called mucosa associated lymphoid tissue or Maltomas. *Helicobacter pylori* gastritis is also now recognised as a risk factor for the development of gastric cancer.

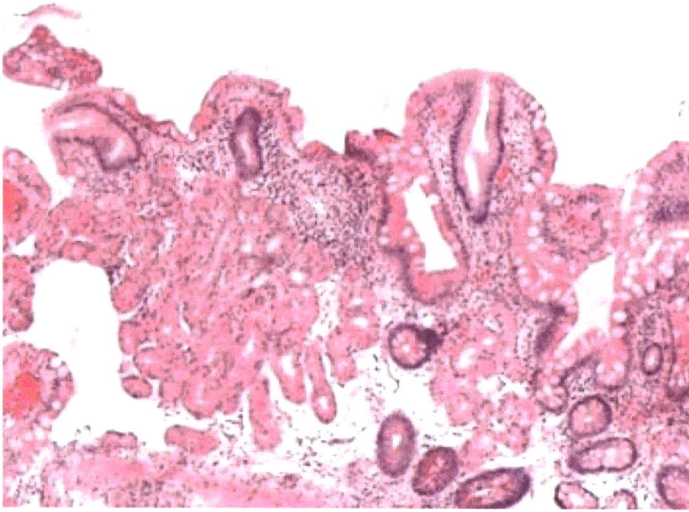

Fig. (2). Autoimmune gastritis with atrophy of specialised mucosa, mild chronic inflammation and intestinal metaplasia.

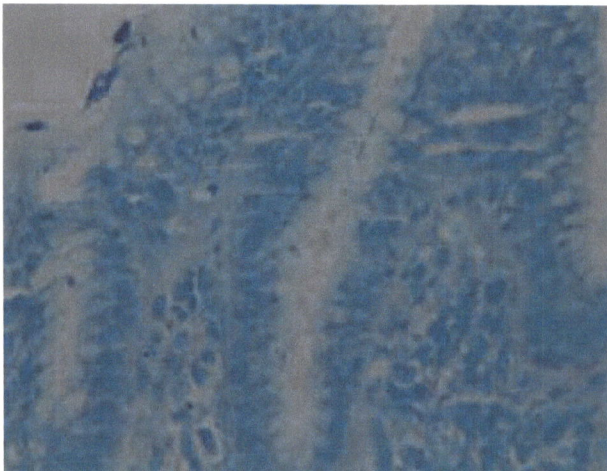

Fig. (3). Modified Giemsa stained slide showing abundant *H. pylori* on the mucosal surface.

Chemical Type Gastritis

Chemical type gastritis or reactive gastritis is probably the commonest type of gastritis within the developed world [8]. It is associated with the presence within the stomach of chemicals, which directly damage the gastric epithelial lining. Causes include non-steroidal anti-inflammatory drugs, bile reflux and alcohol ingestion either alone or in combination with other noxious agents. Direct injury to gastric epithelial cells leads to a regenerative response.

Histopathologically, the changes seen are often most pronounced in the gastric antrum and are characterised by a paucity of chronic inflammation, vascular congestion, loss of epithelial cell cytoplasm, regenerative changes within the gastric pits and upwards spurring of smooth muscle (Fig. **4**). Although histopathologically quite distinct from *H. Pylori* driven gastritis, the pathologist must nevertheless be careful to exclude Helicobacter pylori infection.

Chronic gastritis of either the bacterial or chemical type may be associated with the development of intestinal metaplasia and dysplasia. Intestinal metaplasia is readily recognised by the presence of goblet cells and often also Paneth cells. These cell types are thought to provide a protective response against the chronic continuing injury. Epithelial dysplasia is readily recognisable by the presence of cytological atypia including nuclear hyperchromasia, loss of polarity, nuclear pleomorphism and abnormal mitotic figures. These features alone within a normal architectural glandular context are sufficient to diagnose low-grade dysplasia. Further complex architectural and cytological changes are required for a diagnosis of high-grade dysplasia.

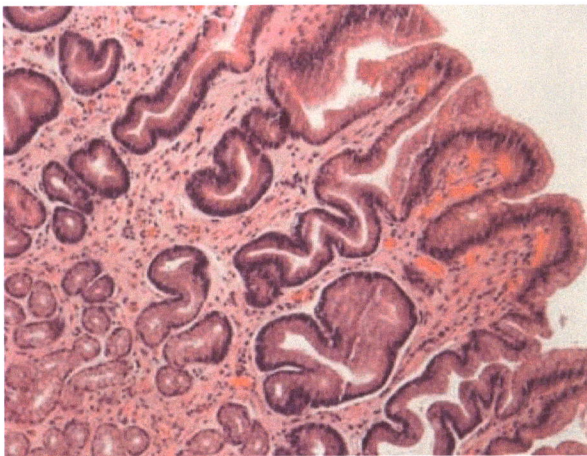

Fig. (4). Extreme epithelial regeneration characterises chemical gastritis.

CARCINOGENESIS IN THE OESOPHAGUS AND STOMACH

Carcinogenesis in the Oesophagus

The aetiology of carcinoma of the oesophagus, either squamous cell carcinoma or adenocarcinoma, has been the subject of intensive research but the precise steps in pathogenesis remains unknown. Although many similarities and overlapping features are thought to be involved in the pathogenesis of both types of oesophageal carcinoma, for the purposes of this chapter they will be treated separately.

Pathogenesis of Squamous Cell Carcinoma

Squamous cell carcinoma of the oesophagus is now known to arise following a step wise pathway from low grade dysplastic change within the squamous epithelium to high grade dysplasia followed by invasive carcinoma [9]. Several pre-disposing factors, which are thought to initiate carcinogenesis, have been studied. These include most prominently alcohol and tobacco consumption. Other pre-disposing factors include dietary problems including vitamin deficiencies such as vitamin A and vitamin C. Infectious agents have also been implicated as initiating factors. Great interest has been focused on a potential role for human papilloma virus infection but its role remains highly controversial. Other associated conditions include achalasia, diverticular disease, Plummer Vinson syndrome and coeliac disease. Although poorly defined, genetic factors, which pre-dispose to oesophageal cancer, may also exist in certain populations. Importantly, as more than one of these suspected pre-disposing factors might be present within any individual or group of individuals within a population, the precise weighting of each factor is difficult to determine.

The stepwise progression from low-grade dysplasia through to invasive squamous cell carcinoma is associated with an accumulation of genetic injury. Important target genes in this process include p53, cyclin D1 and EGFR.

Pathogenesis of Adenocarcinoma

Almost all oesophageal adenocarcinomas are associated with the pre-existing condition of metaplasia (Barrett's oesophagus) [10]. This condition is characterised by the replacement of the normal squamous cell epithelial lining of the lower oesophagus by a columnar lined mucosa variably containing intestinal metaplasia (Fig. **5**). This mucosa, although initially protective against reflux of gastric content, is unstable, and may further alter to produce low-grade epithelial dysplasia followed by high-grade epithelial dysplasia and invasive adenocarcinoma. As with squamous cell carcinoma this stepwise sequence of events has been intensively studied and several associations and risk factors for Barrett's oesophagus and adenocarcinoma are known, although the precise pathogenesis is not. The most important associated risk factor for adenocarcinoma of the oesophagus is obesity, leading to raised intra-abdominal pressure, leading to reflux oesophagitis, leading to a protective Barrett's metaplastic response. Other initiating factors include tobacco and alcohol consumption. The role of inherited factors in the development of adenocarcinoma has begun to be studied. However, familial association with adenocarcinoma is rare. Other rare conditions, which are associated with the development of adenocarcinoma, include achalasia and Zollinger Ellison syndrome. As with squamous cell carcinoma of the oesophagus, progressive accumulation of genetic injury is thought to underpin the development of adenocarcinoma. There is considerable overlap here with mutations in many important tumour suppressor genes and oncogenes common to both types of cancer. Many studies have identified mutations in p53, cyclin dependant kinase inhibitors and EGFR as critical events [11, 12]. Recent studies have also identified mutations in the human epidermal growth factor receptor (HER 2). This latter finding may provide a therapeutic opportunity in the treatment of patients with advanced oesophageal adenocarcinoma [13].

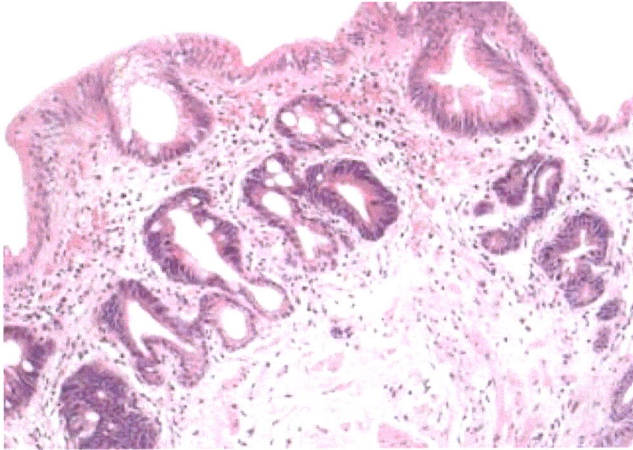

Fig. (5). Columnar lined mucosa with intestinal metaplasia consistent with Barrett's oesophagus.

Lastly, as excessive consumption of tobacco and alcohol together with dietary factors and obesity are all, to some extent, preventable, it may be surmised that with appropriate health strategies centred on prevention, the incidence of adenocarcinoma and squamous cell carcinoma of the oesophagus could be greatly reduced.

Pathogenesis of Gastric Cancer

The precise pathogenesis of gastric adenocarcinoma is not known. However, several associated risk factors are thought to be important in the aetiology of this condition. These may be divided into hereditary and acquired. The relative importance of these is controversial with variation likely within differing geographic populations as well as within individuals.

Inherited Risk Factors for Gastric Cancer

Patients with Lynch syndrome (Hereditary non polyposis colorectal carcinoma), Peutz Jeghers syndrome or Familial Polyposis Coli all have an increased risk of developing gastric carcinoma. The commonest of these conditions is Lynch syndrome. In this disorder an inherited mutation in a DNA mismatch repair genes (MLH1, MSH2, MSH6, PMS2) leads to an accumulation of mutations throughout the cellular genome termed genomic instability [14]. This is manifest by microsatellite instability and loss of expression of mismatch repair proteins within tumour cell nuclei [15]. Familial gastric cancer (Hereditary diffuse gastric cancer) is an autosomal dominant disorder with high penetrance. Approximately 30% of individuals with HDGC have a germ line mutation in the tumour suppressor gene E-cadherin or CDH1. The inactivation of the second allele of E-cadherin through mutation, methylation, and loss of heterozygosity eventually triggers the development of gastric cancer. To diagnose HDGS, two or more cases of diffuse gastric carcinoma in first or second degree relatives must be documented, with at least one diagnosed before the age of 50; or there are three or more documented cases of diffuse gastric carcinoma in first or second-degree relatives, regardless of the age of onset [16].

Non-Inherited Risk Factors

As with oesophageal carcinoma there is a long list of predisposing conditions, which have been associated with the development of gastric adenocarcinoma. These include chronic gastritis whether due to Helicobacter pylori infection or autoimmune disease (pernicious anaemia). In these inflammatory conditions, continuous injury to gastric epithelial cells may be associated with free radical generation and consequent DNA damage, all occurring in the context of a rapidly proliferating epithelial regenerative response.

Dietary factors and vitamin deficiencies have also been implicated. In particular, a meat rich diet or a diet rich in smoked foods have been heavily associated with gastric cancer. Other risk factors include previous gastric surgery, previous peptic ulcer disease and Menetrier's disease. The pathogenesis of gastric carcinoma is thought to be a multistep process from the development of chronic inflammation of whatever cause through the development of intestinal metaplasia as a protective response, then dysplasia and finally invasive carcinoma. The precise contribution of the associated risk factors described above is still the subject of intense debate.

Rare subtypes of gastric carcinoma including gastric carcinoma with lymphoid stroma (medullary type carcinoma) have been associated with Epistein Barr virus infection. Low-grade gastric lymphomas (Maltomas) are also known to be associated with Helicobacter pylori infection. Finally, the commonest sarcoma of the gastro-intestinal tract is a gastro-intestinal stromal tumour (GIST) and is most commonly found within the stomach and is driven by mutations in the KIT gene or the platelet derived growth factor receptor alpha (PDGFRA) gene [17, 18].

PATHOLOGY OF OESOPHAGEAL CANCER

Adenocarcinoma of the Oesophagus

Macroscopically adenocarcinomas of the oesophagus present a wide variety of appearances. Most commonly they appear as an area of ulceration with firm, raised rolled edges. However, more mass-like polypoidal lesions also occur. Either subtype may progress to become circumferential and produce an obstructing stricture. Most are located in the lower oesophagus and it is important to ascertain whether the bulk of the tumour lies within the true oesophagus or across the gastro-oesophageal junction. The cut surface may be firm and white revealing destruction of the oesophageal wall or may more rarely have a glistening appearance if the tumour is of mucinous type. The tumour may or may not involve or extend into surrounding structures such as the diaphragmatic crura, pleura and pericardium and this should be recorded alongside any resection specimen. If the tumour is circumferential, producing a stricture, it may be difficult to open the sectioned specimen fully longitudinally and pathologists are advised to open as close to the tumour as possible longitudinally, from above and below, in order to allow fixation but not to disrupt the circumferential resection margin. Non-mesothelial lined services should be inked prior to fixation to permit accurate assessment of the true specimen margin at microscopy. Serial transverse sectioning will reveal the relationship between the tumour edge and the nearest circumferential margin and its relationship with other structures. Processing the specimen in intact mega blocks will aid in this endeavour and together with photography of transverse slices can permit both surgeon and pathologist to compare the resected specimen with preoperative radiological images (Fig. **6**).

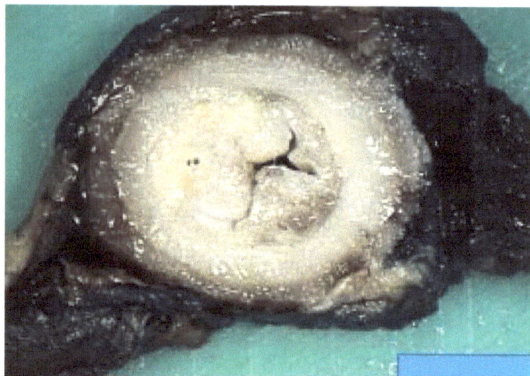

Fig. (6). Adenocarcinoma of the oesophagus producing a tight stricture.

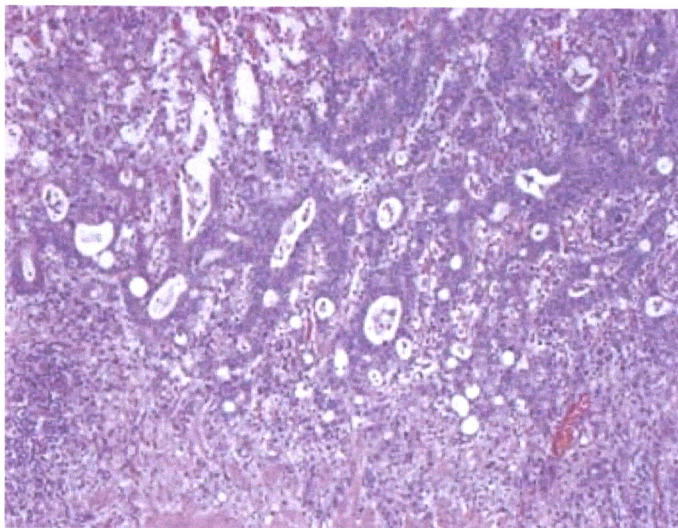

Fig. (7). Moderately differentiated adenocarcinoma of the oesophagus.

Microscopically adenocarcinoma of the oesophagus also shows a variety of appearances according to its differentiation. Well and moderately differentiated tumours show formed glands composed of malignant appearing cells with varying degrees of pleomorphism and mitotic activity (Fig. 7). Mucin production, desmoplastic stroma and necrosis are present to a varying degree. Poorly differentiated tumours may show a solid appearance composed of sheets of malignant cells and distinction from squamous cell carcinoma may sometimes be challenging. Signet ring cell components may be seen but these are quite rare being more commonly associated with upward extension of gastric adenocarcinomas. Tumour may infiltrate deeply involving all layers of the oesophageal wall. Vascular invasion and peri-neural invasion may be prominent. Infiltration of adenocarcinoma underneath normal appearing squamous epithelium is common and may produce a negative superficial biopsy. Submucosal infiltration and extension within submucosal veins and lymphatics may extend proximally for a varying length and occasionally even extend to the proximal margin of resection specimens that appear, on surface examination, normal. In rare cases tumours treated with preoperative chemo radiotherapy may show a total or near total pathological response. This is discussed further below. Oesophageal carcinoma of all types spreads readily to local lymph nodes and then more distant groups. Direct invasion of adjacent organs including bronchus, left atrium and aorta are associated with late presentation and are inoperable. Haematogenous spread to the liver and lungs is common in advanced disease.

Squamous Cell Carcinoma of the Oesophagus

Squamous cell carcinoma of the oesophagus may occur anywhere within the oesophagus but there is a slight preponderance within the middle and upper oesophageal regions by comparison with adenocarcinoma. Macroscopically, these tumours may be grossly indistinguishable from an adenocarcinoma producing a variety of ulcerated, stricturing and polypoidal appearances. Spread is again by direct invasion, lymphatic permeation or *via* the bloodstream to the liver and lungs. Microscopically, squamous cell carcinoma of the oesophagus may exhibit a wide degree of differentiation with well-differentiated forms composed of sheets and islands of invasive squamous cells producing irregular keratin and squamous pearls. Intercellular prickles may be noted between squamous cells. Nuclear pleomorphism and mitotic activity are variable (Fig. **8**). More poorly differentiated tumours may be devoid of such features and distinction from a poorly differentiated adenocarcinoma may be difficult. The presence or absence of dysplasia, whether glandular or squamous, within adjacent mucosa may be helpful in making this distinction. Basaloid squamous cell carcinomas are a rare variant. Very rarely spindle cell squamous carcinomas arise in the oesophagus and these must be distinguished from true sarcomas using immunohistochemical detection of cytokeratin expression. Small cell carcinoma, which is morphologically and immunohistochemically indistinguishable from small cell carcinoma of the bronchus may also occur in the oesophagus.

Effect of Pre-Operative Therapy

The roles of pre-operative radiotherapy and chemotherapy in the management of patients with oesophageal cancer remain subject to debate. While it is common practice in many centres to offer patients pre-operative chemo or radiotherapy or both, the degree and nature of the effect upon oesophageal carcinomas is highly variable. Many tumours show no apparent features of treatment effect while others may show scanty residual carcinoma occurring in a background of dense fibroblastic stroma. Overlying epithelium may show a normal squamous appearance. In some case an almost complete response with apparent eradication of tumour may be seen. The assessment of response to chemotherapy may help predict patient outcome after surgery [19] and help to establish the degree of chemo-sensitivity of the tumour. Accurate prediction of which tumours will respond better to preoperative therapy remains elusive despite several studies of preoperative biopsy material. Adequate representative sampling of tumour tissue with superficial mucosal biopsies is likely to be a confounding problem in these studies.

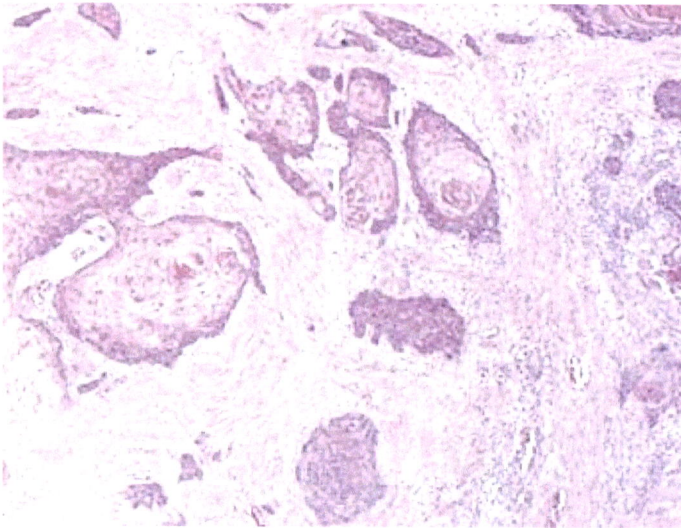

Fig. (8). Moderately differentiated squamous cell carcinoma of the oesophagus.

Molecular Pathology of Oesophageal Neoplasia

In patients with Barrett's oesophagus the diagnosis of dysplasia, which may herald progression to adenocarcinoma, is often challenging. Patients with only low-grade dysplasia may undergo a wide range of treatments including endoscopic mucosal resection for focal lesions or radiofrequency ablation for diffuse areas of dysplasia. Patients with high-grade change may be also have been treated as above or may undergo, in some cases, oesophagectomy. This has led to a search for molecular markers to assist in the diagnosis of epithelial dysplasia in Barrett's oesophagus. Much attention has centred on expression of p53 by immunohistochemistry as an adjunctive marker for dysplasia. Overexpression or total absence of expression may indicate dysplasia, however, histopathological opinion is divided as to its routine use [20]. Additional robust evidence of a higher sensitivity and specificity are required before the pathology community adopts it.

In many solid organs, tumours the identification of molecular pathways underlying carcinogenesis has led to the development of several drugs, which may interfere with tumour survival and shift the benefit balance in favour of patients. Unfortunately, both oesophageal squamous cell carcinoma and adenocarcinoma remain resistant to such approaches and few molecular genetics based therapies are available for these tumours. However, recently, along with gastric adenocarcinoma, palliative treatment with Herceptin is used to treat patients with gastro-oeosphageal adenocarcinomas. Treatment is offered on the basis of tumour expression of the HER 2 new receptor within tumour cells by immunohistochemistry or detection of HER 2 amplification within tumour cells by fluorescent in situ hybridisation (FISH) studies. The decision to treat patients with these novel therapies is a complex one and is often only taken after a full multidisciplinary team discussion [21].

PATHOLOGY OF GASTRIC CANCER

Adenocarcinoma accounts for approximately 95% of all malignant gastric neoplasms. Macroscopically these tumours provide a wide variety of appearances with different growth patterns. For standardization of the common morphologic features of gastric cancers, several classification systems have been proposed. The most widely used classification for macroscopic appearance of gastric cancer is Bormann classification, dividing them into four types:

Type 1: Polypoid: Well circumscribed polypoid tumours.
Type 2: Fungating: Fungating tumours with marked central infiltration.
Type 3: Ulcerated: Ulcerated tumours with infiltrative margins.
Type 4: Infiltrating: Diffusely infiltrated tumours.

The most common macroscopic type is a fungating tumour, which are frequently located in the lesser curvature of the gastric antrum. In contrast, the polypoid and ulcerated types are commonly found in the greater curvature of the gastric corpus. The cut surface, presents as a grey-white to yellow-white solid mass with a firm to hard consistency and frequently contain areas of haemorrhage and necrosis.

Polypoid or mass forming adenocarcinomas are usually gland forming at the microscopic level. However, the diffuse type of gastric adenocarcinoma does not form distinct glands but instead diffusely infiltrates tissue in the form of discohesive signet ring cells characterised by an eccentric nucleus with a predominant cytoplasmic mucinous vacuole. This distinction is emphasised by the "Lauren classification" which divides gastric adenocarcinoma into the intestinal type, which incorporates the polypoid or gland forming variety and the diffuse type which is characterised by signet ring cells (Fig. **9**). Intestinal type adenocarcinoma usually arises in the older people with an increased incidence in men and is frequently associated with chronic atrophic gastritis, intestinal metaplasia and Helicobacter pylori infection. They constitute approximately 60% of gastric carcinoma in high-risk population and occur frequently in the antrum as exophytic bulky lesions. These tumours have a tendency to spread hematogenously and often result in liver metastasis.

Diffuse type adenocarcinoma frequently occurs in younger patients, with equal distribution among men and women. It tends to spread by direct tumour extension, resulting in peritoneal metastasis. When the diffuse type is extensive it may produce a rigid feel (leather bottle) to the gastric wall and has been termed linitis plastica in the past. Some gastric adenocarcinomas do not fit into one of the two types and hence fall into a mixed category. They account for approximately 14% of all gastric carcinoma. Mixed type adenocarcinomas exhibit larger size, deeper invasion, more frequent local invasion, and lymph node metastasis compared to intestinal or diffuse type gastric carcinomas. It has been suggested that mixed type adenocarcinoma of the stomach may have more aggressive behaviour than either of the two pure types and could be separated as a distinct entity.

While other classifications including the Ming (expanding vs infiltrative) and the WHO classification (based on traditional histopathologic features and the degree of differentiation) exist, the Lauren classification retains great utility and is favoured by many pathologists. In addition, has been applied to clinical indications for endoscopic procedure or surgery and has supported unified epidemiologic data collection of gastric cancers by researchers.

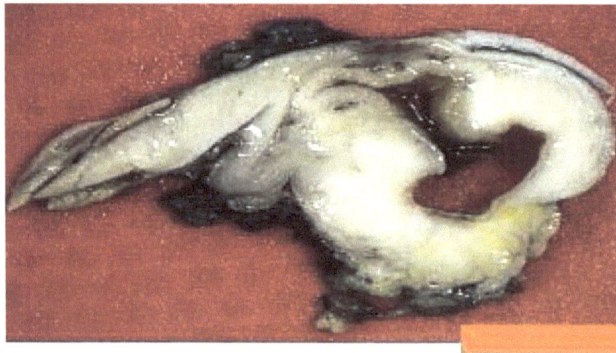

Fig. (9). Intestinal type gastric adenocarcinoma of pyloric antrum.

Generally, all gastric tumours have a propensity to invade within the layers of the gastric wall and in advanced cases may breach the serosal lining of the stomach. Such advanced tumours are commonly associated with disseminated peritoneal disease *via* transcoelomic spread and are usually non-resectable. Gastric adenocarcinomas also metastasise readily to regional lymph nodes. Since the prognosis of gastric cancer depends to a large extent on lymph node metastases, all resected local nodes must be examined for metastatic disease for accurate staging. Spread to distant lymph nodes such as the para-aortic nodes may occur and may also preclude surgical therapy. Direct extension into nearby structures such as pancreas, spleen and liver may also occur. Lastly, as with oesophageal carcinomas, haematogenous spread to the liver and lungs may be a late event and is associated with a poor survival.

The biopsy diagnosis of conventional intestinal type adenocarcinoma of the stomach is relatively straightforward. Biopsy sampling may also include adjacent precursor lesions including high-grade epithelial dysplasia. The microscopic diagnosis of diffuse type gastric cancer may prove more challenging. The number of biopsies taken may have relevance in this regard. In many case, the number of signet ring cells present within the lamina propria may be quite low and therefore difficult for the pathologist to identify. Many pathologists employ a routine mucin stain such as a PAS alcian blue to facilitate the identification of such inconspicuous infiltrates. In cases in which there is a degree of doubt immunohistochemical analysis employing broad spectrum cytokeratins may often prove revealing (Fig. **10**).

In the modern era of endoscopic mucosal resection (EMR) small gastric lesions including adenomas and small adenocarcinomas may be removed without the need for invasive surgery. Such early gastric adenocarcinomas may be accurately staged with regard to depth of invasion and guide the clinician in their decision to pursue further surgery or not. The gross handling of such specimens is of great importance. All such specimens should be received fresh, pinned out to a corkboard, inked on the deep margin, serially sectioned and processed entirely to permit the maximum extraction of information. Staging of gross resection specimens should follow a prescribed pattern utilising a defined dataset such as that produced by the Royal College of Pathologists and the final stage should be annotated according to TNM 7 as developed by the Union for International Cancer Control where T describes the extent of local invasion into the oesophageal wall, N denotes the involvement or sparing of regional lymph nodes and M the presence or absence of distant metastases.

Rare subtypes of gastric carcinoma are known to exist. These include medullary type gastric carcinoma in which large almost blastic appearing malignant epithelial cells are intimately associated with an intense lymphoid reaction. Hepatoid gastric adenocarcinoma in which the tumour morphology is almost identical to a well-differentiated hepatocellular carcinoma rarely occurs. Adenosquamous carcinoma in which a clearly identified squamous cell component is present is rarely reported. Parietal cell carcinoma in which the tumour is composed of malignant oxyntic epithelium is also known to exist. Finally, extremely rare malignant germ cell tumours may occur in the gastric wall, notably choriocarcinoma. In these cases, the diagnosis may only be made by excluding a primary tumour within the gonads.

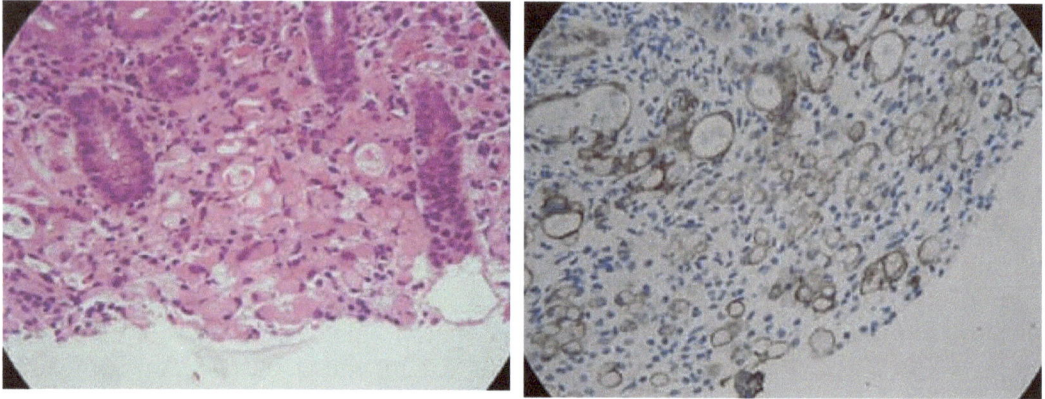

Fig. (10). (a) Occult signet ring diffuse type adenocarcinoma of stomach highlighted by expression of cytokeratin (**b**).

The Molecular Pathology of Gastric Adenocarcinoma

For many years few practical advances in our understanding of the molecular pathogenesis of gastric adenocarcinoma have taken place. This is in great contrast to the situation in colorectal carcinoma where a multistep pathogenesis has been established from the precursor adenoma to colonic adenocarcinoma with a concomitant stepwise alteration in proto-oncogenes and tumour suppressor genes. While a similar step wise progression is thought to occur within gastric epithelial neoplasia the precise sequence of events remains less clear. Key oncogenes and tumour suppressor genes, which are thought to be central in gastric carcinogenesis, include p27, Beta-catenin and p53 [22 - 24].

Despite this, molecular pathological diagnostic tests do have a role in rare types of gastric adenocarcinoma. In hereditary diffuse type gastric cancer mutations in the E-cadherin gene lead to loss of expression of the E-cadherin adhesion molecule from tumour cell junctions and this is detectable by immunohistochemistry. In medullary type gastric carcinoma, in situ hybridisation can demonstrate the presence of Epstein Barr virus within tumour cells, which is felt to be the aetiological agent in these rare tumours. A small subset of gastric adenocarcinomas may be hereditary such as those, which occur in patients suffering from Lynch syndrome. In these tumours it is usually possible to demonstrate micro-satellite instability amplified by the polymerase chain reaction (PCR) and subsequent analysis. In addition, immunohistochemistry may be used to identify absence of mismatch repair protein expression and by inference suggest which mismatch repair gene is responsible for the syndrome. As with Lynch derived colorectal carcinoma the four commonest genes assessed by these methodologies are MLH1, MSH2, MSH6 and PMS2 [25] (Fig. **11**).

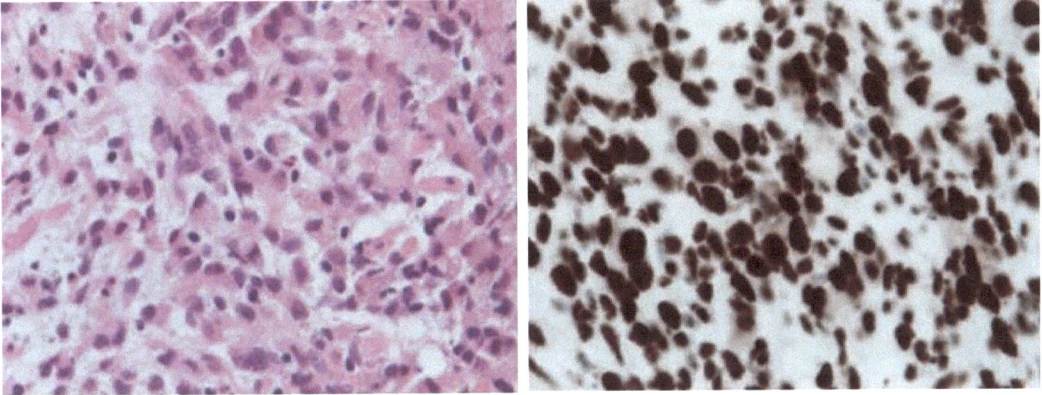

Fig. (11). Diffuse type gastric cancer (**a**) with strong nuclear expression of MLH1 (**b**) in keeping with a mismatch repair proficient phenotype.

Perhaps the most important application of molecular pathology to the treatment of gastric adenocarcinoma is the demonstration of HER 2 gene amplification and protein over-expression in a number of these tumours. Over-expression of HER 2 within a gastric adenocarcinoma provides a potential therapeutic target for treatment with the anti HER 2 antibody Trastuzumab. Approximately, 10-20% of gastric adenocarcinomas demonstrate HER 2 gene amplification with a slightly higher frequency in tumours of the gastro-oesophageal junction region. For the pathologist HER 2 gene amplification may be demonstrated by fluorescent in situ hybridisation (FISH) analysis. Alternatively, over-expression of the protein product may be demonstrated by immunohistochemistry. Various grading schemes, largely derived from previous work on breast cancer, are applied to immunohistochemical assessment of HER 2 within gastric carcinomas. Currently, within the UK, only strong 3+ immunohistochemical expression is felt to correlate best with HER 2 gene amplification. Conveniently, all of these ancillary studies may be performed in routine formalin fixed paraffin embedded tissue sections from biopsy samples [26] (Fig. **12**).

OTHER TUMOURS OF THE OESOPHAGUS AND STOMACH

Mesenchymal Tumours

Spindle cell tumours of the upper gastrointestinal tract have undergone an evolution in both terminology and treatment over the last two decades. The emergence of gastrointestinal stromal tumours (GISTs) as a separate type of spindle cell tumour as distinct from smooth muscle tumours is at the core of this revolution. Gastrointestinal stromal tumours are thought to derive from cells similar to the interstitial cells of Cajal, which are the pacemaker cells of the gastrointestinal tract. They show pathological, immunophenotypic and molecular biological differences from both benign and malignant smooth muscle tumours.

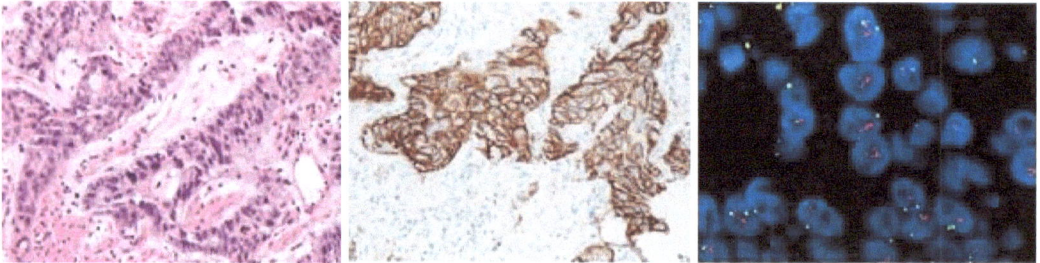

Fig. (12). (**a**) Intestinal type gastric adenocarcinoma (H&E), (**b**) Strong expression of Her-2 by immunohistochemistry and (**c**) Her-2 amplified by fluorescent in-situ hybridisation (FISH).

Gastrointestinal Stromal Tumours

Gastrointestinal stromal tumours are rare in the oesophagus but occur most commonly within the stomach wall. The converse is true of smooth muscle tumours (leiomyoma/ sarcoma), which are commoner in the oesophagus but rare in the stomach. The gross appearances of gastrointestinal tumours, varies considerably but the majority produce a polypoid mass shaped lesion, which extends within the lumen of the stomach arising from its muscle coat (Fig. **13**).

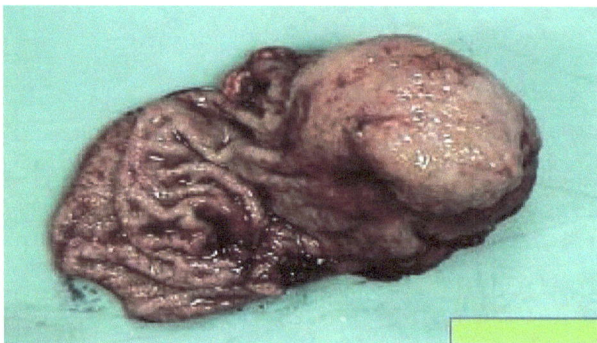

Fig. (13). Gastric GIST producing a massive intramural swelling.

Gastrointestinal stromal tumours may also extend subserosal often producing a pedunculated mass, which appears suspended from the outside of the gastric wall. Some tumours have a characteristic dumbbell appearance with an intraluminal component and an extraluminal subserosal component. Larger tumours are often associated with central areas of mucosal ulceration and may be associated with copious bleeding from this point. Smaller lesions may only show a diffuse submucosal swelling on endoscopy with overlying normal gastric mucosa on routine biopsy. Microscopically gastrointestinal stromal tumours of the stomach show a wide variety of appearances. The commonest type however is the spindle cell form in which tumour cells show an elongated tapering shape with abundant eosinophilic cytoplasm and slender cigar shaped nuclei. A common feature is a pronounced para-nuclear cytoplasmic vacuole. Cellular pleomorphism is highly variable and areas of degeneration are common. Mitotic activity is also variable. The next commonest phenotype is the epithelioid cell variant in which tumour cells show great similarity to standard epithelial cells. This might, in rare cases, lead to confusion with a gastric adenocarcinoma. Lastly, mixed tumours with both spindle cell and an epithelioid differentiation also occur [27].

Immunohistochemistry of GIST

The defining feature of gastric GISTs is strong and diffuse expression of KIT (CD117) (Fig. **14**) and DOG1 (discovered on GIST1). These markers are strongly expressed in 95% of tumours regardless of the morphological subtype of GIST present. Gastrointestinal stromal tumours are also characteristically negative for desmin but may show variable positivity with actin, caldesmon, CD34 and S100 [28].

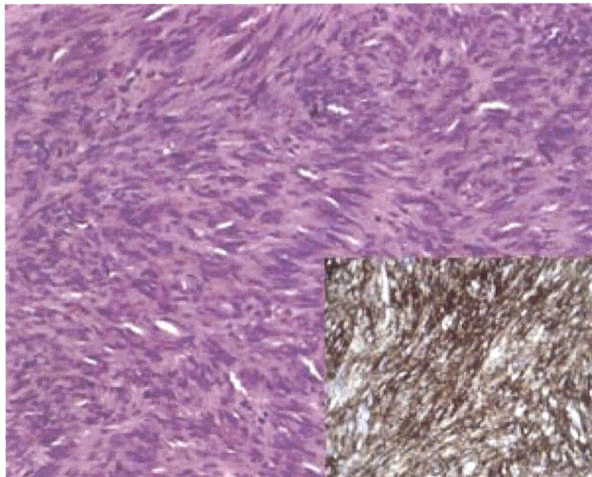

Fig. (14). Typical spindle cell type low grade gastric GIST with strong expression of KIT (insert).

Molecular Pathology of Gastrointestinal Stromal Tumours

Approximately 85% of gastrointestinal stromal tumours harbour driving mutations in the KIT proto-oncogene. This oncogene codes for a transmembrane tyrosine kinase receptor, which is constitutively activated by gene mutation. Hot spots for gene mutation occur in exons 9, 11, 13 and 17 of the KIT gene. Of these, exon 11 mutations are the commonest. A further subset of gastrointestinal stromal tumours (5-10%), are driven by mutations in the platelet derived growth factor receptor alpha gene (PDGFRA). Mutations in this gene occur most commonly in exons 12, 14 and 18. Mutations in exon 18 of the PDGFRA gene are most common. PDGFRA mutant tumours may often by epithelioid in nature. Interestingly, they may also fail to express KIT by immunohistochemistry. As responsiveness to tyrosine kinase inhibitor (TKI) drug therapy is dependent on which mutation is present within a GIST, mutation analysis of both the KIT gene and the PDGFRA gene is now an important part of the standard assessment of these tumours [29].

The behaviour of gastrointestinal stromal tumours is variable and is influenced by its primary site. The risk of progressive disease also increases with increase in tumour size and with increase in mitotic rate [30]. Tumours, which are deemed to be at high risk of progressive disease, may be further treated with tyrosine kinase inhibitor therapy depending on its mutation status. Patients with high-risk tumours are at an increased risk for liver metastases and/or peritoneal deposits despite having a complete (R0) resection.

Smooth Muscle Tumours

Both benign and malignant true smooth muscle tumours of the stomach wall occur. Benign smooth muscle tumours are leiomyomas, which are often incidentally discovered at the time of gastric resection for malignant epithelial disease. These tumours produce a firm often well-circumscribed appearance. They are composed of myoid appearing spindle cells. In contrast to GIST they stain strongly positive with markers of muscle differentiation *e.g.* desmin and actin but are negative for KIT and DOG1. Leiomyosarcomas while extremely rare, also occur within the stomach. These show a similar immunophenotype to benign smooth muscle tumours but also demonstrate characteristic features of malignancy such as cellular pleomorphism, high mitotic rate, necrosis and invasion of other structures.

Lymphoid Tumours

The stomach and oesophagus are unusual sites for primary non-Hodgkin's lymphoma. However, the lymph nodes of both of these organs may be involved by systemic low-grade lymphomas such as chronic lymphocytic leukaemia (CLL). Primary non-Hodgkin's lymphomas of the stomach predominantly low-grade B cell lymphomas, which are derived from mucosa, associated lymphoid tissue (MALT). These tumours are associated with Helicobacter pylori infection and eradication of this infection may lead to elimination of the tumour in low-grade early cases. High-grade non-Hodgkin's B cell lymphomas also occur within the stomach. These may represent evolution from a lower grade pre-existing Maltoma. These tumours are commonly treated by systemic chemotherapy however large obstructing tumours or tumours associated with uncontrolled haemorrhage may be surgically resected. The diagnosis of lymphoma is readily made by endoscopy and biopsy but also requires detailed immunohistochemical and molecular genetic studies.

CONSENT FOR PUBLICATION

Not applicable.

CONFLICT OF INTEREST

The author declares no conflict of interest, financial or otherwise.

ACKNOWLEDGEMENT

Declare none.

REFERENCES

[1]   Winter HS, Madara JL, Stafford RJ, Grand RJ, Quinlan JE, Goldman H. Intraepithelial eosinophils: a new diagnostic criterion for reflux esophagitis. Gastroenterology 1982; 83(4): 818-23. [PMID: 7106512]

[2]   Brown LF, Goldman H, Antonioli DA. Intraepithelial eosinophils in endoscopic biopsies of adults with reflux esophagitis. Am J Surg Pathol 1984; 8(12): 899-905. [http://dx.doi.org/10.1097/00000478-198412000-00002] [PMID: 6517181]

[3]   Fléjou JF, Svrcek M. Barrett's oesophagus--a pathologist's view. Histopathology 2007; 50(1): 3-14. [http://dx.doi.org/10.1111/j.1365-2559.2006.02569.x] [PMID: 17204017]

[4]   Barrett NR. The lower esophagus lined by columnar epithelium. Surgery 1957; 41(6): 881-94. [PMID: 13442856]

[5]   Walsh SV, Antonioli DA, Goldman H, *et al.* Allergic esophagitis in children: a clinicopathological entity. Am J Surg Pathol 1999; 23(4): 390-6. [http://dx.doi.org/10.1097/00000478-199904000-00003] [PMID: 10199468]

[6]   Lewin KJ, Dowling F, Wright JP, Taylor KB. Gastric morphology and serum gastrin levels in pernicious anaemia. Gut 1976; 17(7): 551-60. [http://dx.doi.org/10.1136/gut.17.7.551] [PMID: 964688]

[7]   Warren JR, Marshall B. Unidentified curved bacilli on gastric epithelium in active chronic gastritis. Lancet 1983; 1(8336): 1273-5. [PMID: 6134060]

[8]   Dixon MF, O'Connor HJ, Axon ATR, King RFJG, Johnston D. Reflux gastritis: distinct histopathological entity? J Clin Pathol 1986; 39(5): 524-30. [http://dx.doi.org/10.1136/jcp.39.5.524] [PMID: 3722405]

[9]   Mandard AM, Marnay J, Gignoux M, *et al.* Cancer of the esophagus and associated lesions: detailed pathologic study of 100 esophagectomy specimens. Hum Pathol 1984; 15(7): 660-9. [http://dx.doi.org/10.1016/S0046-8177(84)80292-0] [PMID: 6745909]

[10]   Hamilton SR, Smith RRL, Cameron JL. Prevalence and characteristics of Barrett esophagus in patients with adenocarcinoma of the esophagus or esophagogastric junction. Hum Pathol 1988; 19(8): 942-8. [http://dx.doi.org/10.1016/S0046-8177(88)80010-8] [PMID: 3402983]

[11]   Wongsurawat VJ, Finley JC, Galipeau PC, *et al.* Genetic mechanisms of TP53 loss of heterozygosity in Barrett's esophagus: implications for biomarker validation. Cancer Epidemiol Biomarkers Prev 2006; 15(3): 509-16. [http://dx.doi.org/10.1158/1055-9965.EPI-05-0246] [PMID: 16537709]

[12]   Wong DJ, Paulson TG, Prevo LJ, *et al.* p16(INK4a) lesions are common, early abnormalities that undergo clonal expansion in Barrett's metaplastic epithelium. Cancer Res 2001; 61(22): 8284-9. [PMID: 11719461]

[13]   Thompson SK, Sullivan TR, Davies R, Ruszkiewicz AR. Her-2/neu gene amplification in esophageal adenocarcinoma and its influence on survival. Ann Surg Oncol 2011; 18(7): 2010-7. [http://dx.doi.org/10.1245/s10434-011-1554-1] [PMID: 21267790]

[14]   Leach FS, Nicolaides NC, Papadopoulos N, *et al.* Mutations of a mutS homolog in hereditary nonpolyposis colorectal cancer. Cell 1993; 75(6): 1215-25. [http://dx.doi.org/10.1016/0092-8674(93)90330-S] [PMID: 8261515]

[15]   Walsh S. The pathology of Lynch syndrome. Diagn Histopathol 2015; 21: 161-4. [http://dx.doi.org/10.1016/j.mpdhp.2015.04.007]

[16]   Oliveira C, Machado JC, Carvalho A, Carneiro F, Seruca R, Caldas C. E-cadherin germline mutations in families with diffuse gastric cancer. Mod Pathol 2001; 14: 93A-A.

[17]   Hirota S, Isozaki K, Moriyama Y, *et al.* Gain-of-function mutations of c-kit in human gastrointestinal stromal tumors. Science 1998; 279(5350): 577-80. [http://dx.doi.org/10.1126/science.279.5350.577] [PMID: 9438854]

[18]   Heinrich MC, Corless CL, Duensing A, *et al.* PDGFRA activating mutations in gastrointestinal stromal tumors. Science 2003; 299(5607): 708-10. [http://dx.doi.org/10.1126/science.1079666] [PMID: 12522257]

[19]   Hornick JL, Farraye FA, Odze RD. Prevalence and significance of prominent mucin pools in the esophagus post neoadjuvant chemoradiotherapy for Barrett's-associated adenocarcinoma. Am J Surg Pathol 2006; 30(1): 28-35. [http://dx.doi.org/10.1097/01.pas.0000174011.29816.fa] [PMID: 16330939]

[20]   Kaye P. p53 Immunohistochemistry as a biomarker of dysplasia and neoplastic progression in Barrett's oesophagus. Diagn Histopathol 2015; 21: 89-98. [http://dx.doi.org/10.1016/j.mpdhp.2015.04.001]

[21]   Van Cutsem E, Bang YJ, Feng-Yi F, *et al.* HER2 screening data from ToGA: targeting HER2 in gastric and gastroesophageal junction cancer. Gastric Cancer 2015; 18(3): 476-84. [http://dx.doi.org/10.1007/s10120-014-0402-y] [PMID: 25038874]

[22]   Eguchi H, Herschenhous N, Kuzushita N, Moss SF. Helicobacter pylori increases proteasome-mediated degradation of p27(kip1) in gastric epithelial cells. Cancer Res 2003; 63(15): 4739-46. [PMID: 12907657]

[23]   Franco AT, Israel DA, Washington MK, *et al.* Activation of beta-catenin by carcinogenic Helicobacter pylori. Proc Natl Acad Sci USA 2005; 102(30): 10646-51. [http://dx.doi.org/10.1073/pnas.0504927102] [PMID: 16027366]

[24]   Wei J, O'Brien D, Vilgelm A, *et al.* Interaction of Helicobacter pylori with gastric epithelial cells is mediated by the p53 protein family. Gastroenterology 2008; 134(5): 1412-23. [http://dx.doi.org/10.1053/j.gastro.2008.01.072] [PMID: 18343378]

[25]   Bellizzi AM. Update on immunohistochemistry to identify colorectal tumours with deficient DNA mismatch repair, Diagnostic Histopathology, vol 21, pp 122-130, March 2015 2015.

[26] Hechtman JF, Polydorides AD. HER2/neu gene amplification and protein overexpression in gastric and gastroesophageal junction adenocarcinoma: a review of histopathology, diagnostic testing, and clinical implications. Arch Pathol Lab Med 2012; 136(6): 691-7.
[http://dx.doi.org/10.5858/arpa.2011-0168-RS] [PMID: 22646280]

[27] Doyle LA. Gastrointestinal stromal tumour and other mesenchymal tumours of the GI tract: the role of immunohistochemistry in an evolving era of molecular diagnostics. Diagn Histopathol 2015; 64: 53-67.
[http://dx.doi.org/10.1111/his.12302]

[28] Doyle LA, Hornick JL. Gastrointestinal stromal tumours: from KIT to succinate dehydrogenase. Histopathology 2014; 64(1): 53-67.
[http://dx.doi.org/10.1111/his.12302] [PMID: 24117705]

[29] Heinrich MC, Corless CL, Demetri GD, *et al.* Kinase mutations and imatinib response in patients with metastatic gastrointestinal stromal tumor. J Clin Oncol 2003; 21(23): 4342-9.
[http://dx.doi.org/10.1200/JCO.2003.04.190] [PMID: 14645423]

[30] Miettinen M, Sobin LH, Lasota J. Gastrointestinal stromal tumors of the stomach: a clinicopathologic, immunohistochemical, and molecular genetic study of 1765 cases with long-term follow-up. Am J Surg Pathol 2005; 29(1): 52-68.
[http://dx.doi.org/10.1097/01.pas.0000146010.92933.de] [PMID: 15613856]

CHAPTER 5

Radiological Investigations of Oesophago-gastric Disorders

Robert Foster[1] and **Sami M. Shimi**[2,*]

[1] *Department of Radiology, Ninewells Hospital and Medical School, Dundee, Scotland, UK*

[2] *Department of Surgery, Ninewells Hospital and Medical School, Dundee, Scotland, UK*

Abstract: The contribution of radiological investigations in oesophago-gastric disorders has traditionally been diagnostic and for staging of malignant disease. However, radiological techniques have evolved in recent years into interventional procedures in the management of gastrointestinal bleeding, porto-systemic shunt formation, biopsies, stent placement and in the management of post-surgical complications. Indeed, interventional radiology cover is one of the criteria stipulated in guidelines for a quality oesophago-gastric service.

The evolution of radiological modalities of investigation and staging has brought a larger choice of techniques and more sophisticated equipment, which have impacted, on clinical practice. This has resulted in the requirement for super specialisation amongst radiologists in order to keep abreast of contemporary techniques. "G-I radiologists" have become adept with the nuances of specialist interpretation of radiographic images of the gastro-intestinal tract and have embraced advanced techniques of image acquisition and interrogation to provide maximal information. In addition, some have developed specialised interventional procedures for diagnostic and therapeutic purposes.

Keywords: Diagnostic radiology, Interventional radiology, Computed tomography, Magnetic resonance imaging, PET/ CT, Barium meal, Ultrasound, Cancer staging, Nuclear medicine imaging, Radiological stenting, Image targeted biopsy, Embolization.

PLAIN RADIOLOGY

For oesophago-gastric disorders, endoscopy has become the gold standard diagnostic modality and is significantly more sensitive for the detection of early disease, particularly small or mucosal lesions. Additionally, it affords the opportunity for biopsies and local therapy when this is necessary. However, once

* **Corresponding author Sami M. Shimi:** Department of Surgery, Ninewells Hospital and Medical School, Dundee DD1 9SY, Scotland, UK; Tel: +44 1382 660111; E-mail: s.m.shimi@dundee.ac.uk

the diagnosis of oeosphageal and gastric cancer is established, accurate radiological staging is essential in determining treatment intent, appropriate therapy, planning the surgical approach, and in determining the risk of tumor recurrence and overall prognosis. In addition, a number of non-surgical management approaches have evolved which are in the realm of radiology.

Plain radiology probably offers very little in the management of oesohago-gastric diseases. However, contrast examination of the oesophagus and stomach remains useful in documenting structural topography particularly when endoscopy is difficult to interpret. With dynamic fluoroscopy, this examination provides key functional information on motility, reflux, smooth muscle function and extravasation out with the GI tract when present. Cross sectional imaging builds another layer of image enhancement to demonstrate surgical anatomy and the full extent of the disease. In some instances, this helps in planning the surgical approach or procedure. Contrast enhanced cross sectional imaging improves the definition of structures of interest and in PET CT for example, adds a functional element to enhance the diagnostic ability. Sophisticated ultrasound imaging has been vital for characterising suspicious nodules in the liver. In addition, it provides guidance for percutaneous interventional techniques. Current research on high intensity focussed ultrasound will establish this modality as a therapeutic tool. With advances in image-guided therapy, interventional radiologists can insert fine probes to deliver ablative electric currents in electroporation or guide high intensity focussed ultrasound for energy ablation.

Plain X-Ray radiology is important in the assessment of acute presentations of the majority of surgical patients. Plain X-Rays provide a simple and usually rapid means of confirming or excluding some disease or abnormality on the basis of the learned radio-densities of tissues, fluids and gasses in appropriate locations in the body. Extravasation of gas either in the mediastinum, thorax or in the upper abdomen on plain X-Rays immediately increases the suspicion of a perforated viscus. Accumulation or pooling of fluids in the thorax can also provide corroborating evidence of a perforation with leakage of intra-luminal contents. Foreign bodies can also be seen on plain X-rays and their location estimated depending on their position in the GI tract. This includes therapeutic foreign bodies such as stents when they migrate from their intended position. Finally, Plain X-Rays are important in the short-term assessment of surgical patients when they develop respiratory complications. Other than these acute situations, plain X-Ray radiography has limited contribution in the assessment of oesophago-gastric conditions.

Fluoroscopy and Contrast Examinations

Fluoroscopic and contrast examinations have a definite but limited place in the assessment of oesophago-gastric disorders. Some primary care physicians in remote locations use these investigations in the primary assessment of patients who present with concerning symptoms of malignancy. However, endoscopic visualisation remains the first test of choice for accurate assessment of oesophago-gastric conditions when available. Subsequent enteric contrast studies can prove beneficial in patient management to assess the presence or absence of obstruction and consequently the feasibility of some therapeutic adventures.

Fluoroscopic examination involves ionising radiation with multiple low dose acquisitions obtained in rapid succession to provide a viewable cine sequence. In a similar fashion to plain film radiography an x-ray tube (generator) is on one side of the patient and a detector on the other. Usually, the detector and tube are on a fixed gantry, which move together around a couch/table on which the patient is positioned. The table can move independently from the tube/detector gantry as well as tilt in order to facilitate examinations being performed in various positions (standing/ lying down).

In general, modern systems will have a screening setting which uses lower doses at a consequence of reduced image quality and a second higher dose acquisition with better quality images and higher resolution. Both settings have the capacity to increase or decrease the frame rate. For studies in which there is a greater emphasis on visualising motion, such as a contrast swallow for the investigation of motility disorders a higher frame rate such as 3 - 7.5 frames per second would be used. For other indications such as Barium follow-through for investigation of small bowel transit, a much lower acquisition rate would be satisfactory or even single frame acquisitions at designated time intervals.

Screening is often used for aligning the tube/detector and patient in preparation for the higher dose diagnostic acquisition. Different frame rates for screening and acquisition can be selected. Increasing the frame rate also increases radiation dose due to an increased number of exposures being taken. Most investigations can be performed remotely with the operator standing behind a lead glass shield for radiation protection. Certain investigations necessitate the operator to be in front of the lead shielding. In these cases, lead coats are required.

The choice of contrast to be administered orally depends on the indication. In general, if the contrast is expected to progress intraluminally in the GI tract to demonstrate anatomy and intraluminal disorders, barium provides better resolution being denser and consequently better visualised. Alternatively, if there is suspicion that the contrast may extravasate out with the GI tract, either in the chest or abdomen, a water-soluble contrast should be used. Barium extravasation into the mediastinum or peritoneal cavity, cause an intense inflammatory reaction and is usually incorporated into the tissues permanently making repeat examinations very difficult to interpret. If there has been recent surgical intervention or the suspicion of a leak, a water-soluble contrast such as Gastrograffin is used. In addition, if there is a risk of aspiration in an unwell or neurologically obtunded patient, a water-soluble contrast agent (gastromiro) is commonly used. Gastromiro is less well visualised when compared with the Gastrograffin but is not associated with pulmonary edema if aspirated. Similarly, aspirated Barium is associated with pneumonitis and repeated chest infections since it is difficult to clear. It is possible to use other agents such as those used for vascular or urological studies if the patient is intolerant of the more common enteric agents.

Currently, fewer and fewer enteric contrast swallows and meals are being performed as the primary investigation of potential gastro-oesophageal malignancy in favour of more sophisticated endoscopy and cross sectional imaging. Nevertheless, these studies are still being performed, often to assess the symptomology of suspected benign upper digestive tract conditions. Barium swallows are still relatively commonplace and are being performed primarily for the assessment of dysphagia, usually when there is the suspicion of a motility disorder. On occasion more malignant appearing pathology is encountered. Cine Fluoroscopy is particularly useful to assess the swallowing mechanism in patients with neurological abnormalities or after a cerebro-vascular accident. No other test can provide similar information on the oro-pharyngeal swallowing mechanism and its disorders.

Contrast Swallow

This is the most commonly encountered fluoroscopic examination pertaining to the upper gastrointestinal tract. This examination provides information on abnormalities of the oesophagus and proximal stomach. The patient holds oral contrast in their mouth whilst an acquisition is obtained to visualise the passage of the contrast column through the oesophagus. Essential elements to be assessed during this dynamic investigation include delay or abnormality of the phases of the swallow, delay to passage of contrast through the oesophagus, irregularity of muscular contractions, delayed oesophageal clearing, intraluminal filling defects, mucosal irregularity, strictures, pouches and whether or not there is a hiatus hernia. Irregularity of muscular contractions, inevitably result in delayed contrast clearance. Disorganised contraction without a rhythmic wave results in focal areas of contraction with upstream pockets of hold-up of contrast. In achalasia, there is insufficient relaxation to the distal oesophageal sphincter. The resulting radiological feature is of a length of narrowed lumen that has been described as "birds-beak" in appearance due to a tapered narrowing. The resulting obstruction leads to significant proximal distension that fills with contrast. A hiatus hernia is radiologically evident when there are visible gastric rugae above the diaphragmatic hiatus. In post-operative cases, in which there is suspicion of an anastomotic leak a water-soluble agent is used. It is important in these cases, particularly when there are lots of surgical clips and drains to take an acquisition prior to administration of contrast- a spot film. This allows the determination of whether small densities were present previously. These examinations can be complicated by patient morbidity. Patients are often unable to stand as with a normal swallow but may tolerate being semi-recumbent with a tilted table. The technique is identical to the normal swallow with a particular focus on the anastomosis, often with zoomed views. In cases where there is dubiety, it is not uncommon to subsequently use a cross sectional imaging modality with oral contrast such as oral enhanced CT to confirm the diagnosis. Any contrast material out with the lumen is suggestive of leakage. The dynamic nature of fluoroscopy is beneficial when there are large bore surgical drains next to the anastomosis. Leaking contrast can be seen to pass directly into the drains and then out of the patient in a prompt fashion. CT swallow has the potential to be falsely reassuring in these cases as there is no mediastinal pooling. The classic appearance of a stricturing lesion within a hollow viscus such as the oesophagus, on a contrast swallow, is the so-called "apple-core" lesion. The oesophageal stricturing lesion gives an appearance that is not dissimilar to that is seen more commonly within the colon on Barium enema and now more commonly on CT colonography. Eccentrically located or intra-luminal oesophageal tumours can be identified as fixed filling defects within the contrast column. One benefit to enteric contrast studies is that they provide dynamic assessment of the swallow, contrast passage through the gastro-oesophageal junction and the stomach. This functional assessment can raise the suspicion of conditions such as linitis plastica (leather-bottle stomach), which is non-distensible and non-contractile. By contrast, the non-dynamic nature of CT may give the impression that the stomach is simply collapsed.

Double Contrast Examinations

The initial part of this investigation is identical to the contrast swallow as above. Subsequently, the patient is given more contrast that is not screened as it is ingested. In addition, an agent that produces carbon dioxide is given with the oral contrast to distend the stomach. As the examination proceeds, the patient is asked to roll from the supine position, to their right side, into a prone position, on to their left side and then back to the supine position. This procedure aims to coat the stomach lumen with contrast and minimise the amount that passes through the pylorus so the stomach remains distended. The radiologist observes and provides an analysis of gastric filling defects/intra-luminal masses, strictures and ulcers as well as normal passage through the pylorus. However, the sensitivity for the detection of gastric ulcers is significantly below that of endoscopic assessment.

Contrast Follow-Through Examination (Enteroclysis)

This investigation may include a swallow (depending on the presenting clinical history and indication). The initial part of this examination includes an assessment of the stomach as detailed above. Subsequently, the patient is given additional oral contrast in addition to a gas-releasing agent to distend the bowel. Certain contrast agents, for instance Gastrograffin, also has an effect on increasing gut motility. Consequently, Gastrograffin is commonly combined with a denser contrast agent such as Barium. The patient drinks several cups of contrast and has standard abdominal radiographs at defined intervals depending on the rate of passage though the small intestine. If there are any areas, which do not appear to distend, the patient can be screened on the fluoroscopy machine to visualise the presence or absence of peristalsis. Indications of a follow-through usually relate to possible motility disorders or occlusive disease.

Tubogram/ Squirtogram/ Fistulogram

The great benefit of fluoroscopy is the adaptability for problem solving. Contrast can be injected down in situ drains, fistulas, sinuses etc. in order to assess patency, potential communications or to define anatomy. Tubogram can be performed in patients who have undergone percutaneous intubation to assess patency and passage of the contrast intraluminally. Generally, barium or water-soluble contrast agents are used, the choice of which is often operator dependant.

CROSS SECTIONAL IMAGING

In the context of oesophago-gastric disorders, cross sectional radiological imaging is mainly used in the staging of oesophago-gastric malignancies, in the diagnosis of the full extent of oesophago-gastric injury after trauma and in post-operative diagnosis and often management of complications. Recent advances in medical imaging have established the role of whole-body computed tomography (CT), whole-body magnetic resonance imaging (MRI), and positron emission tomography-computed tomography (PET/CT) in the staging, and long-term monitoring of patients with oesophago-gastric malignancy. Although CT has its limitations, including exposure to radiation doses that can be triple those associated with MRI, it remains more sensitive than MRI for characterizing oesophago-gastric malignancies. In addition, CT is less sensitive for the accurate staging of the T and N status than endoscopic ultrasound. By contrast, MRI is more expensive, requires prolonged scanning times that some patients may not tolerate well in a claustrophobic environment. Combined PET/CT imaging with 18F-FDG tracer, provides superior images of malignant lesions of the oesophagus and has high sensitivity for the detection of isolated focal metastases. Percutaneous ultrasound and MRI have a particular role to play in characterizing small hepatic nodules, which raise suspicion on CT.

Computed Tomography (CT)

Computed Tomography (CT) or Computerized Axial Tomography (CAT) scanning is a technique that uses ionizing radiation. Similar to conventional radiography, CT uses a tube to produce x-rays. The emitted x-rays are collimated or focused to produce a narrow beam that is detected by rows of detector plates on the opposite side of a circular gantry. Unlike radiography, the detector does not produce an image; instead it measures the extent of attenuation of the emitted x-ray by the intervening tissues of the patient. By rotating both the x-ray tube and detectors around the patient the attenuation, and thereby the composition of the body is assessed over a single narrow slice. Moving the patient through the rotating gantry allows multiple slices to be obtained in quick succession. The rotation of the tube and detectors around the patient allows the corresponding attenuation of each x-ray path to be assessed and using complex mathematical algorithms. Both the density and location of the structures can be mapped. Each slice can then be amalgamated to produce a seamless volume that can be reconstructed in any plane.

Density is measured as Hounsfield Units (HU), named after Geoffrey Hounsfield a pioneer in the development of computed tomography. Gas attenuates little to none of the x-ray beam and is assigned -1000 HU and appears as black on the constructed image. Metal is very dense, consequently is highly attenuating and is given the value of 1000 HU and is depicted as white. Other tissues can be mapped to a scale ranging between these two extremes. Simple water has a density which corresponds to ~0 HU, fat is less dense and therefore less attenuating so has a negative value, usually ~-100 HU. Soft tissue attenuates to a greater degree than water and commonly falls within the region of 30-100 HU. Soft tissues and organ structures density inherently varies and becomes more attenuating if the tissue enhances or contrast is administered (depending on the phase of contrast). Contrast agents are typically based on the metal Iodine.

Assuming the absence of contraindications, CT is generally performed with IV iodinated contrast. After intravenous injection of the contrast, scans are obtained after timed intervals. The timing after contrast is injected determines the phase of scanning. An arterial phase scan (contrast within the arteries) would be performed after 30-35 seconds and a venous phase study after 65-70 seconds. The majority of CT scans are performed in the venous or portal-venous phase.

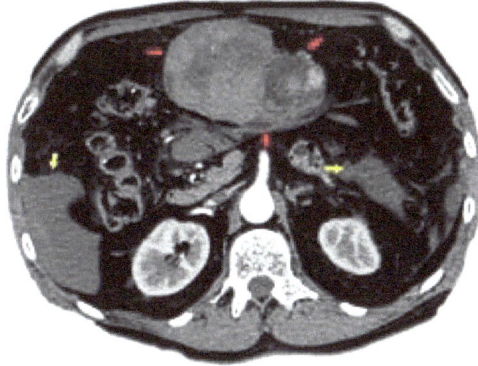

Fig. (1). IV contrast enhanced CT of the abdomen showing a large Gastrointestinal Stromal Tumour with central necrosis. On the left lateral aspect, just below the arrow in the 2 o'clock position there is a small brighter or hyper attenuating area. This region was not visible on the subsequent non-contrast scan and represents haemorrhage. There is fluid within both sides of the abdomen (yellow arrows) that is denser than simple water and represents haemorrhage.

CT is becoming more and more prevalent in all aspects of medicine and surgery. With newer processing techniques and algorithms such as iterative reconstruction, the associated and sometimes prohibitive doses are significantly reduced. Machines have developed significantly from their induction when single slices were obtained at a time. With the current large detectors multiple slices are acquired simultaneously, combined with increased gantry and rotation speeds, scan times are faster and hence more tolerable to patients. The increased sophistication has translated into increased demand for two-dimensional imaging.

CT is used for the assessment, staging and follow-up of both malignant and non-malignant oesophago-gastric conditions (Fig. **1**) [1]. The majority of CT studies are performed either in the outpatient setting, but an increasing number of scans are done on inpatients either awake or anaesthetised and ventilated. Importantly, the availability, speed at which scans can be acquired and the compatibility with non-specialised patient monitoring equipment lend this modality to the assessment of the acutely unwell patient. Emergency oesophago-gastric conditions suitable for CT assessment include oesophageal rupture/tear, upper gastrointestinal bleeding, suspected gastric perforation, gastric volvulus and trauma.

CT in Oesophageal Rupture: The consideration of oesophageal rupture may be as a result of the presence of mediastinal or subcutaneous gas evident on plain film. It is however usually clinically suspected based on the presenting history or other relevant recent interventions. Classically this condition was investigated fluoroscopically with a water-soluble contrast swallow. Enteric swallows provide real-time visualisation of the presence or absence of contrast leaking from the oesophagus and subsequently pooling within the mediastinum. Increasingly, contrast-enhanced CT is the modality of choice for the assessment of these patients. Similar to traditional fluoroscopic swallows the patient ingests a water-soluble contrast medium although the manner in which the test is organised differs. The administered contrast needs to be far more dilute than is typically given for a fluoroscopic examination to prevent significant streak artefact and obscuration of adjacent structures.

Theoretically, administered contrast does not need a density much above that of soft tissue to be identified as separate or out with oesophagus. Typically, a contrast medium containing 300 mg Iodine/ml is diluted to a concentration of 5-10% with sterile water. Several mouthfuls of contrast are swallowed whilst on the table, just before the scan is commenced. An additional mouthful is then held in the mouth until the patient is asked to swallow, immediately prior to the scan being acquired. A real time swallow, similar to fluoroscopic studies is not obtained. Instead the initial swallows allow any contrast to exit any potential defect and pool within the mediastinum. The swallow prior to scan acquisition attempts to opacify and distend the oesophagus.

CT in Anastomotic Leaks*:* In the case of small or sealed leaks, a defect may not always be visible. Contrast seen to be outwith the oesophagus is however diagnostic for a leak. The site, if not seen, is usually directly adjacent to the extra-luminal mediastinal contrast although due to gravity it tends to settle into a dependent position. CT has a far higher sensitivity for the detection of small volumes of extravasated contrast and is able to provide better anatomical localisation compared with fluoroscopy. Similarly, small bubbles of mediastinal gas can be identified that are not visible on other modalities in cases of oesophageal rupture/tear. Small tears that penetrate through the full thickness of the oesophagus appear similar to how they look on traditional fluoroscopy images, as a focus of mural irregularity or a small flap.

CT in Gastric Perforation: Gastric perforation is often difficult to appreciate on a standard CT. Although free intra-abdominal gas may be evident, the site of the defect is often not seen unless very large. Unlike contrast, gas tends not to collect adjacent to defects, instead moving to non-dependent locations. For cases in which there is suspicion of a gastric defect, it can be worthwhile administering a reasonable amount of dilute, water-soluble contrast to fill the stomach before commencing the scan. Contrast, may either fill and opacify the defect or pool locally beside the defect.

CT in Oesophago-gastric Bleeding: Upper gastrointestinal bleeding is usually managed endoscopically in the first instance. Some cases proceed to CT for the assessment of on-going bleeding or re-bleeding following intervention. Alternatively, if the bleeding lesion was not seen or is endoscopically inaccessible, CT angiography is indicated. For these cases, CT angiography can be a useful tool, not only to identify the presence or absence of bleeding but also to help identify the causal vessel to guide any subsequent treatment. A meta-analysis has shown that CT angiography has a high sensitivity and can detect bleeding rates as low as 0.3 ml/min, which is greater than that of conventional angiography (0.5 ml/min) and only marginally behind that of the nuclear medicine test of labelled red-cell scans (0.2 ml/min) [2].

In cases of suspected bleeding, a scan has to be performed with iodinated IV contrast. Several studies are performed in different phases of contrast. Initially a non-contrast study is acquired, as a frame of reference. Acutely clotted blood is hyper dense relative to water. Without the plain study it is not possible to definitively say whether something is enhancing or is simply hyper dense. If an area increases in density following administration of contrast it can be said to be enhancing. The unenhanced study is particularly useful when there is adjacent calcified material, ingested hyper dense foodstuffs and to help identify either intra-luminal or intra-abdominal haemorrhage. Subsequently arterial phases (25-30 seconds post contrast) and portal venous phases (65-70 sec) are acquired. If there are on-going dubiety further image acquisitions can be performed although do contribute to increasing the overall radiation dose.

A point of bleeding appears as a blush of contrast that is out with a vessel and if still bleeding, enlarges on subsequent acquisitions. Typically, arterial bleeds are first visible in the arterial phase and venous bleeding in the venous phase. The slower venous bleeding or oozing can often be difficult to appreciate but is a situation when a more delayed phase comes in useful.

The limitation of CT angiography is that extravasation requires active bleeding at a rate of 0.3 ml/min or greater. If on-going bleeding is below this rate, or there is no active bleeding at the time of scanning, a bleeding source will not be identified. Hyper dense fluid adjacent to a structure may indicate the source. Conversely the presence of large volumes of enteric or intra-abdominal blood, if diffuse, can make pinpointing the source impossible if the bleeding has subsequently subsided.

CT in Perfusion Studies: Studies involving several contrast phases also have a role in the assessment of the oesophago-gastric vascularity. Not only can there be direct visualisation and assessment of the arteries and veins, the way in which the mucosa and wall enhances can give an indication to the likelihood of ischemia. Situations in which this is particularly useful include post oesophagectomy cases where there is a gastric pull-through or with gastric volvulus.

Arterial occlusion or disruption generally results in reduced enhancement of the oesophageal or gastric wall. There is often wall thickening, oedema and there may be the presence of intra-mural and subsequently portal venous gas. Intra-mural gas often occurs with established ischemia when there is mucosal breakdown. Gas then passes into the draining venous system. Intra-mural or portal venous gas does not always indicate ischemia, merely that there has been compromise to the mucosa. Fairly florid portal venous gas can be seen in cases of gastroenteritis, diverticulitis or gastritis. It is also a recognised finding in patients with emphysema. Careful interpretation of this finding is required with correlation to the clinical picture and current patient condition.

Venous occlusion with an intact arterial supply leads to venous congestion. Mural enhancement is often visible although often less than that of the adjacent tissues, although enhancement can be variable. Marked mural thickening and adjacent fat stranding is often evident. Ischemia is often difficult to entirely exclude on CT, particularly when for instance there is a variable occlusion such as with a partial gastric volvulus, which may tort and subsequently resolve. With gastric torsion CT is often capable of differentiating organo-axial rotation from mesenteric-axial although this becomes more challenging when there is increasing dilation. Additionally, CT is often able to indicate whether or not there is frank evidence of ischemia but is not able to exclude it when enhancement is either equivocal or normal.

CT in Post-Operative Complications: Following the significant physiological stresses associated with operative intervention which can often be compounded by patient co-morbidities, it is not uncommon for a patient to make a slower than expected recovery. An important cause of slow recovery can be a result of an operative complication for which CT is an excellent investigative tool. A disproportionate volume of intra-abdominal free gas adjacent to an anastomosis for the time since surgery is often a tell -tale sign for an anastomotic leak which can be confirmed with ingested oral contrast. Small volumes of intra-abdominal fluid are normal, particularly in the immediate post-operative period. Larger collections may undergo organisation with thickened or enhancing walls, particularly when infected. Gas within a collection that does not communicate with another gas filled structure or has not been recently drained should be regarded as infected until proven otherwise.

Over and above the diagnostic indications, CT can be used to facilitate the placement of medical devices with a high degree of accuracy. Common CT guided procedures include drainage of collections, biopsy and ablation of lesions. CT guided procedures all follow the same basic principal of scanning through a small area of several slices in which a needle is being moved. After each movement the same area is re-scanned to determine the new position of the needle tip, allowing step-wise adjustments and manipulation through a safe trajectory down to the target. Once the needle is in position, subsequent steps are indicated by the pathology and the intended procedure.

There are several inherent differences in technique that result from differing scanner capabilities and the operator's preferences; either remaining in the room whilst slices are acquired or vacating it after each needle movement. In all instances where a member of staff remains in the room throughout the procedure, lead protection is mandatory. Newer machines often include the capabilities of what is termed CT fluoroscopy, where the operator remains in the room and is able to scan and move the needle in real time. Machines with CT fluoroscopy facilitate a more dynamic procedure that can account for patient movement and respiratory variation. Although CT fluoroscopy images are of a lower dose than for a diagnostic scan there is an associated radiation dose to all staff in the room that could theoretically become significant if lots of procedures are performed.

3D Imaging

With ongoing advances in 3D post-processing, the plane of imaging has become irrelevant. Image series obtained from high-speed multi-detector CT scanners are now reconstructed as remarkably lifelike 3D volumes for angiographic imaging, cardiac imaging, excretory urography imaging, and a range of endoluminal imaging purposes. Clinicians and, in particular, surgeons have increasingly come to rely on such studies to help with surgical planning. Relatively recently, 3D capabilities are available on workstations throughout Radiology departments, including various service specialized applications to facilitate such reconstruction and display.

Recent advances in computed tomographic (CT) technology including the introduction of multi–detector row CT and the development of three-dimensional (3D) imaging systems have provided the distinct clinical potential for evaluation of various oesophago-gastric disorders, particularly the initial staging of oesophago-gastric cancer. Multi–detector row CT allows thinner collimation, which improves the visualization of subtle tumors as well as the quality of the 3D data sets. Two-dimensional (2D) multi-planar reformation (MPR) and CT gastrography, including virtual gastroscopy and transparency rendering performed with the volume rendering technique, are types of interactive 2D and 3D medical imaging tools that combine the features of multi-planar cross-sectional imaging, gastroscopy viewing, and UGIS images. By using multi–detector row CT, 3D imaging of the stomach becomes more practical and useful in the detection and evaluation of gastric malignancies and the variety of benign conditions that affect the stomach.

PET-CT

Positron Emission Tomography is a nuclear medicine technique that is used to assess or detect areas of increased metabolic activity in conjunction with CT. A radioactive isotope is used that when decaying, does so by emitting positrons, which annihilate when they contact local electrons, the resulting emission of paired gamma rays can be detected by a gamma camera. Computer software is then able to identify the gamma rays origin and subsequently maps this location to a non-contrast CT, performed at the same attendance for the purposes of anatomical reference. Nuclear medicine techniques although sensitive, generally have relatively poor spatial resolution when compared to other modalities. Nuclear medicine relies on the decay of radioactive isotopes administered to the patient. The decaying isotope emits particles/ electromagnetic waves, which register on surrounding detectors. The region of origin of the particles is estimated in order to build an image of the tumour rather than relying on tissue composition as with other modalities.

The most commonly used radioactive isotope in PET-CT is 18F-FDG (2-deoxy-2 (Flourine-18) flouro-D-glucose. This analogue of glucose is taken up by all metabolising cells but in greater concentrations where there is increased metabolic activity such as the case in malignant tissue (Fig. **2**).

Malignant cells typically have greater metabolic demands and cell turnover when compared with normal tissues. Consequently, there is accumulation of greater concentrations of 18F-FDG and consequently a greater number of gamma rays are detected to be arising from this area.

The limitations of this technique are that any focus of increased metabolism will portray increased FDG accumulation, which is not specific to malignancy. Consequently prior to scanning there is a relatively rigorous patient preparation. Scanning is usually delayed at least 72 hours after interventional procedures including biopsies.

Patients require to be fasted for at least 4 hours prior to the examination. Before the injection of the radioisotope they are asked to rest in an area of relative sensory deprivation, for usually 15-20 minutes. Prior to injection of the radio-isotope, (the dosage is calculated based on bodyweight), patients rest for a further

1-2 hours before scanning in order to allow distribution of the tracer throughout the body and accumulation in the relevant areas of high metabolic activity.

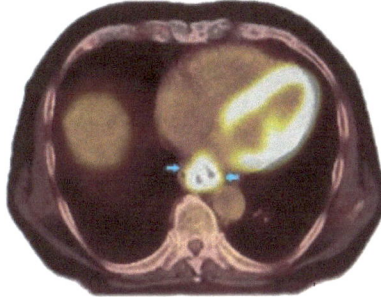

Fig. (2). A fused image combining a non-contrast CT for anatomic reference and PET data to FDG accumulation. Axial reformat. Increased activity displayed by a mid-oesophageal tumour (between blue arrows). Note how the highly metabolically active myocardium of the left ventricle is similarly FDG avid when compared with the adjacent tumour.

PET-CT is now generally indicated in all patients with oesophago-gastric malignancy in which curative intent is being considered [3]. Although PET images are fused with CT, the inherently low spatial resolution of nuclear medicine tests negates the assessment of local invasion of the primary lesion. Similarly, closely approximated nodes are often difficult to differentiate as separate. PET-CT's role in staging is for the detection of distant and otherwise difficult to detect metastases. With small volume metastases, there will be a correspondingly small area of tracer accumulation and PET-CT may be falsely reassuring. This is particularly the case with small peritoneal deposits or lung lesions. Nodes distant from the primary lesion which although not enlarged may have an abnormal nodal morphology and consequently be regarded as equivocal on CT. Assuming there is no local cause such as infection or inflammation, nodes exhibiting increased tracer uptake on PET-CT should be regarded as involved (Fig. **3**).

The great advantages of PET-CT are, wide coverage of a larger volume more than normally covered at CT staging, and is highly sensitive for the detection of distant metastases. The most frequent sites in which metastases are commonly found, but are missed on CT, and subsequently identified on PET-CT are lesions within the liver and spine. Additionally, PET-CT scan aid the identification of metastatic deposits in more uncommon sites such as the brain and skeletal muscles [4].

Two typical PET-CT appearances are described when there are peritoneal metastases. The first is of diffuse spreading activity throughout the abdomen with obscuration of the normal visceral outlines. The second is of discrete nodular foci throughout the abdomen and not related to solid organs or nodal stations. Foci of increased activity often correlate with focal soft tissue nodularity on the non-contrast CT. Small volume disease although evident on CT may fall below the threshold for detection on PET-CT [5]. In cases where there is dubiety about the possibility of mesenteric dissemination, staging laparoscopy is indicated.

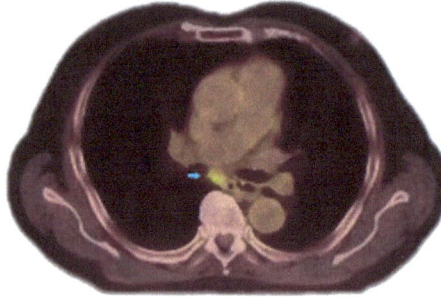

Fig. (3). A fused image combining a non-contrast CT for anatomic reference and PET data to FDG accumulation. Axial reformat. Lying adjacent to the oesophagus there is a lymph node (blue arrow) with greater FDG accumulation than the blood pool (adjacent vessels) suggesting this has increased metabolic activity. This is a case of lymph node metastasis from a more distal oesophageal tumour.

PET-CT findings should be interpreted with caution. Although sensitive it is not very specific. Any form of infection or inflammation will exhibit increased tracer accumulation. Similarly, non-metastatic or pre-neoplastic entities can exhibit increased activity such as polyps. Conversely certain tumour subtypes such mucinous carcinoma, poorly differentiated adenocarcinoma and signet ring cell carcinoma tend to have relatively poor FDG accumulation. The difficulty in these instances arises because like the primary lesion, any metastatic disease would also typically have reduced activity. PET-CT negative nodes and distant lesions in these patients should be highly scrutinised and there should be consideration to the use of other imaging modalities or even biopsy for a full assessment [5].

Magnetic Resonance Imaging (MRI)

Magnetic resonance imaging is a modality that does not require ionising radiation; instead, it uses a strong magnetic field and is able to detect subtle differences in tissue composition to produce an anatomic image. The basics of MRI relate to how the strong magnetic field is able to align the procession of protons (Hydrogen atoms) within the body (or any tissue) to the axis of the magnet. A radiofrequency (RF) pulse is emitted by the scanner at a range of frequencies corresponding to that of the proton procession. The energy delivered by the RF pulse is able to knock the alignment of the Hydrogen atoms procession from the axis of the magnet by varying angles. When the RF pulse is stopped, the protons return to the original alignment at varying rates depending on the tissue they originate within. As they re-align there is a small amount of emitted energy that can be detected by sensor coils. The tiny emitted energies require coils to be as close to the assessed tissues as possible. Coils generally have a specific body part application although some can be used for a number of applications. Coils are generally placed around the patient although endoluminal coils can be used for applications such as rectal or prostate staging. The emitted energies are very small and in order to build up an image the protons are "flipped" multiple times to build up amplified images. Extremely complicated computer processing is required to analyse the emitted energy in order to build up a picture of the tissue structure being analysed.

There are two main types of MRI. Open (or low-field) MRI has a typical magnetic field strength of around 1.0 tesla (T), while Closed (or high-field) MRI is the more powerful at around 1.5 or even 3T. A Closed MRI scan often involves a cylinder-shaped scanner that is uncomfortable for larger patients and leaves some patients claustrophobic. For many patients Open MRI minimizes anxiety and claustrophobia because its 'C' shaped design offers a spacious environment in which patients lie between two plates. They are also used for intraoperative imaging or image- guided interventions where easy access to the patient is required. The main drawbacks of Open MRI are that the sequences needed (length of time to get an image) are longer, the signal-to-noise ratio is lower, and the spatial resolution is poorer. Consequently, for the analysis of small structures such as joints, Closed MRI is recommended because the quality and detail of the image will be superior. Also, the field strength of open magnets is significantly reduced and may be inadequate for some scanning purposes.

While it may have apparent limitations in terms of indications, there are situations that call for Open MRI, which is not reliant on having the patient lie in a long narrow tube. Open MRI can be used where there is the problem of claustrophobia. Furthermore, the increasing number of overweight and obese patients produces more problems for high-field MRI units. A third advantage of low- field MRI is that the images obtained are affected to a much lesser degree by metallic structures that may be present in the body such as implants or metallic foreign bodies. The majority of radiology departments have closed high field MRI scanners with a few units hosting open scanners.

Some sequence acquisitions can take upwards of 10 minutes each with a scan being comprised of multiple sequences. Long scan times may be difficult for some patients to tolerate. As a consequence of the lengthy sequences any significant movement results in significant movement artefact, which can render images non-diagnostic. Although there is the possibility to "gate" (time) to respiratory motion and cardiac motion this increases sequence acquisition time. Sequence time generally increases with increasing number of slices within a volume. Gated sequences are used in cardiac imaging but for the larger field scanning that typically would be used to image the gastro-intestinal tract the sequence lengths would become prohibitive. The angle at which slices are obtained can be done without changing patient position or angling the machine. Other uses of MRI include applications such as functional MRI, which works in a similar fashion to PET-CT whereby MRI is able to detect areas of increased metabolic activity.

Normal medical monitoring devices, and other medical devices such as pumps and ventilators cannot be used in MRI scanners, which limits their usage in acutely ill patients. Modern ceramic instruments and devices have recently been specifically designed for use in MRI scanners, but these tend to be expensive. Metals within the body, as long as they are fixed, such as hip replacement prosthesis are safe. Intra-cranial aneurysm clips, heart valves *etc.* that are not pre designated for use in MRI are absolute contra-indications. Certain metallic implants although technically safe for use in MRI, particularly those that are linear can induce a current and become hot, something the patient has to be aware of and able to indicate to the scanning staff. Significant burns can result from internal metal or indeed leads overlying the patient. Similarly tattoos or cosmetic creams containing metal pigments may heat during the scan.

The main advantage of MRI is that it does not use radiation. Certain sequences can visualise flow within vessels without the need to injected contrast. The range of commonly used contrast agents is greater than that for other modalities with a number of highly specialised indications such as contrast that is taken up by hepatocytes. This favours MRI as an ideal utility to characterise liver lesions. MRI of the liver has a high sensitivity and specificity for the detection and characterisation of liver metastases. Diffusion weighted imaging is a technique that assesses the diffusion of water molecules within a specific volume. Normally, passage of water within tissues is relatively uninterrupted. Certain lesions, particularly tumours, have more tightly packed and irregular cell structure, which impedes water passage and can be identified on MRI. The soft tissue differentiation of MRI is greater than that of CT and conventional radiography and can visualise organ structures not normally accessible to ultrasound. MRI is the ideal modality for assessing the brain, spine and soft tissues.

MRI is used for the assessment of rectal tumours with sensitive differentiation between closely approximated soft tissue structures around the rectum, identifying the rectal wall separately. This provides a relatively accurate indication of the likelihood and extent of invasion of rectal tumours. Currently, MRI has limited clinical use in the assessment of and the local staging of oesophageal and gastric cancer. The proximity to the heart, compounded with respiratory motion artefact and peristalsis make these areas difficult to assess. Although it would be technically possible to obtain sensitive scans of the area, by time gating for cardiac and respiratory movements, the scan times would be prohibitively long. Endoscopic ultrasound provides better spatial resolution and tissue differentiation of the oesophageal and gastric wall than MRI. However, for T4 tumours with invasion of adjacent organs, the tissue differentiation is poorer than it would be for MRI. Current practice is to combine staging modalities including laparoscopic staging for the assessment of oesophago-gastric and gastric neoplasms.

Generally, unless there are contra-indications, MRI is usually performed with post IV contrast sequences. Several different contrast agents are available and have varying indications. Extra-cellular contrast agents, typically Gadolinium based, behave in a similar fashion to contrast administered for CT scans giving vascular enhancement and have subsequent renal excretion. Hepato-biliary specific agents are taken up by hepatocytes and are excreted by the biliary system to varying degrees. There has been significant evolution and refinement of hepatocyte specific agents since their introduction in 1997 (Mangafodipir trisodium) [6]. Multihance (Gadolinium-BOPTA) was introduced in 2004 and although primarily an extra-cellular contrast agent, 3-5% is take up by and excreted by hepatocytes. Primovist or Eovist (Gadolinium-EOB-DTPA) are more hepatocyte specific with greater proportions (approximately 50%) being taken up by hepatocytes. The more hepatocyte specific an agent is, the poorer the extra-cellular or vascular enhancement will be.

Contrast enhanced MRI with a hepatocyte specific agent has a greater sensitivity for the detection of hepatic colorectal metastases (95%) when compared to contrast enhanced CT (63%) and contrast enhanced ultrasound (73%). There is reduced sensitivity for detection of lesions smaller than 10 mm although this remains far greater than with CT or ultrasound [7]. A large meta-analysis found that MRI with hepatocyte specific contrast agents to have a sensitivity of 93% and specificity of 95% for the detection of liver metastases. This sensitivity and specificity is reduced when looking at sub-10 mm lesions [8]. Although the sensitivity for the detection of lesions using MRI with hepatocyte specific contrast agents is greater than MRI with diffusion weighted imaging (DWI) alone (94.4% vs. 78.3%), for the smaller lesions (<10 mm), DWI is thought to be more sensitive (92% vs 98%) [9]. Consequently, these techniques are often performed together as a part of standard MRI liver examinations.

Ultrasound

Ultrasound is a radiological examination that employs sound waves to differentiate between soft tissue structures. The ultrasound probe vibrates emitting sound waves that pass into the patient via a coupling jelly, which bridges the interface between the probe and the soft tissue surface, eliminating the intervening air space. The sound waves pass through soft tissues and are reflected by any interfaces caused by variation in the soft tissue density. Sound waves are not only emitted by, but also detected by the same probe. Depending on the time it takes for a wave to be emitted and received, the depth of the tissue can be calculated by knowing the speed of sound transmittance in the relevant tissue. The received intensity of the wave determines the displayed signal intensity.

Sound waves travel faster through mediums of increased density due to the closer approximation of vibrating molecules. Consequently, the speed of transmission through soft tissues is greater than through gasses. It is important to note that there is a significantly decreased speed of travel in gasses and dispersement of the wave when encountering a soft tissue to gas interface. It is for this reason that it is difficult to see beyond gas filled body structures which appear as an echo-bright surface closest to the probe with a large area of shadowing beyond.

Between each soft tissue interface there is a resultant echo that is detected by the probe. Deeper structures necessitate the wave to travel further both towards and then back to the probe. The result is that the echo takes longer to be received and delays the subsequent transmission of new echoes. Consequently, the rate at which the image refreshes (temporal resolution), is reduced. Additionally, in order to view deeper structures a lower sound wave frequency is required. The lower the frequency the better the tissue penetration but is at the cost of reduced temporal and spatial resolution. High frequency ultrasound is used to view structures that are close to the probe and has a high resolution, capable of resolving subtle differences in soft tissue composition. Applications such as endoscopic ultrasound use high frequency probes for the assessment of tumour extension through the closely approximated oesophago-gastric wall. The high frequency and resulting high spatial resolution inherently limit assessment of deeper extension such as potential T4 tumour invasion.

Ultrasound is often the index examination, as it does not rely on ionising radiation. It often incidentally identifies lesions within the liver as part of a routine abdominal ultrasound. Metastases often appear as solid, hypoechoic lesions with evidence of mass effect (displacing adjacent structures or vessels). Percutaneous ultrasound is not routinely used in the staging of oesophago-gastric tumours. Occasionally it may be used to further categorise a liver lesion seen on CT, determining whether or not it is solid or cystic.

Intra-operative ultrasound has a number of applications. The advantages over percutaneous ultrasound, is that the probe can be directly applied to the organ or structure in question. The result is that there is reduced tissue penetration allowing use of higher frequency probes that afford increased spatial and temporal resolution. Additionally, it is possible to negate the problem often when scanning percutaneously when there is obscuration of the target organ as a result of overlying loops of bowel. A recent technical innovation uses High Intensity Focussed Ultrasound for the ablation of hepatic metastases particularly those that are not surgically palpable, usually due to the depth within the liver. Additionally, smaller lesions may be visible and better targeted due to the benefits of using a higher frequency probe.

Contrast enhanced ultrasound is being used with increasing frequency although not commonly employed as part of standard staging. This technique visualises micro-bubbles that are injected intravenously. The reflection of the delivered sound waves as a result of the gas filled bubbles within vascular structures improves the resolution. Lesions with vascularity "enhance" in a similar fashion, as they would do on either CT or MRI [10]. Not all ultrasound machines have the required software capabilities to allow the use of ultrasound contrast agents.

Ultrasound and even contrast enhanced ultrasound, relative to CT or MRI is a cost-effective and relatively quick non-invasive test without radiation burden. The limitations of ultrasound are that it is an operator and patient dependent technique. The liver can often be difficult to visualise adequately in patients with a high BMI, particularly those with central abdominal obesity. Additionally, when there is intra-hepatic fatty infiltration the liver appears diffusely bright and there is reduced ultrasound penetrance making visualising the whole liver difficult. A further advantage to ultrasound is that it is a dynamic examination and as a result allows the targeting of small lesions for biopsy, which would be difficult on CT.

Ultrasound is able to visualise the manipulation of medical devices in real time and is an excellent modality for most guided interventional procedures. It is particularly helpful when the patient has difficulty remaining still or is taking varied respiratory efforts given the more dynamic nature of the procedure. The limitations are that when there are adjacent or overlapping gas-containing structures the ultrasound wave is largely reflected and consequently deeper structures are poorly visible. Very deep structures can also be quite difficult to identify and in such cases CT is the preferred modality.

NUCLEAR MEDICINE IMAGING

The basic principles to the majority of nuclear medicine tests, PET-CT included, is that a radioisotope is administered to the patient and the emitted radiation is detected and measured. Depending on the injected agent, the isotope accumulates in the corresponding organ or tissues, and detected by the gamma cameras or detectors to identify these areas as regions of increased activity. PET-CT makes up the majority of nuclear medicine techniques employed for the staging of oesophago-gastric cancer. Whilst other nuclear medicine tests exist they often have a far more specific indication.

Bone scans, use the radioisotope Technetium 99 m, combined with methylene diphosphonate (MDP) and accumulate in areas of increase osteoblastic/osteoclastic activity. Although a bone scan could be used to identify bony metastases, PET-CT will also identify these lesions as areas of increased metabolism as well as the primary tumour and other metastases.

Beyond staging, nuclear medicine has uses for providing dynamic and functional assessment with indications such as motility disorders of the oesophagus or stomach such as gastroparesis. Unlike with bone scans and PET-CT where the radioisotope is injected intravenously, functional oesophago-gastric tests such as gastric emptying studies are done with the patient ingesting the radioisotope. Gastric emptying scintigraphy is the gold standard method for assessment of gastric emptying.

Gastric Emptying Studies

Two tests are usually carried out, one for liquid gastric emptying and one for solid gastric emptying. The main indication is suspicion of delayed gastric emptying with repeated nausea and vomiting in the absence of a structural abnormality. Normally, the patient is fasted prior to the examination. Similar to a number of nuclear medicine tests, the radioactive isotope Technetium 99 m is used and for gastric emptying studies is combined with Sulphur colloid. The administered dose is calculated based on the patient's weight. As the study aims to provide a functional assessment of how the stomach empties normally, the radioisotope is mixed with either milk for liquid gastric emptying studies or foodstuff such as scrambled eggs or rice for solid gastric emptying studies.

Imaging is performed immediately and at delayed intervals for several hours measuring the detected radioactivity in the stomach. A correction is made for the expected reduction in activity due to decay of the radioisotope based on the known half-life. A further reduction in activity from the region of interest (stomach) occurs as a consequence of passage of the radiolabelled foodstuffs into the small bowel. Consequently, the rate of emptying can be quantified and compared with standardised normal values [11].

Oesophageal Transit Studies

These tests are usually carried out as a substitute to manometric studies of the oesophagus due to patients' intolerance or lack of appropriate equipment.

Occasionally, they are requested when other tests have not reached a diagnosis. Unlike other tests, they are specific for measuring the transit times through different segments of the thoracic oesophagus. Similar to gastric emptying studies, the patient is fasted prior to the examination. The radioactive isotope Technetium 99 m is used and mixed with scrambled eggs. The administered dose is calculated based on the patient's weight [12].

Imaging is performed immediately and at delayed intervals for several minutes, measuring the detected radioactivity in regions of interest, which correspond to the different segments of the thoracic oesophagus. A correction is made for decay of the radioisotope and for reduction in activity due to the passage of the radiolabelled foodstuffs into the stomach. The transit times through different segments of the oesophagus, for the whole oesophagus and the pattern of transit are quantified and compared with standardised normal values (Fig. **4**).

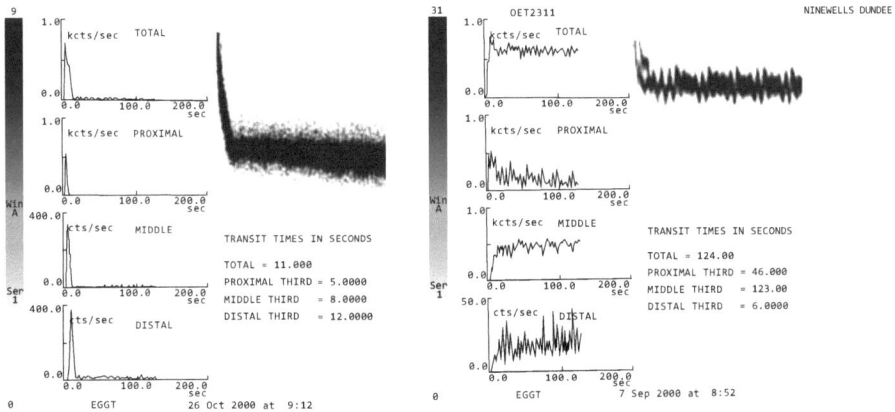

Fig. (4). Oesophageal Egg Transit Studies using Tc99 scrambled egg. The study on the left is showing a normal motility pattern and the one on the right showing prolonged oesophageal transit typically found in achalasia.

STAGING OF OESOPHAGO-GASTRIC NEOPLASMS

In contrast to conventional gastroscopy and upper gastrointestinal series (UGIS) images of the stomach, CT provides information about both the gastric wall and the perigastric extent of disease. Endoscopic ultrasonography (US) provides the most useful information regarding tumor location, horizontal extension of the tumor, the depth of mural invasion, and perigastric lymphadenopathy. Endoscopic US allows reliable distinction between an intramural lesion and extrinsic compression. In comparison with endoscopic US, multi–detector row CT is able to demonstrate not only the immediate vicinity of the stomach but also more distant regions, such as para-aortic lymphadenopathy and abdominal organs.

Small and early gastric cancer is often harder to appreciate radiologically when compared with oesophageal lesions, particularly when there is poor gastric distension. T1, T2 and even small T3 lesions can be difficult to appreciate. The lesions can often, be masked by gastric rugal folds. Small oesophageal lesions can often be seen as concentric mural thickening with associated upstream oesophageal dilation, gastric lesions have to be far larger to create similar effects in the stomach.

In general, oesophageal and gastric tumours can be staged with reference to the classification of AJCC-UICC TNM staging manual [13]. Some difficulty arises with tumours of the oesophago-gastric junction in terms of assigning them to oesophageal or gastric origin. This is often difficult with CT particularly in the presence of a hiatus hernia and is best assessed endoscopically. Tumours arising either at the gastro-oesophageal junction or those within the proximal 5cm of the stomach but crossing the gastro-oesophageal junction are staged as per oesophageal staging in the current 7th edition of TNM staging. Currently, this is not universally adopted and a future edition of the TNM staging is likely to change this position.

Staging currently uses the seventh edition of the AJCC-UICC TNM system with revisions. The current staging framework includes new definitions and classifications of both T*is* and T4 disease. Furthermore, there is sub categorisation of regional nodal disease, simplification of what is termed metastatic disease and consideration of factors such as histological grade and cell type.

T Staging

This is based on the depth of tumour invasion and the involvement of local surrounding structures (Table 1). CT does not have the spatial resolution or the soft tissue differentiation to definitively assess accurately the local stage of either oesophageal or gastric lesions. Endoscopic ultrasound remains the gold standard in local tumour staging. This is particularly so for the oesophagus. For the stomach, laparoscopy is an essential adjunct investigation to inform the T and M staging. In addition, peritoneal cytology could be obtained at the same time.

Table 1. T Category definitions, Oesophageal and junctional cancers (TNM 7th Edition) [14].

T category	Features
TX	Primary tumor cannot be assessed
T0	No evidence of primary tumor
Tis	High-grade dysplasia
T1	Tumor invades lamina propria, muscularis mucosae, or submucosa

(Table 1) contd.....

T category	Features
T1a	Tumor invades lamina propria or muscularis mucosae
T1b	Tumor invades submucosa
T2	Tumor invades muscularis propria
T3	Tumor invades adventitia
T4	Tumor invades adjacent structures
T4a	Resectable tumor invading pleura, pericardium, or diaphragm
T4b	Unresectable tumor invading other adjacent structures, such as the aorta, vertebral body, and trachea

Oesophageal Tumours

<u>*Oesophageal T1 and T2 Tumours:*</u> In the presence of a well distended oesophagus, a wall thickness of 3 mm or less is considered to be normal and abnormal when thickness is equal to greater than 5 mm [14]. In practice the oesophagus is often poorly distended or collapsed and consequently smaller or early disease is often not seen.

<u>*Oesophageal T3 Tumours:*</u> These tumours are generally visible on CT even with a poorly distended oesophagus, appearing as either eccentric or circumferential focal wall thickening, with or without a visible endoluminal component (Fig. **5**). The absence of a substantial serosa around the oesophagus facilitates early malignant extension into the adjacent fat and accounts for the reason a significant proportion of lesions are staged as T3 or greater at the time of diagnosis.

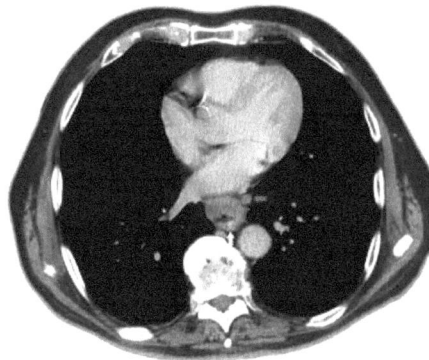

Fig. (5). IV contrast enhanced CT of the chest. Axial reformat. Eccentrically thickened mid oesophagus secondary to tumour (yellow arrow). The oesophageal wall is thickest anteriorly, the point at which the tumour likely originated. At this point the outer aspect of the oesophagus is ill defined with haziness to the peri-oesophageal fat. There remains a discernible fat plane lying between the oesophageal tumour and the posterior aspect of the left atrium (between green arrows). Lying to the left lateral aspect of the tumour there is a rounded, homogenous and abnormal peri-oesophageal lymph node (red arrow).

Disease classified at T3 indicates direct tumoral extension beyond the adventitia. On CT, this appears as ill-defined strands of soft tissue or even subtle haziness within the peri-oesophageal fat. The limitations being that any form of local inflammation or desmoplastic reaction can mimic T3 disease. Tumours associated with esophagitis or arising on a background of Barrett's esophagitis can be extremely difficult to locally stage accurately with CT and is this is a particularly where endoscopic ultrasound, which has better spatial resolution and tissue differentiation is extremely useful. However, this technique is operator and patient dependent, and can also over stage the local extent of a tumour in the presence of local inflammation or oedema. A designation of T3 implies that the tumour is resectable pending the N and M designation and the condition of the patient.

Oesophageal T4 Tumours: With the 7th edition of TNM staging, T4 disease is sub-classified into disease, which is technically resectable (T4a), and disease, which is deemed to be unresectable (T4b). T4a represents direct invasion of the pleura, pericardium or diaphragm including diaphragmatic crura. Although these structures are technically resectable, this by no means implies that a resection should be undertaken particularly if several of these structures are involved indicating circumferential involvement. In this scenario, the tumour is described as locally advanced but resectable. T4b disease indicates invasion of the aorta, trachea, vertebral column or frank cardiac invasion (Figs. **6** and **7**). In these circumstances, the tumour is technically not resectable and for staging purposes described as unresectable by the designation of T4b status.

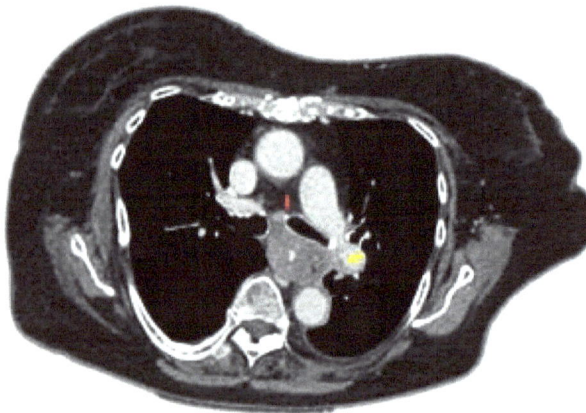

Fig. (6). IV contrast enhanced CT of the chest. Axial reformat. Locally advanced T4b oesophageal tumour with marked mural thickening. The anterior aspect the tumour extends into the mediastinum beneath the carina and surrounds the proximal bronchi (red arrow). On the left lateral aspect, the tumour contacts and invades the left main pulmonary artery. At the point of contact, the vessel is distorted with a bowed contour (yellow arrow).

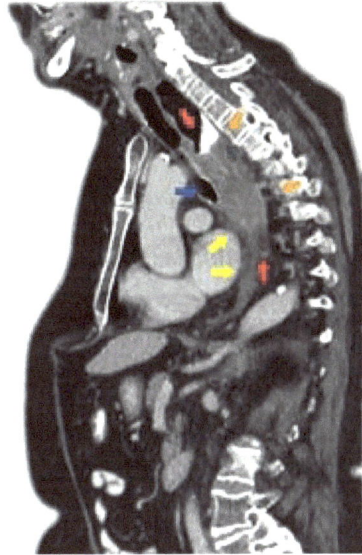

Fig. (7). IV contrast enhanced CT of the chest and abdomen. Sagittal reformat. Depicted between the red arrows there is a large and locally advanced T4b oesophageal lesion with associated obstruction. Above the tumour there is oesophageal dilation and pooling of oral contrast. The tumour surrounds the bronchi (blue arrow), invades the heart (yellow arrows where it abuts the left atrium) and the vertebral bodies (orange arrows).

CT is considered the better modality when assessing the invasion of local structures over endoscopic ultrasound (Fig. **5**). Although the resolution of endoscopic ultrasound is better this is only true over a very shallow depth [15]. Direct invasion appears as a loss of the intervening fat plane between the tumour and adjacent organs/structures. Particularly with mid oesophageal lesions where there is inherently limited surrounding fat, identification of a clear fat plane can often be difficult to assess and approaches the limits of CT resolution. This inherent difficulty can often be compounded when the patients have either lost weight as a result of dysphagia or indeed malignancy itself. Features supporting extra-organ extension include; a large plane of contact with the adjacent organ with no perceptible intervening fat plane, local soft tissue thickening (pericardium, diaphragm etc.), bowing or indentation of the structure, vascular encasement, intra-vascular tumour thrombus or visible fistulation. Tumours arising either at the gastro-oesophageal junction or those within the proximal 5 cm of the stomach but crossing the gastro-oesophageal junction are staged as per oesophageal staging [16].

Gastric Tumours

Gastric T1 and T2 Tumours: These lesions are confined to the gastric wall. T1 disease involves the lamina propria or muscularis mucosae (T1a) or the submucosa (T1b). T2 staging reflects involvement of the muscularis propria. These lesions are endoscopic entities and are not seen on CT. Infrequently, indeterminate localised gastric wall thickening due to peri-tumoral oedema may be seen particularly in the presence of ulcerated tumours. However, these appearances are non-specific.

Gastric T3 Tumours: Extension beyond the gastric wall as a result of penetration of the subserosa, without visceral peritoneal involvement is classified as T3. Radiologically T3 disease appears as loss of clarity or haziness to the outer gastric wall often with spiculation or stranding within the perigastric fat. Involvement of the gastro-colic, gastro-hepatic ligaments, extension into the lesser or greater omentum also reflects T3 disease as long as there is no involvement of the visceral peritoneum (T4 disease). Distinction between T3 and T4 disease has significant implications and has to be made carefully since it determines potential treatment options and prognosis (Table **2**).

Table 2. T Category definitions, gastric cancer (TNM 7th Edition) [16].

T category	Features
TX	Primary tumour cannot be assessed
T0	No evidence of primary tumour
Tis	Carcinoma in situ: intraepithelial tumour without invasion of the lamina propria
T1	Tumour invades lamina propria, muscularis mucosae, or submucosa
T1a	Tumour invades lamina propria or muscularis mucosae
T1b	Tumour invades submucosa
T2	Tumour invades muscularis propria
T3	Tumour penetrates subserosal connective tissue without invasion of visceral peritoneum or adjacent structures. T3 tumours also include those extending into the gastro-colic or gastro-hepatic ligaments, or into the greater or lesser omentum, without perforation of the visceral peritoneum covering these structures
T4	Tumour invades serosa (visceral peritoneum) or adjacent structures
T4a	Tumour invades serosa (visceral peritoneum)
T4b	Tumour invades adjacent structures such as spleen, transverse colon, liver, diaphragm, pancreas, abdominal wall, adrenal gland, kidney, small intestine, and retroperitoneum

Gastric T3 Tumours: Extension beyond the gastric wall as a result of penetration of the subserosa, without visceral peritoneal involvement is classified as T3. Radiologically T3 disease appears as loss of clarity or haziness to the outer gastric wall often with spiculation or stranding within the perigastric fat. Involvement of the gastro-colic, gastro-hepatic ligaments, extension into the lesser or greater omentum also reflects T3 disease as long as there is no involvement of the visceral peritoneum (T4 disease). Distinction between T3 and T4 disease has significant implications and has to be made carefully since it determines potential treatment options and prognosis.

Gastric T4 Tumours: Without direct extra-organ spread, tumour involving the visceral peritoneum signifies T4a disease. Tumour extension along the gastro-hepatic or gastro-colic ligaments predisposes to direct extension to the liver and colon respectively. Additionally, extension into the lesser sac affords direct access to the pancreas. With direct organ extension staging is classified at T4b disease. Assessment is made to determine whether or not a discernible fat plane can be identified between the primary tumour and adjacent structures. Generally, there is a greater volume of peri-gastric than peri-oesophageal fat making this process easier. The exception being when there is associated gastric outflow obstruction and the gross distension distorts anatomy and pushes the diseased gastric wall against adjacent local structures. Adjacent peritoneal thickening, nodularity, or a large plane of contact with or bowing of local structures favours involvement.

Nodal Status

The nodal status in oesophago-gastric cancer is a significant prognostic factor, which determines treatment intent, treatment options and ultimate survival. The extensive submucosal lymphatics of the oesophagus and stomach predispose to early regional and metastatic nodal spread. Endoscopic ultrasound has better resolution in assessment of para-oesophageal nodes and those in the coeliac axis.

The 7th edition regards all para-oesophageal nodes between the cervical/supraclavicular and celiac stations as regional. 1-2, 3-6 and 7+ nodes when involved by tumour constitute N1, N2 and N3 disease respectively (Table 3). Similarly, N-stage in gastric cancers is also based on the number of regionally involved nodes. 1-2, 3-6 and 7+ involved nodes indicate N1, N2 and N3 disease, respectively.

Table 3. N Category definitions, oesophageal and gastric cancer (TNM 7th Edition) [16].

N category	Features
NX	Regional lymph node(s) cannot be assessed
N0	No regional lymph node metastasis
N1	Metastasis in 1 to 2 regional lymph nodes
N2	Metastasis in 3 to 6 regional lymph nodes
N3	Metastasis in 7 or more regional lymph nodes

In oesophago-gastric cancer, radiological staging is not definitive in assessing the presence or absence of tumour within lymph nodes, although PET-CT does have a high sensitivity and specificity for identifying abnormal nodes. Ultimately pathological assessment is necessary to determine final nodal stage. Radiological staging provides an informed best guess to determine treatment intent and options. This is based on the shape and size of the lymph nodes. Normally lymph nodes are ovoid in shape, have a smooth contour and a discernible fat containing hilum. Abnormalities of shape, contour and spatial pattern are taken together to predict involvement. Mediastinal and lower cervical lymph nodes are considered of a normal size when they measure 10 mm or less in their short axis diameter. Porta-hepatis nodes are generally larger and would be considered enlarged when they measure over 12 mm in short axis (Fig. **8**). Unfortunately size alone is an unreliable predictor of nodal involvement. Any local or regional node that has any abnormal features should be regarded as suspicious. Involved nodes generally if large enough, exhibit increased tracer uptake on PET-CT scanning. However, reactive lymph nodes in the presence of local inflammation can also exhibit tracer uptake on PET-CT. Ultimately pathological assessment would determine the final nodal staging.

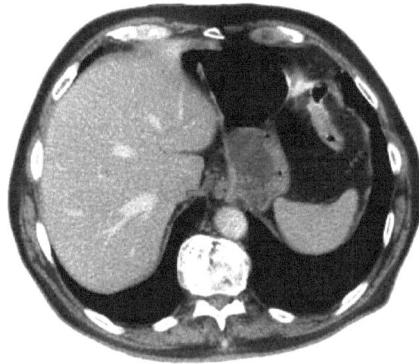

Fig. (8). IV contrast enhanced CT of the abdomen of patient with mid-oesophageal adenocarcinoma. Axial reformat. Adjacent to the gastric cardia on the lesser curvature of the stomach there is an irregular enlarged lymph node with loss of the normal fatty hilum (red arrow).

Metastatic Disease

Previous TNM staging of oesophageal lesions included subdivisions of M staging with M1a indicating nodal metastases, either supraclavicular or celiac and M1b disease when there was overt distant disease. The 7th edition includes only M1 or M0 to indicate presence or absence of metastatic disease, respectively.

Oesophageal tumours metastasise preferentially to the liver, lungs, bony skeleton and the adrenal glands (decreasing frequency). Gastric tumours are less commonly associated with solid metastases at the time of diagnosis but most frequently spread to the liver due to venous drainage via the portal vein. Less commonly they spread to lungs, adrenals, bony skeleton and ovaries (Krukenberg tumours).

Hepatic metastases are best depicted in the portal venous phase where they appear as hypo attenuating (lower density) and often ill-defined lesions. Compared with simple hepatic cysts, metastases generally are less well defined and of slightly higher attenuation (soft tissue compared with water). Smaller lesions, particularly those that are sub 1 cm, are difficult to confidently characterise and in these cases ultrasound or MRI of the liver are better modalities. Alternatively, small lesions can be differentiated from cysts and other more benign liver lesions on the routinely performed staging PET-CT. Assuming the primary lesion is metabolically active, metastases would also generally exhibit tracer uptake. Smaller lesions or those from a primary that does not exhibit significant FDG uptake cannot reliably be discounted.

Lung metastases typically manifest as smooth rounded soft tissue density nodules. Small or single lesions are more difficult to categorically classify as metastases on CT. Larger or multiple rounded pulmonary nodules can be predicted as metastases with greater certainty. Occasionally, it can be difficult to differentiate metastatic disease in the lung from primary lung tumours although primary lung cancer is more commonly solitary and has spiculated margins. The most common differentials for small pulmonary nodules include intrapulmonary lymph nodes (usually peripheral, lying on fissures or flat in appearance), granulomata (may contain calcification) or hamartoma (may have visible internal fat +/- calcification). PET-CT can sometimes help by detecting increased metabolic activity although for smaller lesions, the sensitivity decreases. Small lesions that do not appear to have increased activity on PET-CT cannot be discounted as benign, particularly if the primary tumour does not have significant tracer uptake. Ultimately smaller nodules may require follow up scans to determine their involvement.

Adrenal metastases often appear as focal heterogeneous enlargement of the gland. When staging oesophago-gastric cancers it is important to differentiate adrenal metastases from the more frequently encountered adrenal adenomata. Typically, adenomas are small (<3cm) and of homogenous low density. Most contain fat and identification of fat density material on CT is highly specific for adenomata. If not identified on CT, MRI sequences can be performed to assess the presence of fat by a phenomenon known as chemical shift artefact. Lipid poor lesions are harder to diagnose and generally have a density approaching that of soft tissue. Adenomas tend to enhance and then rapidly washout whereas non-adenomas on the whole washout more slowly. By performing contrast enhanced CT with several acquisitions at differing times the degree of washout can be quantified and the likelihood of adenoma assessed. Alternatively, on PET-CT, the vast majority of adrenal adenomata are non-functioning and unlike metastases, do not exhibit increased activity.

Bony metastases can either present as sclerotic or lucent lesions. Compounding features include destruction of the bony cortex, an associated soft tissue mass and bony fractures. Smaller lesions can be difficult to detect. The sensitivity of CT for detection of bony metastases is less than that of bone scans, MRI and PET-CT.

Peritoneal disease is less commonly encountered than solid organ metastases although is an extremely bad prognostic feature and indicates incurable disease. The most common finding is of intra-abdominal free fluid although attempts should be made to differentiate peritoneal disease from other causes of intra-abdominal fluid accumulation. CT on the whole is relatively good at the identification of peritoneal dissemination, which may appear as mesenteric stranding, peritoneal nodularity or thickening which in some cases can be fairly gross. Serosal deposits may appear as discrete soft tissue deposits, a focal point of obstruction or distortion of the bowel. The limitations of CT are reached in patients in whom there is a paucity of intra-abdominal fat or where there is co-existing ascites. PET-CT can often be beneficial in identifying disease in patients where there is limited fat or where disease is subtle but relatively diffuse.

Ovarian metastases or Krukenberg tumours are of soft tissue density or solid adnexal lesions. If there is dubiety as to whether or not an ovarian lesion is solid or may simply appear to be hyper-dense for other reasons such as internal cystic haemorrhage, vaginal ultrasound may prove to be of value. Alternatively, PET-CT can depict increased tracer uptake in case of ovarian metastases.

CT remains the modality of choice for the follow up of patients with oesophago-gastric malignancy, whether the treatment is surgical, oncological or multi-modality. Routinely, a standard CT of the chest, abdomen and pelvis is performed following IV contrast (portal venous phase). If there is dubiety regarding disease recurrence such as equivocal liver lesions further imaging may be tailored to suit the findings, such as MRI of the liver.

INTERVENTIONAL RADIOLOGY PROCEDURES

The majority of interventional procedures pertinent to the oesophagus and stomach are performed using fluoroscopy for guidance. Fluoroscopy provides real time 2-D visualisation of the movement of medical instruments *in-situ*. For endovascular techniques in which a wire is negotiated along blood vessels, fluoroscopy is able to produce what is known as a "road-map". With the injecting of intra-vascular iodinated contrast, vessels can be defined and the image stored. The stored image can be superimposed onto the screen while manipulating the guide-wire allowing anatomical vascular navigation. Although a valuable technique, this can often be difficult due to patient movement. Although a form of fluoroscopy is available with some CT scanners, the complexity to the manipulations associated with the interventional procedures requires long screening times that would result in prohibitive doses of radiation. Interventional procedures are minimally invasive and particularly suitable for acutely ill patients who are unable to withstand general anaesthesia and surgery. The procedures can be done under local anaesthesia and analgesia with or without minimal sedation. Although percutaneous procedures are minimalist in access, they should achieve the same end result. It is increasingly recognised that these "minimalist" procedures are very effective.

Management of Bleeding

This is a commonly encountered endovascular procedure in patients bleeding from the gastro-intestinal tract. The procedure is used to minimise potential bleeding for subsequent operative intervention, or to control active bleeding. The techniques broadly revolve around the occlusion or embolisation of vessels, which are either bleeding themselves or supplying the bleeding lesion or by reducing the pressure in a high-pressure venous system (portal hypertension).

Embolisation can either be done selectively or non-selectively. For a single bleeding vessel, attempts will focus on selective occlusion of the vessel. If the exact vessel could not be identified or if it is too small to reach with catheters, an attempt to devascularise the region by occlusion of a larger feeding vessels, can be done. The same principle applies to when a lesion is to be devascularised to minimise blood loss if a subsequent operation is planned. Occluding the larger feeding vessel carries the risk of devasculrising other structures, which derive their blood supply from the same feeding vessel. Hence, non-selective embolisation is only considered as a final resort or when the patient's clinical condition necessitates prompt management such as with massive haemorrhage. Embolisation is most commonly achieved with either prothrombotic small particles or metallic coils to occlude and thrombose the vessel(s).

Trans jugular Intrahepatic Porto-systemic Shunt (TIPS) is a radiological procedure that uses imaging guidance to percutaneously create a connection within the liver between the portal and systemic circulations. It is placed to reduce portal pressure in patients with complications related to portal hypertension. The goal of TIPS placement is to divert portal blood flow into the hepatic vein, so as to reduce the pressure gradient between portal and systemic circulations. TIPS may successfully reduce variceal bleeding in the stomach and esophagus in patients with cirrhosis. Shunt patency is maintained by placing an expandable metal stent across the intrahepatic tract.

A small catheter is passed through the external jugular vein down to the level of the hepatic vein. With image guidance and using contrast, a needle is used to make a passage between the hepatic and portal veins inside the liver. A catheter is advance down the track and the passage between the hepatic and portal veins is dilated with a balloon. A vascular stent is then deployed in the passage and the high pressure in the portal circulation will drive blood through to the systemic circulation. The reduced pressure in the portal circulation should reduce variceal bleeding. Occasionally, additional manoeuvres such as embolization of bleeding varices may be necessary to stop the bleeding completely. The whole procedure can take up to 3 hours. It is usually carried out either general anaesthesia or heavy sedation.

Management of Ischaemia

Acute or chronic ischaemia of the native oesophagus and stomach are extremely rare due to the multiple blood supply of these organs. However, the transposed stomach after oesophagectomy can undergo ischaemic changes in the early post-operative period, due to insufficiency of its vascular channels. The role of radiology in this situation is to assess the gastric perfusion in unwell post-operative patients referred for CT scans. Ideally, these patients should have had an endoscopy to assess the perfusion of the transposed stomach. However, in the absence of endoscopy or if endoscopic images were equivocal, IV contrast enhanced CT should provide an assessment of gastric perfusion.

Oesophageal, Gastric and Pyloric Stenting

Stenting of the oesophagus, stomach or pylorus are indicated in the presence of a malignant obstruction interfering with the passage of food in patients whose survival is expected to be more than a few weeks. In practice, radiological screening is essential for accurate positioning of stents. In addition, some long or tortuous malignant strictures require radiological screening with steerable guide wires to traverse the obstructing lesion. Whether stenting is done by a radiologist, or an endoscopist depends on available facilities and expertise. In essence, a guide-wire within a catheter is passed orally through the obstructing lesion. In conjunction with any available cross sectional imaging, water-soluble contrast is administered to delineate the location as well as the expected length of the obstruction. A decision is then made as to the length and type of stent required. Stents can be broadly classified as either covered or non-covered. A covered stent has a silicone membrane covering either partially or fully, which prevents tumour in-growth through the metal wire wall. The disadvantage to covered stents is that they have a tendency to migrate distally. This is particularly problematic when the tumour shrinks as a result of oncological therapy.

The selected stent on and its delivery device is then railroaded over the placed guide wire. Due to the calibre of the delivery device and the fact that it is not entirely flexible the patient will likely require some form of sedation and possible analgesia. The delivery devices have radio-opaque markers for the proximal and distal ends of the stent. Using the information gained from administered oral contrast, the stent is deployed under direct image guidance to cover the area of stenosis. Stents fully deployed in the incorrect location can sometimes be difficult to retrieve or reposition radiologically and may require endoscopic support.

Naso-jejunal Tube Insertion

This is indicated in malnourished (multiple causes) patients who are at risk of gastro-oesophageal reflux. A feeding tube is inserted via the nose into the stomach. Subsequently, the stiffening wire and weighted tip can be manipulated under fluoroscopic guidance to the duodenal-jejunal flexure. In the majority of cases, this placement can be done using knowledge of the expected anatomy. With distorted anatomy or when there is difficulty in the passage, it may be necessary to administer a small volume of dilute oral contrast. This outlines the anatomy and induces peristalsis, which can help the passage of the feeding tube through the pylorus and duodenum.

Radiologically Inserted Gastrostomy (RIG)

A RIG is indicated in patients with proximal oesophageal obstruction where a stent is contra-indicated. A stent placed in the proximal oesophagus can overlap with the proximal oesophageal sphincter (crycopharyngeus) and cause pain and choking episodes, which can often be intolerable. The RIG can be used for feeding and administration of fluids and medication while the tumour can be managed by oncology if appropriate. In this technique, a steerable fine catheter can be negotiated per-orally through the obstruction tumour into the stomach using image guidance with injections of contrast through the catheter as appropriate. Once the catheter is in the stomach air is injected into the stomach to distend it and bring the gastric wall nearer to the anterior abdominal wall (below the ribs), in the process pushing bowel loops inferiorly and out of the way. The radiologist can then insert a needle percutaneously into the distended stomach. A guide wire is then inserted through the needle into the stomach. The needle is then withdrawn and serial dilators railroaded over the guide wire to progressively dilate the percutaneous gastrostomy track. Eventually a "button" gastrostomy is railroaded over the guide wire and the retention device deployed in the stomach.

This technique can be challenging in patients who have had previous abdominal surgery due to intra-peritoneal adhesions restricting bowel movement. The procedure is usually done under local anaesthesia applied at the site of insertion of the RIG.

Drainage of Focal Collections

Focal septic collections in the chest or abdomen, discovered on CT in septic unwell patients in the post-operative period can be drained percutaneously by interventional radiology with image guidance without need for further surgery. The technique involves localisation of the collection and identification of a straight trajectory for a percutaneous route to the collection, which avoids bowel loops, solid organs and blood vessels. With image guidance using Ultrasound or CT, a needle can be inserted into the collection along the mapped trajectory. Aspiration of septic material should confirm that the tip of the needle is within the septic collection. A guide wire is inserted through the needle, which is withdrawn and replaced by a wide (7 FG) pigtail catheter railroaded over the guide wire. The source of sepsis will also need to be separately managed if appropriate. Systemic antibiotics can also be prescribed guided by the microbial sensitivities of the organisms isolated from the collection.

FUTURE PROSPECTS IN RADIOLOGY

Over the last few years, there have been significant advances in CT scanner technology with falling doses and scanning times. Newer scanners offer better spatial resolution, tissue definition at significantly reduced patient doses due to new image reconstruction techniques. The demand for CT is constantly increasing and will continue to do so. Concern still remains that despite scanners offering lower dose techniques, the increased reliance on CT to provide quick, cheap and diagnostic studies, results in patients having serial examinations resulting significant radiation doses. Consequently, manufacturers continue to attempt further dose reductions whilst maintaining image quality. As a result, particularly for imaging of the gastrointestinal tract, CT will probably replace plain film abdominal radiographs.

The field that has the greatest potential for significant expansion is MRI. The lack of ionising radiation makes this an appealing modality for use when serial examinations are required. One of the current and probably most significant limiting factors is the significantly longer scanning times. This reduces patient throughput and scanner availability. With installation of more powerful magnets (3-Tesla and beyond) there would be a reduction in scan time whilst maintaining the signal to noise ratio (image quality). MRI whole body staging for the detection of metastatic disease is already in use although is less well recognised than PET-

CT. Whole body diffusion weighted imaging is able to detect areas of restricted diffusion, a phenomenon often encountered with malignancy to a good degree of accuracy.

The most exciting likely development is the general introduction of functional MRI beyond that of research. Whilst maintaining the anatomical data of current MRI, it offers better soft tissue differentiation than CT, and provides co-existent functional information. Specific biomarkers are currently in development, which are capable of producing an imaging phenotype of a disease process at a cellular level, similar to genetic typing of tumours. The result would be "personalised imaging" based on characteristics of the pathological process, allowing guidance and early assessment of delivered therapies before significant anatomical change. Currently, MRI sequences under development can analyse axonal structure of the brain based on the known tissue histopathology. Techniques are likely to be expanded to assess malignant cell traits, detect cancer pre-cursors as well as disease activity by looking at neutrophil density as an example [17].

Another exciting area within the realm of interventional radiology is irreversible electroporation. With this technique, superfine insulated electrodes are inserted percutaneously into solid organ tumours or metastases. Pulsed super voltage current is passed between the electrodes to ablate the tumours. Although this technique remains experimental at this stage, encouraging results have been obtained in the palliation of symptoms from recurrent gastric and pancreatic tumours and hepatic metastases [18]. Functional imaging is an exciting new avenue, already with multiple sites acquiring MRI-PET scanners combining anatomy with functional imaging. New cellular genetic and molecular biomarkers should expand this field further. In combination with developments of the already widely used diffusion weighted and perfusion imaging (assessment of cell density and vascularity), MRI is well placed to eventually supersede CT for staging and cancer follow up. Finally, open MRI scanners are likely to be used in image-guided minimally invasive biopsies and therapy.

CONSENT FOR PUBLICATION

Not applicable.

CONFLICT OF INTEREST

The authors declare no conflict of interest, financial or otherwise.

ACKNOWLEDGEMENT

Declare none.

REFERENCES

[1]　Parry K, Haverkamp L, Bruijnen RCG, *et al.* Staging of adenocarcinoma of the gastroesophageal junction. Eur J Surg Oncol 2016; 42(3): 400-6.
[http://dx.doi.org/10.1016/j.ejso.2015.11.014] [PMID: 26777127]

[2]　Wu LM, Xu JR, Yin Y, Qu XH. Usefulness of CT angiography in diagnosing acute gastrointestinal bleeding: a meta-analysis. World J Gastroenterol 2010; 16(31): 3957-63.
[http://dx.doi.org/10.3748/wjg.v16.i31.3957] [PMID: 20712058]

[3]　Lin J, Kligerman S, Goel R, Sajedi P, Suntharalingam M, Chuong MD. State-of-the-art molecular imaging in esophageal cancer management: implications for diagnosis, prognosis, and treatment. J Gastrointest Oncol 2015; 6(1): 3-19.
[PMID: 25642333]

[4]　Hong SJ, Kim TJ, Nam KB, *et al.* New TNM staging system for esophageal cancer: what chest radiologists need to know. Radiographics 2014; 34(6): 1722-40.
[http://dx.doi.org/10.1148/rg.346130079] [PMID: 25310426]

[5]　Lim JS, Yun MJ, Kim MJ, *et al.* CT and PET in stomach cancer: preoperative staging and monitoring of response to therapy. Radiographics 2006; 26(1): 143-56.
[http://dx.doi.org/10.1148/rg.261055078] [PMID: 16418249]

[6]　Lafaro KJ, Roumanis P, Demirjian AN, Lall C, Imagawa DK. Gd-EOB-DTPA-enhanced MRI for detection of liver metastases from colorectal cancer: A surgeon's perspective! Int J Hepatol 2013; 2013: 572307.
[http://dx.doi.org/10.1155/2013/572307] [PMID: 23653860]

[7]　Muhi A, Ichikawa T, Motosugi U, *et al.* Diagnosis of colorectal hepatic metastases: comparison of contrast-enhanced CT, contrast-enhanced US, superparamagnetic iron oxide-enhanced MRI, and gadoxetic acid-enhanced MRI. J Magn Reson Imaging 2011; 34(2): 326-35.
[http://dx.doi.org/10.1002/jmri.22613] [PMID: 21780227]

[8]　Chen L, Zhang J, Zhang L, *et al.* Meta-analysis of gadoxetic acid disodium (Gd-EOB-DTP-)-enhanced magnetic resonance imaging for the detection of liver metastases. PLoS One 2012; 7(11): e48681.
[http://dx.doi.org/10.1371/journal.pone.0048681] [PMID: 23144927]

[9]　Löwenthal D, Zeile M, Lim WY, *et al.* Detection and characterisation of focal liver lesions in colorectal carcinoma patients: comparison of diffusion-weighted and Gd-EOB-DTPA enhanced MR imaging. Eur Radiol 2011; 21(4): 832-40.
[http://dx.doi.org/10.1007/s00330-010-1977-2] [PMID: 20886339]

[10]　Chaubal N, Joshi M, Bam A, Chaubal R. Contrast-Enhanced ultrasound of focal liver lesions. Semin Roentgenol 2016; 51(4): 334-57.
[http://dx.doi.org/10.1053/j.ro.2016.05.018] [PMID: 27743569]

[11]　Camilleri M, Shin A. Novel and validated approaches for gastric emptying scintigraphy in patients with suspected gastroparesis. Dig Dis Sci 2013; 58(7): 1813-5.
[http://dx.doi.org/10.1007/s10620-013-2715-9] [PMID: 23695877]

[12]　Stacher G, Bergmann H. Scintigraphic quantitation of gastrointestinal motor activity and transport: oesophagus and stomach. Eur J Nucl Med 1992; 19(9): 815-23.
[http://dx.doi.org/10.1007/BF00182825] [PMID: 1396878]

[13]　Berry MF. Esophageal cancer: staging system and guidelines for staging and treatment. J Thorac Dis 2014; 6 (Suppl. 3): S289-97.
[PMID: 24876933]

[14]　Li Z, Rice TW. Diagnosis and staging of cancer of the esophagus and esophagogastric junction. Surg Clin North Am 2012; 92(5): 1105-26.
[http://dx.doi.org/10.1016/j.suc.2012.07.010] [PMID: 23026272]

[15] Kim TJ, Kim HY, Lee KW, Kim MS. Multimodality assessment of esophageal cancer: preoperative staging and monitoring of response to therapy. Radiographics 2009; 29(2): 403-21.
[http://dx.doi.org/10.1148/rg.292085106] [PMID: 19325056]

[16] Washington K. 7th edition of the AJCC cancer staging manual: stomach. Ann Surg Oncol 2010; 17(12): 3077-9.
[http://dx.doi.org/10.1245/s10434-010-1362-z] [PMID: 20882416]

[17] Helbren EL, Plumb AA, Taylor SA. The future developments in gastrointestinal radiology. Frontline Gastroenterol 2012; 3 (Suppl. 1): i36-41.
[http://dx.doi.org/10.1136/flgastro-2012-100121] [PMID: 28839691]

[18] Al Efishat M, Wolfgang C L, Weiss M J. Stage III pancreatic cancer and the role of irreversible electroporation, Bmj-British Medical Journal, vol 350, Mar 18 2015
[http://dx.doi.org/10.1136/bmj.h521]

CHAPTER 6

Benign Disorders of the Oesophagus

Sami M. Shimi[*]

Department of Surgery, Ninewells Hospital and Medical School, Dundee, Scotland, UK

Abstract: The prime function of the oesophagus is the transfer of ingested food from the pharynx to the stomach. This is facilitated by its structure. The oesophagus traverses the posterior mediastinum to emerge through the diaphragmatic hiatus into the abdomen. The structure, function and disorders of the diaphragm directly affect oesophageal function. Diaphragmatic hiatal herniae, affect food transport through the oesophagus and is one of the causes of gastro-oesophageal reflux. Chronic reflux contributes to oesophagitis and peptic strictures.

Congenital, traction and pulsion oesophageal diverticula can also affect food transport across the oesophagus and be responsible for dysphagia. Muscular and mucosal rings, cysts and duplications can also affect oesophageal function and cause disordered swallowing. Traumatic and spontaneous oesophageal injuries and perforations can be life threatening and the emphasis is on early diagnosis, prompt resuscitation and antibiotic cover followed by definitive surgical treatment.

Oesophageal variceal haemorrhage can be catastrophic and with significant mortality. It tends to occur in patients with liver disease. Urgent resuscitation, evaluation and appropriate management are all too essential. Patients should be enlisted in surveillance and therapeutic programs to prevent further bleeds. A number of endoscopic and surgical techniques have evolved to manage all these benign disorders of the oesophagus.

Keywords: Benign, Structure, Function, Diaphragm, Hiatal herniae, Gastro-oesophageal reflux, Diverticula, Rings, Perforations, Varices.

MANIFESTATION OF OESOPHAGEAL DISORDERS

Benign oesophageal disorders are very common. They account for up to 20% of consultations in the primary care setting with resultant loss of sleep, social functioning and productivity in a significant proportion of these patients. The oesophagus is a muscular conduit with the primary function to transfer ingested food into the digestive and absorptive parts of the gastrointestinal tract. Disorders

---
[*] **Corresponding author Sami M. Shimi:** Department of Surgery, Ninewells Hospital and Medical School, Dundee DD1 9SY, Scotland, UK; Tel: +44 1382 660111; E-mail: s.m.shimi@dundee.ac.uk

in this part of the pathway, impact significantly on the functioning of the whole individual. Most living species require daily repetitive provision of sustenance to function. Daily repeat ingestion of fluids and food is primarily to provide sustenance to enable the primal individual to perform the required societal functions. Eating and drinking have evolved into pleasurable activities enabling in many situations, social interactions through gatherings besides the primary purpose of sustenance. As such, disorders of structure or function of the oesophagus not only can potentially deprive the individual of the necessary fuel to function but also affect their psyche. In order to fully understand oesophageal disorders and their clinical manifestations, it is essential to have a clear knowledge of the structure and physiology of the oesophagus. This will provide a support to understand deviations from the 'norm' but is also essential for surgical treatment of these disorders.

Structure of the Oesophagus

The oesophagus is a hollow muscular tube, which is about 25 cm long, and connects the pharynx to the stomach. *The cervical part* (5 cm long) is behind the trachea and attached to it by loose areolar tissue. It commences with cricopharyngeus muscle at the inferior portion of the inferior pharyngeal constrictor. Just above cricopharyngeus, the transition between the oblique fibres of the inferior constrictor muscle and the transverse fibres of cricopharyngeus creates a point of potential weakness termed Killian's dehiscence, which is the site of origin of a pharynogo-oesophageal (Zenker's) diverticulum. *The thoracic oesophagus* runs in the superior mediastinum between the trachea and the vertebral column. The upper thoracic oesophagus extends from below the level of cricopharyngeus to the level of the carina. The middle thoracic oesophagus extends from the level of the carina to halfway between the carina and the oesophago-gastric junction and the lower thoracic oesophagus from halfway between the carina and the oesophago-gastric junction to include the lower third of the oesophagus. *The abdominal oesophagus* emerges from between the diaphragmatic crura. The oesophagus consists of four layers. The fibrous adventitia is irregular, and consists of loose, areolar connective tissue containing elastin fibres. The muscular layer is composed of an outer thicker longitudinal and inner circular layer. The submucosa is very loose in order to permit dilatation of the oesophagus during swallowing. The mucosal layer consists of the lining epithelium, connective tissue with papilli (lamina propria) and non-striated muscularis mucosa. The Oesophago-gastric junction consists of the supra-diaphragmatic portion, the inferior oesophageal constriction, the vestibule (intra-abdominal oesophagus), and the cardia. A zone of junctional epithelium is interposed between the squamous lining of the oesophagus and the gastric mucosa.

Physiology of the Oesophagus

The basic function of the oesophagus is to transport swallowed material from the pharynx into the stomach. Conventionally, swallowing has been divided into three stages. The *voluntary stage* initiates the swallowing process by propelling a food bolus into the pharynx. Subsequently, the process of swallowing becomes automatic and involuntary. The *pharyngeal stage* constitutes the passage of food through the pharynx into the oesophagus and involves a high level of coordination of different structures. The *oesophageal stage* is also involuntary and promotes passage of food from the pharynx to the stomach when food is propelled down the oesophagus by peristaltic waves. The swallowing process is coordinated centrally so that the next phase starts appropriately when the previous phase had delivered the fluid or food bolus to the next part of the chain.

Symptoms of Oesophageal Disease

The presentation of oesophageal disease is often typical with one or more of the well-known classic symptoms. Atypical presentation is not, however, infrequent and oesophageal disease may be mistaken for cardiac and pulmonary disorders. In these patients, differentiation is only possible after specialised investigations are carried out. A small cohort of patients with oesophageal symptoms has no abnormality on physical examination and intensive investigations. In some, but not all of these patients, the symptoms reflect a psycho-neurotic state. The typical symptoms of oesophageal disease are: dysphagia; regurgitation; odynophagia; chest pain and water brash.

Dysphagia

Difficulty in swallowing or a sensation of food bolus arrest or delay during swallowing may be due to mechanical obstruction or functional disorder [1]. The patient feels the food sticking and often points to a particular site on the sternum although this does not correlate well with the exact anatomical location of the obstruction. Dysphagia for solids implies significant disease, which may be mechanical or functional whereas dysphagia for liquids only is more likely to be functional (oesophageal motility disorder). In the latter, difficulty with swallowing may be intermittent or its severity variable with exacerbations and periods of relative remission. Some patients with dysphagia find that food transit through the oesophagus can be facilitated by sipping fluid after each solid bolus or by repeated swallows and various postural manoeuvres such as expiration against a closed glottis (Valsalva) *etc*. On the other hand, persistent and progressive dysphagia indicates mechanical narrowing of the oesophageal lumen. This is usually associated with regurgitation and is not relieved by sipping fluids or repeated swallowing. Eventually, with progression to total dysphagia, the patient is unable to swallow saliva and exhibits constant drooling. In obstructive dysphagia, the symptom begins when 20-30 % of the oesophageal lumen is lost and patients usually present when 50 % of the oesophageal lumen is compromised.

The Sensation of a Sub-Sternal Lump (Globus)

When this is present a short period after eating or when fasting it is termed 'globus hystericus'. It is a neurotic symptom in patients with emotional instability but requires thorough examination to exclude organic disease. Dysphagia is never an expression of a purely psychiatric disorder. However, some patients with well-established oesophageal disease may report that their dysphagia is worse during severe emotional periods.

Regurgitation

This symptom results from regurgitation of gastric or oesophageal fluid into the throat accompanied by a sour taste in the mouth. It is often postural and occurs predominantly in the supine position especially at night, with the regurgitated material often staining the pillow. Postural regurgitation which is a very common symptom of reflux disease, is precipitated by meals and activities associated with a rise in the intra-abdominal pressure i.e. bending and straining. Regurgitation may also occur as an overflow phenomenon due to the accumulation of food in the oesophagus proximal to a stenosing lesion. This spillback into the pharynx and mouth at night may lead to aspiration pneumonitis. In oesophageal motility disorders both overflow and postural regurgitation may occur, although the former is more commonly encountered in these conditions.

Odynophagia

This complaint consists of localised pain, usually in the lower sternal region, which occurs immediately on swallowing certain foods or liquids. It always indicates organic disease, most commonly oesophagitis. Hot drinks, acid citrus beverages, coffee and heavily spiced foods are among the most frequent dietary items which induce this symptom. It can be severe enough to condition patients not to eat or drink the offending item, or food in general. Odynophagia can be seen after involvement of the mucosa by reflux, radiation, viral or fungal infections. Less commonly odynophagia can be a manifestation of ulceration or cancer of the oesophagus.

Heartburn

This is the most common manifestation of oesophageal disease and may occur in up to 50% of the population. It is due to reflux of gastric juice, which is injurious to the oesophageal mucosa. The chemical injury is accentuated by a defective clearing of the refluxate by the oesophagus consequent on an impaired motility. This increases the contact time of the acid and any other injurious substance (*e.g.* bile salts) with the oesophageal mucosa. Some patients complain of severe heartburn, yet on endoscopy there is little or no evidence of inflammation. Some do not even respond to traditional acid suppression. This is termed functional heartburn [2]. These individuals may still have reflux with an abnormal oesophageal mucosal sensitivity. Heartburn is often worsened by recumbency, increases in intra-abdominal pressure, and may follow fatty meals or alcoholic beverages. Heartburn is usually relieved, even temporarily, by taking antacids. This symptom can increase in intensity until it is perceived as chest pain.

Chest Pain

Oesophageal anterior chest pain is often described as a tightening or gripping pain, which closely simulates angina pectoris. Thus it may radiate to the back, jaw, arm and ear and may even be relieved by sublingual nitrates. This type of pain is commonly found in patients with reflux oesophagitis or oesophageal motility disorders. It may occur in association with meals when it persists for about an hour after, but is also experienced in the fasting state and is frequently precipitated by emotion and exercise.

Water Brash

This symptom is uncommon and is restricted to patients with reflux disease. It is due to excessive salivation, the mouth becoming full of fluid, which has a salty taste, clear and frothy.

Atypical Presentation of Oesophageal Disease

Patients with oesophageal disease may present with anaemia due to chronic blood loss and, less commonly, with acute upper gastro-intestinal bleeding (haematemesis, melena). Chronic blood loss is usually due to erosive oesophagitis and active bleeding results from the Mallory-Weiss Syndrome or peptic ulceration in a hiatus hernia. Incarceration and strangulation of a para-oesophageal hernia, and spontaneous perforation of the oesophagus (Boerhaave Syndrome), present acutely as a severe life-threatening illness.

Reference has already been made to the frequently encountered difficulty in distinguishing oesophageal from cardiac pain. Often, patients are treated for angina for a while until persistence / aggravation of symptoms indicates the need for coronary angiography. Approximately 20 to 40% of patients with chest pain and normal coronary angiography are subsequently found to have oesophageal disease.

Presentation with pulmonary symptoms is common. These include attacks of coughing, choking and repeated chest infections due to aspiration pneumonitis in patients with overflow or postural regurgitation [3]. The chest radiograph shows areas of consolidation, abscess formation and pleural effusion. Furthermore, intrinsic asthma is often exacerbated by gastro-oesophageal reflux with aspiration particularly in infants and children. Effective treatment of the reflux disease is often followed by a considerable improvement in the asthmatic condition of these patients.

Physical Signs

The oesophagus is a mediastinal structure and is inaccessible to physical examination. However, patients presenting with oesophageal diseases may have physical signs, which should be sought during the examination. These include: evidence of weight loss; pallor due to anaemia; swelling in the neck due to pharyngeal pouch; enlarged lymph nodes in the left supra-clavicular or cervical regions. Chest signs on auscultation and percussion of the lung fields, epigastric mass due to carcinoma of the cardia enlarging downward, hepatomegaly with or without clinical jaundice. Tylosis of the hands and / or feet can be associated with malignant disease of the oesophagus in a familial condition.

THE DIAPHRAGM

The diaphragm (Fig. **1**) is a dome shaped musculotendinous structure, which separates the thoracic from the abdominal cavity. It is attached anteriorly to the lower sternum, laterally to the costal margins and posteriorly (crura) to the first three lumber vertebrae. The aortic hiatus (median arcuate ligament) is situated posteriorly in front of the twelfth thoracic vertebra and through it pass the aorta, the thoracic duct and the azygos vein. To the left and anteriorly is situated the oesophageal hiatus at the level of the tenth thoracic vertebra. In the majority of individuals, the oesophageal hiatus is formed entirely by the fibres of the right crus which is more substantial than the left and arises from the bodies of the first three lumber vertebrae and intervertebral discs. It is connected to the left curs by the median arcuate ligament after it arches over the aorta. The most common arrangement found in up to 60% of individuals are for the right crus to split in to a large right (anterior) and a smaller left (posterior) limb. The splitting is in the ventro-dorsal rather than the sagittal plain, which results in a waistcoat effect and the creation of an obliquely disposed oval diaphragmatic canal rather than an orifice [4].

The vagus nerves, oesophageal branches of the left gastric artery, veins and lymphatics accompany the oesophagus through the hiatus. Slightly to the right of the midline at the level of the ninth thoracic vertebra, is the vena caval foramen in the central tendon. This allows the passage of the inferior vena cava and small branches of the right phrenic nerve. The arterial blood supply to the diaphragm comes from the phrenic arteries and the lower intercostal arteries, which arise directly from the aorta and the terminal branches of the internal mammary arteries.

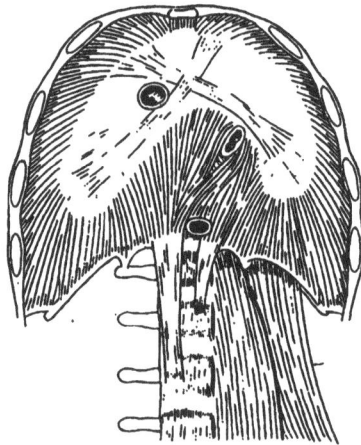

Fig. (1). Schematic diagram showing the inferior surface of the diaphragm as viewed from the abdomen.

Several other structures pass through the diaphragm. The splanchnic nerves pierce each crus, the sympathetic trunks pass behind the medial arcuate ligament, and the subcostal nerves and vessels pass behind the lateral arcuate ligament, while the left phrenic nerve pierces the left dome of the diaphragm to supply its abdominal surface. There is a rich communication between the lymphatic vessels of the posterior mediastinum and the upper abdominal lymph channels.

Congenital Diaphragmatic Herniae

The development of the diaphragm is usually complete by the 8th - 10th week of intrauterine life. Complete absence of the diaphragm occurs rarely. Congenital hernias are the result of maldevelopment of the septum transversum. The prevalence of the condition can be up to 1 in 2100 births and the male to female ratio is 2:1. Approximately 80 % of foetuses with congenital diaphragmatic herniae also have polyhydramnios and most cases can now be diagnosed by ultrasonography by the 25th week of gestation. Attempts at intrauterine diaphragm repair have had some success in specialised units. Attempts to temporarily occlude the main bronchus of the hypo plastic lung have also had limited success. The sites of congenital herniation have long been recognised (Fig. **2**).

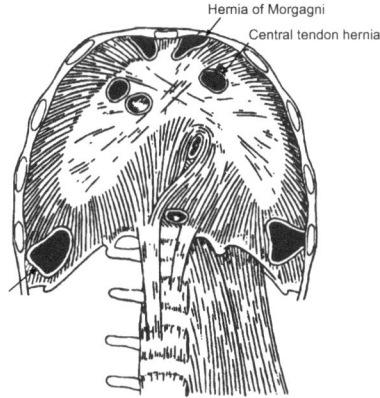

Fig. (2). Schematic diagram showing the sites of congenital diaphragmatic herniae.

In general, 30% of foetuses with congenital diaphragmatic herniae are still born. Fifty per cent of those born alive with a congenital diaphragmatic hernia also have other congenital malformations, most frequently of the nervous system. The association with trisomy 18, 20 and 21 and with Pierre Robin Syndrome is also documented. The majority of diaphragmatic herniae are left-sided (75%), some are right-sided (22%) and few are bilateral defects (3%). The commonest type of diaphragmatic defect is a postero-lateral hernia (90%), followed in frequency by eventration of the diaphragm (5%), and the least common defect being a retrosternal hernia (2%) [5]. Some cases of congenital diaphragmatic hernia are unrecognised until adult life when discovery is incidental. Once discovered, it makes common sense to repair these.

Posterolateral Hernia (Through Foramen of Bochdalek)

These herniae are posteriorly situated and are due to persistence of the pleural-peritoneal canals, which are the last part of the diaphragm to close. The hernia, which is usually left-sided, presents acutely with respiratory distress in the neonatal period. In adults most of these are asymptomatic. Symptomatic patients, present with digestive symptoms due to herniation of the colon, stomach or small bowel.

Parasternal Hernia (Through Foramen of Morgagni or Magendie)

The diaphragmatic hernia described by Morgagni in 1761 is a rare diaphragmatic anomaly that is nearly always congenital. This hernia is more common on the right and occurs through a triangular anterior defect lateral to the sternum between the sternal and costal attachments of the diaphragm where the superior epigastric artery, veins and lymphatics pass from the chest to the abdomen. It is usually asymptomatic in the first years of life. It may be discovered incidentally on a routine radiograph or cause problems in adult life with episodes of pain and tenderness in the right subcostal region and intermittent obstructive symptoms. Complete intestinal obstruction may supervene. The PA chest film in these patients shows a rounded gas containing shadow to the right of the cardiac outline. This shadow is seen to lie behind the sternum on lateral chest films. In doubtful cases, CT with contrast can confirm the diagnosis. Surgical treatment is recommended in all cases because of the risk of intestinal obstruction and strangulation. The best approach is through an upper abdominal incision or by laparoscopy. After reduction of the contents in to the abdomen, the sack, which is usually present is excised and repair, is performed by approximating the two diaphragmatic edges with non-absorbable interrupted sutures. Closure with a synthetic mesh is necessary for large defects. This hernia can be associated with cardiac anomalies as in the pentalogy of Cantrell.

Herniation Through the Central Tendon

The deficiency in the central tendon may be situated at the apex of the right or left cupola or involve the central part in relation to the pericardium. On the right side, a hernia through the central tendon usually contains a mushroom shaped portion of liver parenchyma, which grows through the opening and enlarges on the thoracic surface of the diaphragm. The condition is usually discovered incidentally on a routine chest radiograph. It can be easily differentiated from a primary tumour of the diaphragm by ultrasound scanning or other three-dimensional imaging. In left-sided hernias the fundus of the stomach usually protrudes as an air- containing cyst on top of the diaphragm. A central hernia is usually associated with a defect in the pericardium, and small intestine can herniate in to the pericardial cavity [6].

A small defect in the central tendon on the right side does not require any treatment. However, surgical repair of the other two defects is usually recommended because of the risk of mechanical gastric or intestinal complications.

Congenital Hiatal Hernia

This is usually the sliding type and is associated with gastro oesophageal reflux. More rarely the hernia is of the para oesophageal variety. Both can present in infancy and childhood.

Congenital Short Oesophagus

In the absence of congenital defects, gastro oesophageal sphincter incompetence is often present in the neonate. The condition corrects itself spontaneously during the first few months of life, probably by further development of the intra-abdominal oesophagus. True congenital shortening of the oesophagus in infancy and childhood is very rare. In this condition, the cardia and a large portion of the fundus of the stomach are situated in the mediastinum covered by the phreno-oesophageal membrane, without any obvious hernia sack or sliding.

Most instances of congenital shortening of the oesophagus are acquired and result from prolonged pathological reflux with fibrosis, ulceration and stricture formation. The fibrosis draws the stomach further in to the chest and the oesophageal stricture may be situated at the level of the aortic arch.

Regardless of the aetiology, the most common symptoms are those of spontaneous regurgitation when the infant or child is in the reclining position, recurrent attacks of chest infection or 'asthma'. Aspiration may also result in the development of a lung abscess. The condition requires treatment with an anti-reflux procedure. Most authorities favour a Collis type gastroplasty with a partial fundal wrap. Others recommend an intra-thoracic Nissen fundoplication.

Eventration of the Diaphragm

Anomalous congenital development of the diaphragm or its innervation may result in unilateral elevation of the diaphragm. Alternatively, phrenic nerve injury at birth or later, or injury to the diaphragm, may result in the same problem. Differentiation between eventration of the diaphragm and a large congenital hernia, especially of the Bochdalek type, may be difficult or impossible until surgical exploration.

Eventration of the diaphragm has clinical significance only if it is associated with symptoms or when it cannot be differentiated form other serious conditions. The symptoms of eventration, which are identical to those of large congenital diaphragmatic herniae may occur in the neonatal period and include respiratory distress and tachycardia with impaired cardiac function. In older children, digestive and respiratory symptoms are aggravated by obesity.

In adult patients, the symptoms may be minimal and management is conservative. Surgical treatment is necessary if symptoms are severe or disabling. Approach is through a left thoracotomy. There are several procedures, which can be used to restore the diaphragm to its normal position (Fig. **3**). They include incision or partial excision with plication of the diaphragm. In severe cases, prosthetic replacement of a very attenuated diaphragm with a synthetic mesh is required.

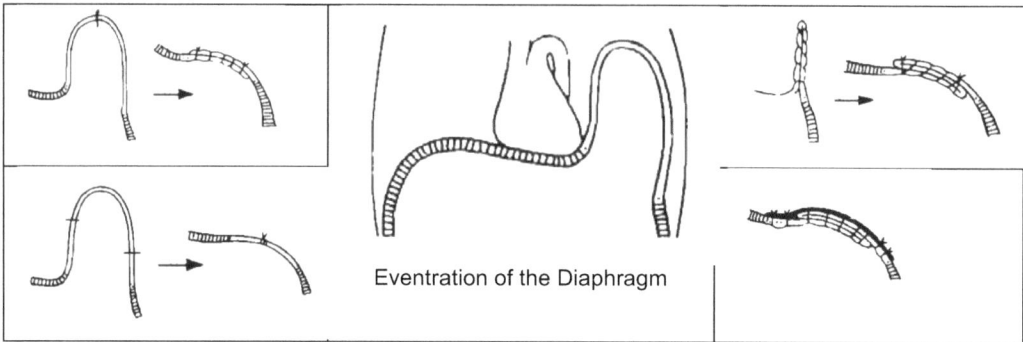

Fig. (3). Schematic diagrams showing techniques for surgical correction of eventration of the diaphragm.

Traumatic Diaphragmatic Hernia

Traumatic rupture of the diaphragm may result from penetrating (25 %) or blunt (75 %) trauma to the abdomen and chest. The tendinous portion, especially on the left side, is the usual site of rupture (68 %) as the liver protects the right side of the diaphragm from most injuries except the penetrating type. The rupture is associated with herniation of abdominal contents and may present acutely following the injury or escape detection until several months to years later. The herniation of abdominal viscera may occur acutely at the time of the injury or be delayed until sometime later. The symptoms are related to the size of the herniated contents and to the onset of mechanical complications such as intestinal obstruction, strangulation, and haemorrhage or progressive cardio respiratory insufficiency.

The diagnosis is usually established on plain chest and abdominal films when a space occupying lesion or bowel gas shadow is seen in the chest. If the omentum spleen or liver is the main herniated structure, the shadow appears solid (Fig. **4**). The herniated spleen is usually ruptured and accompanied by severe haemorrhage. This may result in total opacification of the left chest (haemothorax). Otherwise, air fluid levels may be observed indicative of herniation of hollow viscera (colon, small bowel). Passage of a nasogastric tube identifies a herniated stomach above the diaphragm. CT with contrast radiological studies may be needed to confirm the diagnosis. A significant proportion (40 %) of traumatic diaphragmatic hernia does not produce any visible effects on plain chest radiography. Three-dimensional imaging using CT, or MRI, especially in the setting of trauma is more appropriate. The rupture may be discovered by laparoscopy, thoracoscopy or at laparotomy for associated injuries or subsequently on repeat investigations or as a result of bowel obstruction or strangulation.

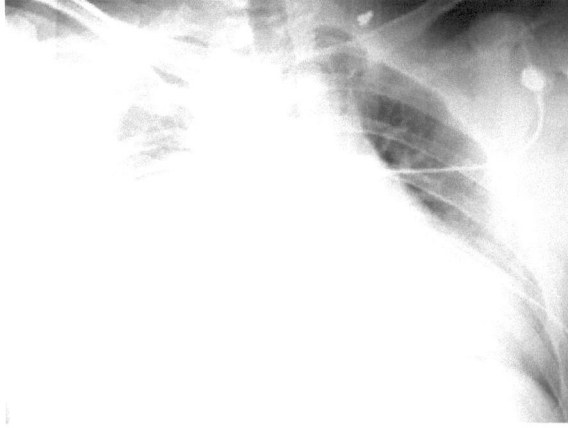

Fig. (4). Plain chest X Ray showing liver herniation through the ruptured right hemi-diaphragm.

In acute rupture, there are often associated injuries, which take precedence over the diaphragmatic injury. However, repair of the acute tear should be performed at the same sitting whenever possible. Elective repair of a traumatic diaphragmatic hernia may be performed through either a left thoracotomy or an upper abdominal approach. In delayed cases, the operation may be difficult due to the presence of adhesions and/or atrophy of the damaged diaphragm. Primary repair is usually possible using interrupted non-absorbable sutures. Otherwise closure with prosthetic mesh is performed.

HIATAL HERNIA

The oesophageal hiatus is an elliptical opening in the muscular part of the diaphragm. The crura arise from the anterior surface of the first four lumbar vertebrae on the right and from L2 and L3 vertebrae on the left to insert anteriorly into the transverse ligament of the central tendon of the diaphragm. There is some reported variability in the configuration of the oesophageal hiatus. The diaphragmatic crura are thick, musculotendinous bundles that become more tendinous and more muscular near their vertebral origins. The lowermost portions of the oesophagus and the gastro-oesophageal junction are held in place through the hiatus by the phreno-oesophageal membrane. With age, the phreno-oesophageal membrane becomes less definite and more fatty. It is also virtually non-existent in patients with long-standing hiatal hernia. This condition is commonly encountered from the fifth decade onwards in the western world and there is a strong aetiological association with obesity. In some cases, the hernia enlarges sufficiently to enable the whole stomach and other intra-abdominal organs to herniate into the chest [7]. Excessive body weight has been found a significant independent risk factor for hiatal hernia. Hiatal hernia, however, is not synonymous with gastro-oesophageal reflux. A hiatus hernia can exist without any symptoms. Further, gastro-oesophageal reflux and reflux oesophagitis can occur in the absence of a hiatus hernia. However, in the presence of hiatus hernia there is a higher chance of developing gastro-oesophageal reflux and oesophagitis. It is possible that in the presence of sphincter dysfunction, a hiatus hernia exacerbates reflux disease and its symptoms are worse than in the absence of such a hernia. There are rare instances of post-traumatic herniation of the stomach through the hiatus and these must be differentiated from traumatic rupture of the diaphragm. In the vast majority of cases, however, the development of hiatus hernia is spontaneous. Gallstones and colonic diverticular disease are commonly present in patients with a hiatus hernia (Saint's Triad) and difficulty may be encountered in establishing which of the three disorders accounts for the patient's symptoms.

Pathology

Conventionally, three types of hiatal herniae are recognised. Type 1: axial, sliding, type 2: para-oesophageal and type 3: mixed.

Axial (Sliding) Hernia

This accounts for the majority (70 to 80%) of cases. The gastro-oesophageal junction and a variable portion of the adjacent stomach slide upwards into the mediastinum carrying with them a peritoneal sac (Fig. **5A**). This results in loss of the cardiac angle of His and, commonly, incompetence of the cardio-oesophageal junction. There is no uniform definition of what constitutes a sliding hiatus hernia. Surgeons, anatomists, radiologists and endoscopists all differ slightly in their views and this must be taken into account when evaluating a symptomatic patient. The symptoms and complications of this type of hernia are those, which are consequent on gastro-oesophageal reflux and reflux oesophagitis (chronic blood loss, stricture formation, Barrett's epithelium *etc.*).

Para-oesophageal Hernia

In this type, the fundus of the stomach rotates in front of the oesophagus and herniates through the hiatus into the mediastinum (Fig. **5B**). As the cardio-oesophageal junction remains in-situ within the abdomen (except in large herniae) sphincter incompetence and reflux are not usually encountered. This type of hernia accounts for up to 10% of cases and is found predominantly in the elderly [8]. In large hernias, the entire stomach and pylorus may be found within the chest inside a large hernia sac, which may also contain the spleen and hepatic flexure of the colon. These large herniae are prone to incarceration and strangulation with infarction and perforation of the stomach. Large hernias can also progress to complete volvulus, which results in pyloric or duodenal obstruction. In patients with chronic blood loss, this is due either to chronic gastric ulceration in the intrathoracic stomach or to an erosive gastritis in a congested and strangulated organ. The majority of uncomplicated para-oesophageal herniae can be easily reduced through the abdomen.

Mixed Hernia

This resembles a large para-oesophageal hernia but the gastro-oesophageal junction is also herniated above the diaphragm (Fig. **5C**). It has features and complications of both types 1 and 2 herniae. It is found in up to 15% of patients. This type of hernia is generally considered to be a late stage of the para-oesophageal variety.

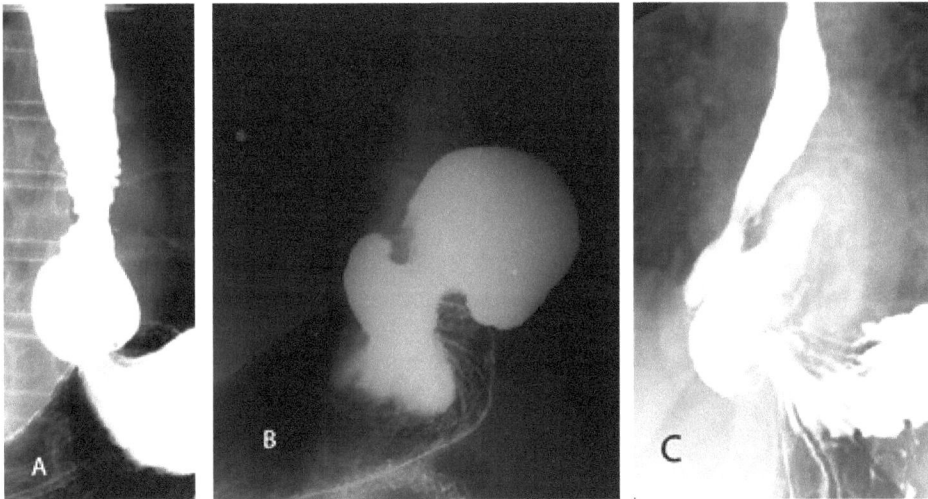

Fig. (5). Barium swallow images of different types of hiatal herniae. A) Axial (sliding) hiatal hernia, B) Para-oesophageal hiatal hernia, C) Mixed type of hiatal hernia.

Clinical Features

In many cases, a hiatal hernia is asymptomatic. In general, the clinical features depend on the type of hernia and the onset of acute life-threatening complications, which can occur with the para-oesophageal and mixed varieties.

Axial (Sliding) Herniae

The condition may be asymptomatic, particularly in elderly patients with limited activity and a sedentary lifestyle. When symptoms occur, they are largely due to gastro-oesophageal reflux and reflux oesophagitis. Chronic blood loss resulting in iron deficiency anaemia is common but active haemorrhage is rare. Some patients may present with dysphagia due to stricture formation without a preceding symptomatic history. Others present with dysphagia secondary to obstruction by diaphragmatic impingement on the herniated stomach. Respiratory compromise can supervene if the whole stomach has herniated into the chest. Post-prandial regurgitation can be a feature in some patients.

Para-Oesophageal and Mixed Herniae

The symptoms of para-oesophageal herniae are due to the pressure effects of the herniated stomach especially when it becomes distended with food or gas. Reflux is rare occurring in only 3% of individuals unless the hernia is or becomes mixed. Common symptoms include pain, dyspnoea, feeling of distension and tiredness, which are precipitated by meals, bending and stooping. The pain is sharp, situated beneath the lower sternum and radiates to the back. It is often accompanied by a bloated sensation, anxiety, palpitation and dyspnoea. The attacks may closely simulate angina pectoris and cardiac arrhythmias may be present during an episode. Belching or vomiting, however, often relieves the pain. Dysphagia is found in 20% of patients with para-oesophageal hernia.

Acute Presentation

Approximately 20% of patients with large para-oesophageal / mixed herniae may present acutely with severe upper gastrointestinal haemorrhage or strangulation / infarction / perforation of the intra-thoracic stomach. In the latter instance the patient develops severe retrosternal pain and shock, which are often mistaken for myocardial infarction. A chest radiograph shows a large gastric gas / fluid shadow overlying the heart. A contrast enhanced CT scan is diagnostic. With gastric infarction and perforation, mediastinal widening and emphysema, left basal collapse and pleural effusion may be outlined by this investigation. Gastric infarction and perforation carry a high mortality rate from septic mediastinitis and bacteraemia.

Treatment

Clinical assessment and appropriate investigations must establish that the symptoms are due to the hiatal hernia. In elderly patients and in individuals with co-morbid disease, case selection for surgery requires astute clinical judgement based on the severity of the symptoms and cardio-respiratory reserve. Middle-aged patients with significant coronary artery disease may require myocardial revascularisation before surgical treatment of the hiatal hernia.

Type 1, axial herniae are treated by reduction with an anti-reflux procedure. This is best achieved by a laparoscopic procedure in the majority of patients [9]. The majority of uncomplicated para-oesophageal herniae can also be approached similarly and are easily reducible via this approach. Following reduction of the hernia, a small and moderate sized hiatus is repaired with interrupted non-absorbable sutures and the gastro-oesophageal junction fixed beneath the diaphragm after restoring the oesophago gastric angle (Allison's Repair). Some surgeons advocate a Nissen fundoplication in addition to reduction and crural repair of these herniae. If the hiatal defect is large, a synthetic mesh can be fashioned around the oesophagus and sutured to the edge of the large defect. However, this is rarely required and mesh repairs can cause a number of complications. In addition to the above, some surgeons advocate a gastropexy in the form of a tube-gastrostomy or otherwise to prevent recurrence. Experienced surgeons using the laparoscopic approach can manage these patients. They are, however, challenging cases in time and effort.

Patients presenting with persistent bleeding from a chronic gastric ulcer in an intra-thoracic stomach may require emergency partial gastrectomy and repair of the hernia. Strangulated / infarcted para-oesophageal and mixed herniae require an emergency laparotomy. If the stomach is viable it is unrotated and reduced into the abdomen and crural repair is performed. If the herniated stomach could not be reduced through laparotomy, a thoracotomy may be required. A Belsey anti-reflux procedure is unwise in this situation as it may lead to gastric / oesophageal perforation. Resection of the infarcted stomach with mediastinal and pleural toilet is necessary for those patients presenting with this serious complication.

OESOPHAGEAL STRICTURES

Peptic strictures of the oesophagus result from chronic reflux esophagitis. They account for 90% of benign esophageal strictures and, arise as a result of exposure to acid and/ or bile. Physiological gastro-oeosphageal reflux is rapidly cleared by normal esophageal peristalsis. Excessive reflux leads to prolonged esophageal exposure to acid, pepsin, and possibly bile and pancreatic enzymes. This leads to inflammation (oesophagitis) in the lower oesophagus. Stricture formation occurs in 7-23% of patients with reflux esophagitis. The process is progressive, beginning with mucosal edema and inflammatory cell infiltrates of the lamina propria. Chronic esophagitis progresses transmurally, into peri-oesophageal tissues, with subsequent fibrosis and scarring leading to luminal compromise and esophageal shortening.

The normal esophagus measures up to 30 mm in diameter. A symptomatic stricture is an esophageal narrowing, usually 13 mm or less in diameter, and causes dysphagia. Peptic strictures occur usually just above the squamo-columnar junction and measure 1-4 cm in length. Significant predictors of stricture formation in patients with gastro-oeosphageal reflux include a lower esophageal sphincter pressure of less than 8 mmHg, impaired esophageal motility, duodeno-gastric reflux and a hiatus hernia.

Diagnosis

The main aim in diagnosis is to characterize the stricture and rule out the presence of malignancy. *Endoscopy and biopsy* are the minimum diagnostic tests in patients presenting with dysphagia. Endoscopy can characterize the diameter and contour of the oesophagus. Endoscopy can also detect evidence of oesophagitis, the presence of Barrett's metaplasia, and can rule out malignancy through biopsy. Frequently however, the presence of a stricture will have deterred further reflux and oesophagitis is not detected on endoscopy. Additional tests such as manometry and pH metry can provide prognostic and aetiological indicators but are not essential in the majority of patients. They are however important in refractory strictures.

Management

The aims of management are to relieve dysphagia and to prevent recurrence of the stricture. *Oesophageal dilation* is the initial means of relieving dysphagia. Dysphagia resolves when the stricture can be dilated to above 14 mm. Mercury filled rubber bougie (Maloney, Hurst) and wire-guided dilators (Savary-Gilliard) are no longer popular. Polyethylene pneumatic balloon dilators are in mainstream use. In theory they are better than wire-guided dilators since they exert no longitudinal shearing force on the esophagus. Two different varieties are available including through-the-scope (TTS) and over-the-wire (OTW) balloon dilators. TTS dilators enable dilation under direct vision and are more popular for this reason. Balloon dilators vary in length and inflated diameter but are commonly 10 - 15 Cm long and 20 mm in diameter. Some manufacturers produce variable diameter balloons dependent on the inflation pressure. After initial stricture dilation, 80% of patients report initial relief of dysphagia. However, 30-50% will require repeat dilation within one year despite adequate acid suppression. Dilation to 20 mm carries a 0.1-0.4% risk of esophageal perforation with each treatment [10]. More recently, self-expanding stents have been used to manage refractory strictures in the oesophagus. The risk inherent in stents is facilitation of reflux and further stenosis above the stent. Some stents have built-in anti-reflux valves. Biodegradable stents with short duration of action have also been used. However, no conclusive results have emerged to recommend the use of self-expanding stents of any variety so far for benign strictures of the oesophagus [11].

Proton Pump Inhibitors (PPI)

These are the most efficacious and cost effective medical therapy for preventing recurrent stricture formation. Long-term PPI maintenance therapy, in conjunction with lifestyle modification is essential to prevent recurrent esophagitis and stricture formation. Enhancing esophageal and gastric emptying with motility agents can be helpful for recurrent strictures.

Surgery

Surgical intervention in patients with peptic stricture is indicated for: 1) inability to dilate the stricture, 2) frequent recurrence of dysphagia, 3) esophagitis refractory to medical therapy, 4) extra-esophageal manifestations such as aspiration pneumonia, and 5) consideration of cost and long term side effects of medical therapy in young patients. For dilatable strictures, the healing of esophagitis is promoted with a standard anti-reflux procedure. The most common anti-reflux procedures are partial (Toupet) or complete (Nissen) fundoplication. Of these, the Nissen fundoplication is the most popular. Patients with undilatable strictures are candidates for trans-hiatal esophageal resection with replacement by stomach, colon or jejunum.

OESOPHAGEAL DIVERTICULA AND CYSTS

Oesophageal Diverticula

Oesophageal diverticula may be congenital or acquired. Congenital diverticula are very rare and are due to incomplete duplication of the oesophagus. Acquired diverticula are classified into pulsion and traction varieties. Pulsion diverticula arise as a consequence of pathological elevation of the intra-luminal oesophageal pressure causing herniation of the mucosa through a weak area in the muscular wall. Traction diverticula are the consequence of inflammatory adhesions between the oesophagus and mediastinal structures, particularly lymph nodes. The subsequent fibrous contracture pulls the oesophageal wall (mucosa and muscle) to form a pouch.

Pseudo-diverticula

These result from dilatation of the oesophageal racemose glands and are confined to the submucosal layer of the oesophagus. They are rare, usually multiple and are often associated with the extensive strictures or motility disorders. Candidosis frequently complicates the clinical picture. The disorder is most commonly encountered in late middle age and a higher incidence has been reported in individuals with chronic alcoholism, immune deficiency and tuberculosis. The aetiology of oesophageal pseudo-diverticulosis is obscure. The most consistent symptom of the disorder is dysphagia, which becomes very painful when monilial infestation supervenes. The clinically important oesophageal diverticula are:

1. Pharyngo-oesophageal diverticulum (Zenker's diverticulum) (65 %).
2. Mid-thoracic diverticula (15 %).
3. Epiphrenic diverticulum (20 %).

Pharyngo-oesophageal (Zenker's) Diverticulum

This diverticulum is of the pulsion variety and is usually secondary to cricopharyngeal dysfunction and less commonly to an oesophageal motility disorder. It develops as a midline mucosal out pouching on the posterior aspect of the pharyngo-oesophageal junction between the fibres of the inferior pharyngeal constrictor and the transverse fibres of the cricopharyngeus and usually manifest on the left side. The anatomical defect in this area, first described by Killian, is triangular in shape and is further accentuated by the absence of the longitudinal fibres of the oesophagus as they sweep anteriorly prior to their insertion into the posterior surface of the cricoid cartilage. As the spine limits posterior extension, the enlarging diverticulum, comes to lie to the side (usually left) as well as behind the oesophagus. There is evidence that more than one type of motility disturbance may be responsible for the development of a pharyngo-oesophageal diverticulum. Most commonly, cricopharyngeal dysfunction is the cause although controversy exists as to its exact nature. Some ascribe it to failure of relaxation of the cricopharyngeus with swallowing (cricopharyngeal achalasia), others to premature contraction of this upper oesophageal sphincter before the pharyngeal contraction is complete and yet another theory postulates a hypertonic sphincter secondary to excessive gastro-oesophageal reflux. In some patients, the diverticulum is secondary to oesophageal motility disorders such as achalasia or diffuses oesophageal spasm and some reports have documented an association between the development of pharyngo-oesophageal diverticulum and gross gastro-oesophageal reflux with or without hiatal hernia.

The diverticulum consists mainly of mucosa and submucosa with a sparse and incomplete muscular coat. As it enlarges, the pouch tends to assume a vertical lie, which compresses and displaces the oesophagus such that its axis becomes in line with the pharynx (Fig. **6**). Ingested food then enters the pouch more readily than the oesophagus.

Symptoms such as coughing and spluttering with meals become more marked and the risks of aspiration are increased. In addition, there is a great danger of iatrogenic perforation of the diverticulum at endoscopy, as the endoscope tends to enter the diverticulum rather than the oesophagus.

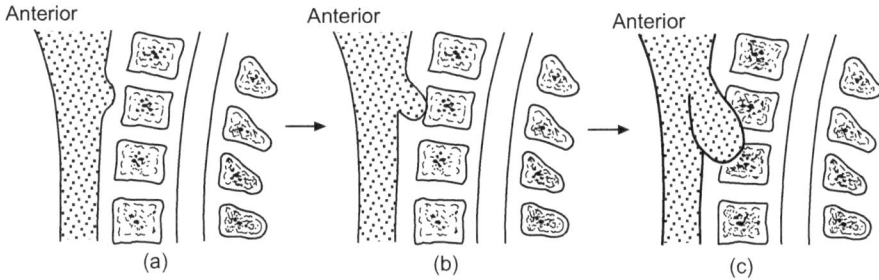

Fig. (6). Schematic diagram showing development and progress of a pharyngo-oesophageal diverticulum. (a) Mucosal herniation between the oblique fibres of the inferior constrictor and transverse fibres of cricopharyngeus, (b) enlargement of the pouch is limited posteriorly by the spine, (c) The pouch becomes dependent and bulges lateral to the oesophagus (usually, the left side).

The main complications of pharyngo-oesophageal diverticulum are:

1. Pneumonitis, lung abscesses, pulmonary collapse.
2. Bleeding from the diverticulum (rare).
3. Perforation (usually iatrogenic).
4. Development of carcinoma (0.3%).

Clinical Features

Pharyngo-oesophageal diverticulum is three times more common in males than females and usually occurs in late middle age and in the elderly. Occasionally the development of the diverticulum is preceded by a period of high dysphagia characterised by difficulty in the transfer of food from the pharynx to the oesophagus. As the condition progresses, the patients complain of regurgitation, constant throat irritation, gurgling noises during swallowing, chronic cough and recurrent chest infections due to aspiration. With compression of the oesophagus, dysphagia becomes more severe and attacks of coughing and spluttering are experienced with each meal. Other symptoms include halitosis, hoarseness and anorexia. These patients typically require a long period to eat even a small meal. The regurgitated material is non-acidic but may contain fermented food. Rarely, the pouch enlarges sufficiently to become clinically palpable in the neck. More usually, a gurgling sound can be elicited on palpation/massage of the left side of the neck at the level of the cricoid performed after the patient is asked to swallow several gulps of air.

A barium swallow best confirms the diagnosis. The lateral films demonstrate the diverticulum better and outline its neck and any oesophageal compression (Fig. 7). It is important that a full barium swallow investigation is performed to exclude gross oesophageal motility disorders and a hiatal hernia. Endoscopy is not necessary for the diagnosis and carries a risk of iatrogenic perforation, especially if the pouch is dependent and in line with the pharynx. If endoscopy is considered necessary, an experienced endoscopist should do it and the introduction of the endoscope from the level of the cricopharyngeus onwards should be performed under vision. Oesophageal manometry, including pressure profiles of the cricopharyngeus should be done to exclude an oesophageal motility disorder. Prolonged pH monitoring is advisable in patients with hiatal hernia and those with reflux symptoms or endoscopic evidence of oesophagitis.

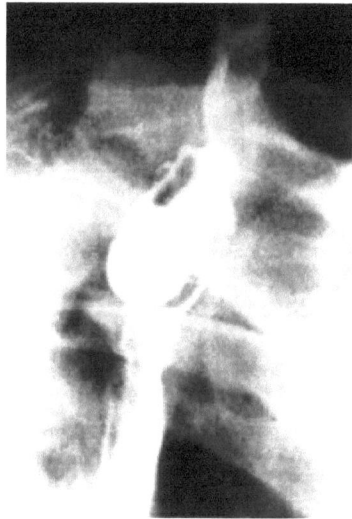

Fig. (7). Barium swallow demonstrating a pharyngeal pouch.

Treatment

The management of pharyngo-oesophageal diverticulum is usually by surgical intervention through either an open approach along the anterior margin of the left sternomastoid from the level of the hyoid bone to the anterior end of the clavicle or endoscopically. There are several surgical options (Fig. **8**), which should be tailored to the clinical findings [12].

1. Cricopharyngeal myotomy: this is suitable for small non-dependent diverticula.
2. Diverticulectomy: this is necessary for large dependent pouches and should be combined with a cricopharyngeal myotomy.
3. Diverticulopexy: this consists of invagination and plication of the pouch. It is suitable for moderate sized pouches, which are not grossly infected or adherent to adjacent structures and is often combined with cricopharyngeal myotomy.
4. Endoscopic division of the septum: in patients with a large dependent diverticulum, endoscopic electrocautery, laser and stapled division of the septum formed by the opposed walls of the diverticulum and the oesophagus is

increasingly popular and should be done under regional anaesthesia. Some surgeons prefer staged division of the septum.

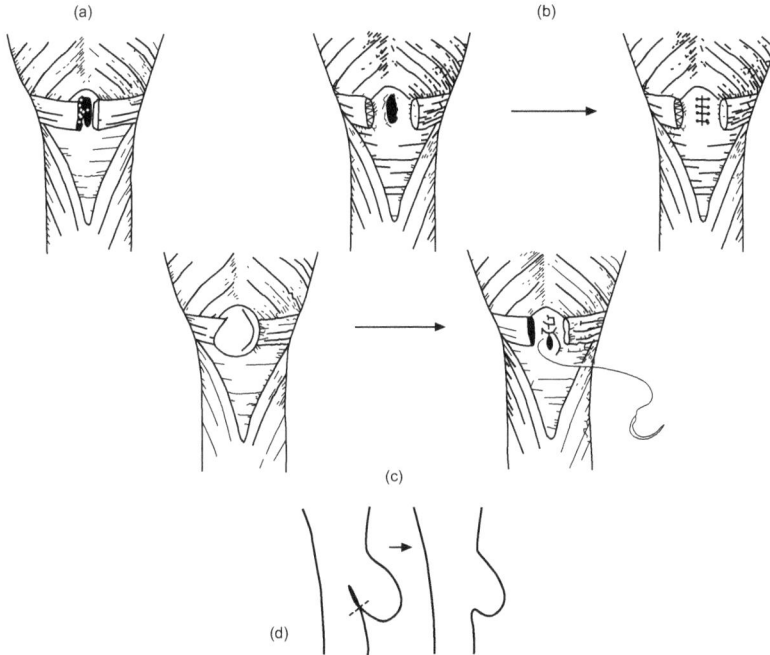

Fig. (8). Surgical procedures to manage pharyngo-oesophageal diverticulum. (a) Cricopharyngeal myotomy, (b) Excision of diverticulum with cricopharyngeal myotomy, (c) Plication of diverticulum and cricopharyngeal myotomy, (d) Endoscopic division of the septum between the pouch and the oesophageal lumen.

Mid-thoracic Diverticula

These are of three kinds: congenital, traction and pulsion. The congenital and traction varieties have a similar radiological appearance (tented triangular shape with a wide neck) and possess a muscular coat. The congenital ones are thought to represent foregut duplications and the traction types are secondary to fibrous adhesions to healed tuberculous lymph nodes. Both the congenital and traction mid-oesophageal diverticula are rare, and the vast majority of pouches in this region of the oesophagus, are secondary to a specific (diffuse oesophageal spasm, high-amplitude peristaltic contractions) or non-specific oesophageal motility disorders which cause a persistent elevation of the oesophageal intra-luminal pressure with subsequent mucosal herniation through a weak defect. These pulsion diverticula are usually narrow-necked and globular in shape and do not possess a muscular coat. The complications of mid-oesophageal diverticula are inflammation and perforation, usually by a swallowed fish bone or foreign body leading to abscess formation and tracheo/broncho-oesophageal fistula. The surgical approach to symptomatic or complicated mid-thoracic diverticula is through a right thoracotomy or thoracoscopy. Excision of the sack (diverticulectomy) is followed by layered closure of the oesophagus. Asymptomatic mid-thoracic diverticula do not require any active treatment.

Epiphrenic Diverticula

Although a few are congenital, the vast majority of epiphrenic diverticula are acquired and of the pulsion variety. The raised intra-luminal pressure being secondary either to a specific motility disorder, usually diffuse oesophageal spasm or achalasia, or to a hiatal hernia and gastro-oesophageal reflux. The symptoms are largely due to the underlying disorder although ulceration is known to occur in the diverticulum and to be a rare cause of haematemesis, which may be severe. Halitosis, anorexia and obscure chest pain are reported to be specific features of epiphrenic diverticula. Although carcinoma has been reported in these pouches, it appears to be rare. The treatment of symptomatic patients is that of the underlying disorder. If the pouch is small, it usually resolves after successful therapy of the motility disorder or reflux disease. Excision of the diverticulum in addition to surgical correction of the underlying disorder is indicated if the pouch is dependent and has a narrow neck such that it cannot drain adequately, or if the sack is inflamed or is compressing the oesophagus by virtue of its size [13].

Sideropenic Dysphagia (Patterson-Kelly, Plummer-Vinson Syndrome)

This syndrome is usually associated with iron deficiency anaemia but may persist for long periods after adequate replacement therapy. It affects predominately post-menopausal females and consists of dysphagia, microcytic, hypochromic anaemia, glossitis, atrophic inflammation of the mucosa of the pharynx and upper oesophagus with areas of hyperkeratosis, ulceration and the formation of high, usually anteriorly placed, oesophageal webs. Other features include dry skin and eyes, koilonychias, splenomegaly and angular stomatitis. Cases associated with reflux oesophagitis have been described, as have rare instances of the condition after gastric surgery. The oesophageal webs are flimsy and can be seen endoscopically or demonstrated by barium swallow. They are easily missed and are readily ruptured at endoscopy. The dysphagia is thought to result more from oesophageal spasm associated with the inflamed atrophic mucosa than partial obstruction due to the oesophageal webs. The anaemia is usually accompanied by a low serum iron concentration. Patients with this condition require long-term follow up because of the substantial risk of the development of upper oesophageal cancer, usually in the post cricoid region. The incidence of oesophageal cancer in these patients is variously reported at 10-30%.

Muscular and Mucosal Rings in the Oesophagus (Schatzki's Rings)

These rings in the lower oesophagus are common and up to 15 % of patients may have them. However, the majority are asymptomatic. These rings may be symptomatic or asymptomatic, depending on the luminal diameter. Most symptomatic patients, present in the fifth decade of life. Most patients present with intermittent, episodic, non-progressive dysphagia to solids. Dysphagia to liquids is usually not present. Dysphagia predictably occurs in patients with a luminal diameter less than 13 mm and may vary between 13-20 mm, depending on the size and type of bolus. Bread and meat frequently precipitate symptoms. Patients often present after rapidly eating meat and drinking alcohol at a restaurant. Some authorities equate Schatzki ring to the "steakhouse syndrome". Two types of rings have been identified in the distal esophagus. The muscular ring, or A ring, is a thickened symmetric band of muscle that forms the upper border of the esophageal vestibule and is located approximately 2 cm above the gastro-oesophageal junction. This type of ring is rare and rarely causes dysphagia. On the other hand, the mucosal ring, or B ring, is quite common. The B ring is a diaphragm-like, thin mucosal ring usually located at the squamo-columnar junction.

The ring is composed of the mucosa and submucosa and does not contain the muscularis propria. Occasionally, the lamina propria may contain fibrous tissue. The ring is usually located at the squamo-columnar junction. Consequently, the upper surface of a Schatzki ring is covered by squamous epithelium, and the lower surface is covered by columnar epithelium.

The pathogenesis of these rings is not clear. Some authorities believe them to be congenital or idiopathic. Others have reported on their association with gastro-oesophageal reflux, eosinophilic or pill-induced oesophagitis [14]. Diagnosis is by endoscopy or a barium contrast swallow. Compression of the abdomen during endoscopy can demonstrate them easily. Food debris may be seen above the ring. Most patients respond well to dilatation therapy. A single episode of pneumatic dilation usually ruptures the mucosal rings. Muscular rings require repeated dilations. In the presence of gastro-oesophageal reflux or motility disorders, it makes sense to correct these medically or surgically. A small number of patients have refractory rings that require more aggressive endoscopic or surgical intervention. Localised resection of the oesophago-gastric junction with re-anastomosis has been described for dilation resistant rings.

Oesophageal Duplication Cysts

Oesophageal cysts are very rare and may be acquired or congenital. The acquired variety is retention cysts of the sub mucous racemose glands and usually occur at the lower end of the oesophagus. They are rarely symptomatic but if large, may cause dysphagia [15]. Removal is achieved through an oesophageal myotomy over the lesion, which shells out easily and without incurring a breach of the oesophageal mucosa.

Congenital (enterogenous) cysts and re-duplications share the same developmental origin and represent embryonic rests within or attached to the oesophageal walls. The cysts are most commonly lined with ciliated columnar epithelium. They usually present in infancy and childhood with pressure effects, i.e. dysphagia, and bronchial obstruction with respiratory distress as they expand within the confined space of the mediastinum. Whenever possible, enucleation of the cyst is performed without resection of the oesophagus but this is not always possible as the cyst may be densely adherent to the oesophageal mucosa as a result of previous inflammatory episodes. Re-duplications are elongated structures, which possess a muscular coat and are lined with squamous epithelium.

OESOPHAGEAL PERFORATIONS

Perforation of the oesophagus constitutes a serious life threatening condition, which is accompanied by a high morbidity, prolonged hospital stay and an appreciable mortality. Survival depends on prompt recognition and early surgical intervention for the majority of cases, although there is a place for non-operative management in selected patients.

Pathophysiology

The categories of oesophageal perforations are outlined in (Table 1). The commonest cause of oesophageal perforations is trauma during endoscopy especially when associated with therapeutic endoscopic measures such as dilatation and / or intubation of strictures. The incidence of oesophageal perforation after rigid endoscopy is 0.5% as opposed to 0.05% after flexible endoscopy. Dilatation considerably increases the risk, the incidence of perforation varying from 0.1% with the Maloney dilators, 0.3% with the Eder-Puestow metal olives and 1-5% after pneumatic dilatation for achalasia using 3.5 - 4 cm balloons. Post-operative perforations refer to oesophageal damage sustained during para oesophageal surgery *e.g.* Nissen fundoplication, repair of hiatus hernia and bariatric surgery. The risk factors for oesophageal iatrogenic perforation during upper abdominal surgery include oesophagitis, scleroderma, poor surgical exposure and poor nutritional status.

Penetrating trauma such as gunshot wounds of the oesophagus are common in certain parts of the world. The cervical oesophagus is the segment most commonly involved. Most cervical oesophageal injuries due to external trauma are associated with the injuries to adjacent structures: spinal cord, thyroid gland, jugular vein, carotid arteries, larynx *etc*.

Overall, the thoracic oesophagus (lower end) is the most commonly affected segment (55 %) and the left side is more commonly affected than the right side. Thoracic injuries also carry the worst prognosis. From the clinical standpoint, oesophageal perforation is classified into early (acute) and late. An acute perforation is one, which presents and is recognised within 4 hours of its occurrence. It carries a good prognosis with a reported mortality of 10% as sepsis is not established and repair is feasible since oedema of the oesophageal wall is minimal. Late perforations include late presentations and missed injuries, which are diagnosed beyond 24 hours of onset. By then, there is considerable trans mural oedema of the oesophagus and significant established contamination of the mediastinum and pleural cavity. The patient's cardiovascular state is unstable from sepsis. The reported mortality of late perforations ranges from 40-60%.

Clinical Features

The early manifestations of an oesophageal perforation are pain, tachycardia and fever. The site of the pain and its radiation vary with the oesophageal segment involved. The pain is, however, always severe. Patients with cervical injuries often develop a nasal voice and may have dysphagia or odynophagia. Hematemesis may also be reported in cervical perforations. This is also a feature of incomplete injuries of the thoraco-abdominal segment. Supraclavicular swelling and crepitus (subcutaneous emphysema) are observed in 60% of cervical and 30% of thoracic-oesophageal injuries. In thoracic injuries, respiratory distress is common and is accompanied by dullness on percussion and diminished air entry and breath sounds on the affected side (effusion/ hydrothorax). Upper abdominal tenderness with rebound and infrequent or absent bowel sounds indicates perforation of the abdominal segment of the oesophagus. However, these abdominal signs may be absent with small perforations (*e.g.* guide wire - induced small unrecognised tears during endoscopy) and the first intimation of this complication may be the development of a sub phrenic abscess.

In late perforations, clinical evidence of established sepsis is present with fever, cardiovascular instability or fully developed septic shock. The infection is polymicrobial with aerobic, anaerobic and fungal organisms. The diagnosis is confirmed by plain and contrast radiology. Plain radiographs (neck, PA and lateral chest) are frequently diagnostic but may not accurately localise the perforation. The radiological features include presence of surgical emphysema in the mediastinum or neck, widening of the mediastinum and an increased distance between the trachea and the vertebral column. Irregularity of the mediastinal air interface is a radiological sign of mediastinitis. Free air beneath the diaphragm may be detected in patients with injuries to the abdominal oesophagus.

A water-soluble contrast swallow (either independently or preferably with CT) is always required in patients with suspected oesophageal perforation. This is to confirm the perforation and to localise it. In addition, it will indicate to which side of the chest the perforation has occurred although that may be evident from plain radiography. Endoscopy is not required for the diagnosis of complete injuries but is indicated when clinical suspicion persists despite negative contrast studies. Its main indications are:

1. Diagnosis of incomplete (intramural) perforation and Mallory-Weiss syndrome.
2. Retrieval of foreign bodies and endoscopic control of bleeding.

Neonatal and Paediatric Oesophageal Perforations

Neonatal perforations are rare and may be traumatic or spontaneous. Both occur more commonly in premature babies and are attended with a substantial mortality, 19% for the traumatic variety and 33% for spontaneous perforation. The two conditions differ in certain distinguishing features (Table 1).

Table 1. Distinguishing features of traumatic and spontaneous oesophageal perforation in neonates.

	Traumatic	Spontaneous
Site	Hypo-pharynx and cervical oesophagus	Distal oesophagus
Prematurity	30 - 35 %	20 %
Gender	Mainly females	Equal distribution
Aetiology	Trauma: intubation, oral suction	Unknown
Clinical features	Difficulty in oesophageal intubation, oral drooling of secretions.	Respiratory distress.
Radiographic findings	Non-specific changes on plain films. Leak may be demonstrated on contrast films.	Pneumothorax, hydrothorax or pneumomediastinum
Mortality	10 %	35 %

Oesophageal injuries in children are either iatrogenic following dilatation or result from ingestion of foreign bodies and corrosive agents. The range of foreign bodies swallowed is extreme and includes coins, pins, aluminium can top, alkaline pencil batteries *etc*. Unless corrosive in nature, the symptoms following ingestion of foreign bodies, may be delayed several weeks to months. The swallowed object gradually burrows through the oesophageal walls and adjacent tissue often leading to the development of a tracheo-oesophageal fistula and respiratory infection. Pyrexia and persistent cough are common presenting features and paradoxically, dysphagia is rare. Endoscopy often fails to reveal the foreign body but may show an area of granulation tissue. Confirmation of the diagnosis is best achieved by radiology.

Spontaneous Oesophageal Injuries in the Adult:

Traditionally, three conditions come under this category:

1. Intramural hematoma (incomplete perforation).
2. Mucosal laceration (Mallory -Weiss Syndrome).
3. Complete spontaneous perforation (Boerhaave Syndrome).

Intramural Hematoma

This lesion, which is extremely rare, arises as an oesophageal mucosal tear associated with submucosal bleeding with dissection of this plain by the expanding intramural hematoma. The clinical picture is said to be distinctive with a history of gagging or choking while eating, followed by sharp mid epigastric/lower retrosternal pain radiating to the back and associated with haematemesis. A contrast radiological swallow demonstrates a double barrel oesophagogram. The condition is self-limiting in the majority of cases and there have been no reported incidences of progression to a complete perforation. Rarely, endoscopic incision of the septum between the true and false lumens of the oesophagus is required.

Mallory - Weiss Syndrome

This syndrome consists of painless haematemesis after vomiting, retching and straining induced by usually excess alcohol intake. However, there are notable and frequent exceptions to this definition. In particular, there is a high incidence of associated gastro-oesophageal disease. The Mallory Weiss Syndrome is common and accounts for 5-10% of patients undergoing endoscopy for haematemesis.

The lesion consists of a longitudinal mucosal tear involving the mucosa alone or the mucosa and submucosa on the gastric side of the oesophago-gastric junction. The tear, which may be single or multiple, is located on the lesser curve side in the majority of cases (85%). Associated lesions are found in 75% of patients and include hiatal hernia, oesophagitis, oesophageal varices and duodenitis/peptic ulceration. Although the bleeding stops spontaneously in the majority of patients, it may be severe and recurrent.

The condition is more often found in males (70%) and a history of large alcohol intake is frequently present (40-70%) but not invariable. Hypovolaemia requiring blood transfusion is found in one in ten patients. The diagnosis is confirmed by upper gastrointestinal endoscopy, which is delayed until resuscitation with blood transfusion is achieved in all shocked patients. The treatment is conservative with gastric acid suppression and antacids. Endoscopic electro coagulation is reserved for patients with actively bleeding tears at the time of endoscopy. Percutaneous radiological embolisation of the feeding (left gastric) artery is used in poor risk patients such as cirrhotic individuals. Surgical treatment is only indicated for those patients who continue to bleed or in whom the haemorrhage recurs after the above measures. It consists of suture ligation of the bleeding mucosal tears through a generous gastrotomy.

Boerhaave Syndrome

The fatal condition of acute gastric distress, forceful vomiting, severe chest pain and collapse due to a complete tear of the lower thoracic oesophagus, just above the cardia, was first described by Herman Boerhaave, a Dutch sea admiral. This aristocratic gentleman succumbed in this way following a bout of over indulgence of food and drink. However, only a minority of complete spontaneous perforations of the lower thoracic oesophagus fit the classical description of Boerhaave. The condition is uncommon and occurs usually between the ages of 40-60 years with a male to female ratio of 2:1. There is frequently a long history of indigestion and chronic gastrointestinal disease such as duodenal ulcer, reflux oesophagitis and hiatal hernia. Apart from over eating, other pre-disposing factors include neurological disorders, tumours and gastrointestinal obstruction. Boerhaave Syndrome has also been reported during childbirth, severe convulsions and even straining during defecation.

The clinical manifestations consist of sudden severe epigastric pain radiating to the left chest and shoulder and upper abdomen, which develops after a violent retching episode or straining. Dyspnoea and shock rapidly supervene. The correlation between retching/vomiting and the onset of pain is only encountered in 40% of patients. Aside from shock, physical findings include surgical emphysema in the neck, dullness and diminished air entry over the base of the left lung, tenderness and guarding in the upper abdomen and absent or infrequent bowel sounds. The condition may very closely simulate myocardial infraction, perforated peptic ulcer, pulmonary embolism, dissecting aortic aneurysm and severe acute pancreatitis with any of which it is often misdiagnosed [16]. The chest radiograph can show a left sided plural effusion and oral contrast enhanced CT or contrast swallow radiology establish the diagnosis.

Management of Oesophageal Perforations

The management of oesophageal perforations consists of simultaneous diagnosis and resuscitation for these severely ill patients at presentation. Anti-fungal and antibiotic therapy with broad-spectrum antibiotics, which includes anaerobic cover, should be commenced as soon as the diagnosis is made. Monitoring of vital signs, which include central venous pressure must accompany intravenous fluid resuscitation. Inotropic support may be necessary at the outset in a proportion of patients. After a period of optimisation, the vast majority of patients require management directed at the perforation. There are however certain specific indications for adopting conservative management:

1. Incomplete injuries: traumatic perforation of the neonate, intramural hematoma and the Mallory-Weiss Syndrome.
2. Complete injuries: these include minor guide-wire induced sub diaphragmatic perforation and certain thoracic perforations. The accepted criteria for a conservative approach in thoracic injuries are a localised perforation contained within the mediastinum or between the mediastinum and the visceral pleura, the cavity drains easily in to the oesophageal lumen, minimal symptoms are present, and clinical sepsis is minimal.

Conservative management entails cessation of oral intake, antibiotic and anti-fungal therapy, nasogastric aspiration, nutrition (parenteral or enteral), and underwater seal pleural drainage in the presence of a pleural effusion. The condition of the patient should be monitored closely and frequently and surgical intervention is undertaken if there is lack of progress or deterioration in the development of clinical sepsis.

Several options for the management of the perforations are available. Once the diagnosis is confirmed, treatment should be tailored to the individual patient and factors such as delay in presentation, underlying oesophageal disease, location of the perforation and cause of the perforation all influence the method of management. The overall aim of treatment is to seal or control the leak while maintaining gastrointestinal continuity, drain the infected or contaminated area, diversion of oesophageal (or gastric) contents, aggressive antibiotic therapy to treat sepsis and nutritional support (intravenously or through a feeding gastrostomy/ jejunostomy) until the perforation has healed and the patient is able to resume oral nutritional support. Depending on the condition of the patient and the treatment modality, some patients may require additional measures such as respiratory, cardiovascular or renal support.

Cervical oesophageal perforations usually respond to simple treatments including surgical drainage alone or closure of the perforation with or without drainage along with general supportive measures. Larger perforations which are usually the result of trauma may be treated with a sternocleidomastoid muscle flap [17].

Abdominal oesophageal perforations are primarily treated by surgery, drainage, and lavage of the contaminated abdomen together with primary closure of the perforation and buttressing the closure with viable adjacent tissue such as stomach (fundoplication or a Thal patch), omentum or both.

Thoracic oesophageal perforations carry the highest rate of mortality and morbidities. They have the highest variation in methods of treatment among surgeons.

Endoscopic Treatment of Oesophageal Perforations

Sealing the leak can be achieved by the endoscopic application of fibrin glue sealant or cyanoacrylate. This however is limited to small perforations. The implantation of completely covered self-expanding metal or plastic stents (SEMS or SEPS) is the endoscopic method that has been most extensively studied and has proven to be effective in 67%-100% of cases. Stents can be used for early and late diagnosed perforations and for small or large tears [18]. They are however limited to perforations in the thoracic oesophagus.

Another method, which has been described, is the closure of intrathoracic anastomotic perforations by endoscopic placement of a vacuum-assisted closure (EndoVAC) system [19]. Endoscopically accessible perforations can be plugged with polyurethane foam sponges, connected to a drainage tube, which can be brought out through the nose. The sponges of variable sizes are placed endoscopically through the perforation to lie in the peri-oesophageal tissue. Negative pressure is applied to the drainage tube. Use of the sponge leads to formation of granulation tissue, while the vacuum removes secretions, reduces oedema, and consequently improve blood flow. This results in a clean wound base. The sponges need to be replaced regularly depending on the amount of contamination. Initially twice weekly changes are required reducing to once every two weeks [20]. This method was originally described for the management of post-operative anastomotic leaks with moderate success. However, it tends to be labour intensive and expensive. It may be indicated for perforations in the cervical oesophagus or proximal thoracic oesophagus.

Temporary drainage of gastric contents can be achieved by a percutaneous endoscopic gastrotomy, which can be performed at the same sitting and through this aperture a jejunal feeding tube can be introduced and directed through the pylorus for nutritional support. The additional measures of antibiotics and percutaneous chest drainage when there is contamination are mandatory in all cases. Percutaneous chest drainage can be via large bore chest drains inserted into the pleural cavity (pleural drainage), by image guided drainage of localises abscesses or mediastinal collections or a combination.

Surgical Treatment of Oesophageal Perforations

The best results are obtained with early perforations, the mortality rising 4 to 5 folds if the perforation is treated surgically beyond 24 hours of onset. The approach depends on the segment of oesophagus involved: cervical injuries are approached through an incision along the anterior border of the left sternomastoid muscle, thoracic injuries through a right or left thoracotomy (depending on the exact level) and lower end/abdominal injuries through a left thoraco-abdominal approach.

Early perforations: The surgical treatment depends on whether the perforation has occurred through an otherwise normal oesophagus or it is associated with significant oesophageal disease, *e.g.* carcinoma, stricture. In the absence of significant oesophageal disease, the perforation is closed in layers with non-absorbable sutures and drainage established. This is sufficient for early cervical injuries but for thoracic perforations most surgeons recommend additional buttressing with pleural or intercostal flaps for high lesions and a diaphragm flap (Fig. **9**), pericardial patch, or omental patch for low lesions. Alternatively, the latter may be reinforced by a Thal fundal patch or a Nissen fundoplication, which is particularly useful in posterior injuries of the abdominal segment.

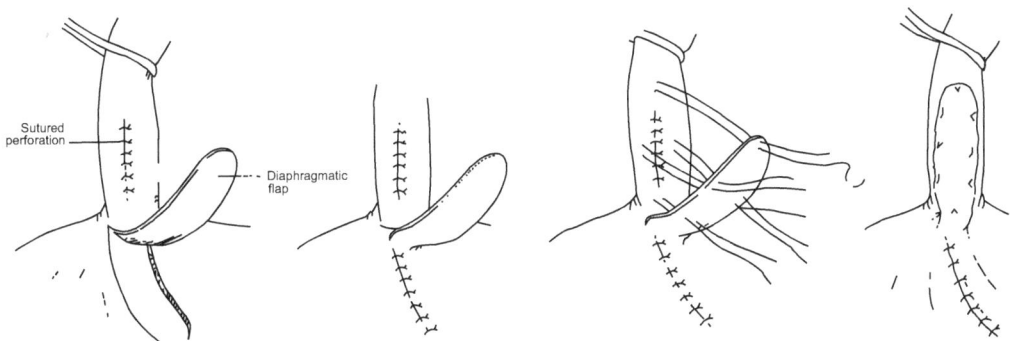

Fig. (9). Technique of diaphragmatic flap reinforcement of sutured early oesophageal perforation.

If the perforation is associated with significant oesophageal disease, endoscopic measures are preferred. Resection (usually oesophago-gastrectomy) with primary reconstruction can be performed. However, these procedures are often associated with an unacceptable mortality and morbidity in this group of patients. In these circumstances, the reconstruction is better delayed in which case a totally diverting cervical oesophagostomy is carried out (see below) and the stomach end is closed.

Late perforations: If the diagnosis of the injury is delayed, direct suture of the oesophageal tear is not possible due to the severe trans mural oedema. The options available are the following:

1. Endoscopic management.
2. T-tube drainage of the perforation.
3. Closure of the defect with a suitable flap of gastric fundus.
4. Oesophageal diversion with or without exclusion.

Oesophageal intubation with a covered self-expanding metallic stent is indicated in late diagnosed perforations in patients who will have often deteriorated with sepsis increasing their surgical risk. The stent could be placed endoscopically or radiologically. The choice is determined by available expertise and equipment, by the size of the perforation and by the condition of the patient. Additional measures to drain sepsis should be undertaken preferably by image guided percutaneous routes.

T-tube drainage of the perforation entails a thoracotomy or a thoracoscopy, pleural drainage and the insertion of a large T tube (preferably silicon, size 22-24 French) in to the oesophageal lumen through the perforation. Drains are also left to the mediastinum and the pleural cavity. Some surgeons advocate the repeated endoscopic application of cotton wool pledgets soaked in 20% sodium hydroxide followed by 30% acetic acid to the edges of the perforation.

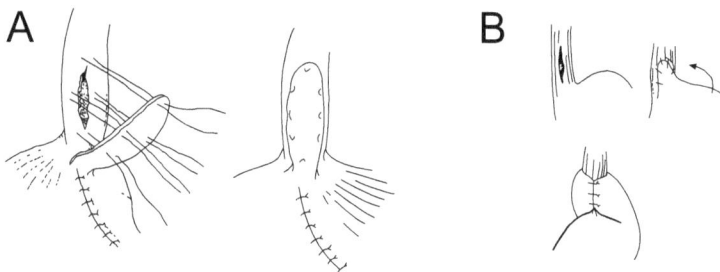

Fig. (10). Techniques for closure of lower oesophageal perforation. A) a diaphragmatic flap is used to seal the tear. B) A Thal fundic patch is used to seal the tear and reinforced by a fundoplication.

Closure of the defect should be attempted in lower thoracic and abdominal perforations by the use of diaphragm flap, omental patch or gastric fundus. In either event, no attempt is made to suture the perforation, the gap is either covered with a diaphragmatic flap, which is sutured to healthy oesophageal wall beyond the tear (Fig. **10A**) or plugged with a Thal fundal patch over which a fundoplication is fashioned (Fig. **10B**).

Diversion is appropriate for high thoracic injuries. After pleural toilet and insertion of drains down to the perforation and in the pleural cavity, the chest is closed and a cervical oesophagostomy is performed by the technique described by Ergin (Fig. **11**). Some advocate diversion with exclusion for late perforations. A cervical oesophagostomy is performed and, through a thoracotomy, the oesophagus is banded with Teflon distal to the perforation. Definitive treatment is carried out at a later stage if the patient survives. The disadvantage of exclusion is that a second thoracotomy is always necessary to remove the band even if the patient does not require oesophageal resection.

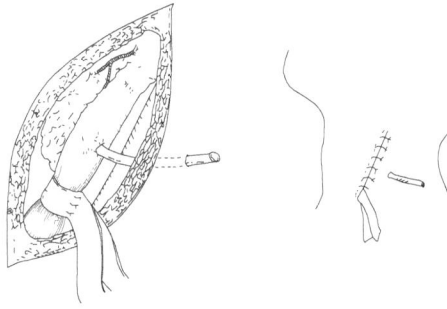

Fig. (11). Surgical technique for a temporary diverting cervical oesophagostomy.

VARICEAL HAEMORRHAGE

Varices are the cause of bleeding in around 11% of patients presenting with upper GI haemorrhage, and in the majority of patients the varices are oesophageal. In cirrhosis, oesophageal varices tend to develop when the hepatic venous pressure gradient (HVPG) is above 10 mm Hg (normal <5 mm Hg). The mortality of variceal bleeding remains high at between 15% and 20%, and the outcome closely correlates with the severity of the underlying liver disease. This can be assessed by evaluating the Child-Pugh score (Table **2**).

Table 2. Child-Pugh classification of chronic liver disease.

Parameter	1 Point	2 Points	3 Points
Ascites	Absent	Slight	Moderate
Bilirubin (micromole/L)	< 11	11-45	> 45
Albumin (g/L)	> 35	28-35	< 28
Prothrombin time (Seconds over control)	< 4	4-6	> 6
Or INR	< 1.7	1.7-2.3	> 2.3

(Table 2) contd.....

Parameter	1 Point	2 Points	3 Points
Encephalopathy	None	Grade 1-2	Grade 3-4
Total score of 5-6 = Grade A (well compensated disease) Total score of 7-9 = Grade B (significant functional compromise) Total score of 10-15 = Grade C (decompensated liver disease)			

Patients presenting with upper GI bleeding with stigmata of liver disease where variceal haemorrhage is a possibility, should be assessed, resuscitated and risk-stratified as for non-variceal haemorrhage. Additional attention should be given to the correction of coagulopathy and thrombocytopenia, as this is frequently present in those with advanced liver disease. Prompt liaison with the hepatology service is important to adequately optimise patients for early endoscopy.

Endoscopic Therapy

Endoscopic therapy, involving either injection sclerosis or band ligation, is considered the intervention of first choice for acute variceal bleeding. This however may be combined with pharmacologic agents to reduce portal blood pressure. Emergency endoscopic therapy requires skilled endoscopists with experience in various modes of therapy. Experienced staff to monitor and resuscitate patients who are often unstable as they continue to bleed must be available to support the endoscopy unit. The initial procedures and resuscitation are similar for patients with oesophageal or gastric variceal bleeding. Control of varices however is different.

Oesophageal Varices

Variceal band ligation is superior to injection sclerotherapy in terms of rebleeding rate, mortality rate and rate of death due to rebleeding. Band ligation requires fewer endoscopic sessions to achieve variceal obliteration and is also associated with fewer adverse events such as sepsis, oesophageal ulceration and stricture formation. Due to these reasons, band ligation is the therapy of choice for the management of oesophageal variceal bleeding.

Gastric Varices

Gastric varices can be classified according to their location and relationship to oesophageal varices. Those that continue from oesophageal varices and extend for <5 cm along the lesser curvature of the stomach are termed gastro-oesophageal varices (GOV) type 1. Those that continue from oesophageal varices but extend towards the fundus along the greater curvature are GOV type 2. Isolated gastric varices (IGV) are not in continuation with oesophageal varices and can be in the fundus (IGV type 1) or anywhere distally (IGV type 2) (Fig. **12**). Although gastric varies seem to bleed less frequent than oesophageal varices, the intensity of the bleeding and trans- fusion requirements are often greater, which lead to a higher mortality once bleeding has occurred. For gastric varices, irrespective of type, cyanoacrylate superglue injection is more effective than band ligation in terms of initial haemostatic control, rebleeding rate, need for blood transfusion and treatment-induced ulcer bleeding. Gastric variceal glue injection is not without risk as it can be associated with glue embolisation to the lungs with haemodynamic compromise and hypoxia. Glue injection requires an experienced team for both endoscopic skill and excellent coordination between the endoscopist and assisting nursing staff to minimise the risk of damaging the endoscope permanently with glue or gluing the endoscope or injector needle onto the varicose vessel itself. Thrombin injection of gastric varices has also been used similarly with promising results [21].

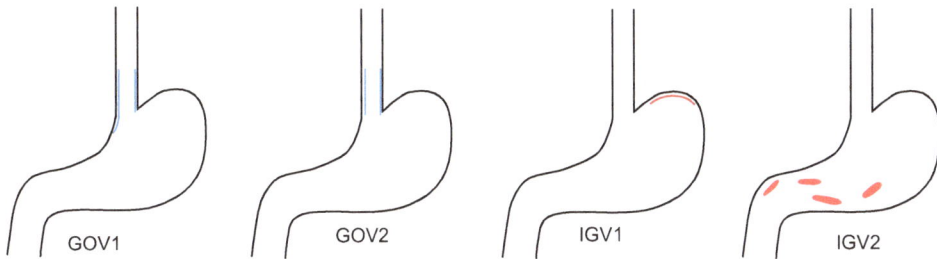

Fig. (12). Classification of gastric varices.

Pharmacotherapy for Variceal Bleeding

Pharmacologic agents have been shown to be highly effective as adjuncts in the control of the bleeding episode. In patients with acute variceal bleeding, pharmacologic agents improve the efficacy of endoscopic therapy to achieve initial control of bleeding and 5-day hemostasis, but generally fail to affect mortality.

Vasoactive Therapy

Vasoactive drugs reduce portal hypertension by decreasing portal blood flow. Terlipressin is preferred over somatostatin or its analogues (such as octreotide) as it is the only one to have shown a reduction in mortality, with numbers of patients needed to treat (NNT) of 8.3 to prevent one death. A typical terlipressin dosing regimen starts with 2 mg given intravenously followed by 1-2 mg every 4-6 hours. Terlipressin should be started promptly if variceal bleeding is suspected and continued after endoscopy for at least 48 h. Beneficial effects have been demonstrated for both pre- and post-endoscopic diagnosis or therapy.

Antibiotic Therapy

Bacterial infections are common in cirrhotic patients with variceal bleeding and manifest in around 66% within 2 weeks. In 30%-40% of patients, an infection is present on admission. It has been hypothesised that sepsis-induced systemic endotoxin release promotes an increase in portal pressure due to local vasoconstriction and a rise in intrahepatic vascular resistance. Accordingly, sepsis has been implicated in precipitating variceal bleeding. Cirrhotic patients with variceal bleeding, who either have sepsis on admission or who go on to develop it, have high rates of failure to control bleeding, and increased rebleeding and mortality. Prophylactic antibiotic use has been shown to significantly reduce mortality in cirrhotic patients with variceal bleeding, and thus antibiotics should be promptly commenced on admission for cirrhotic patients. Broad-spectrum antibiotics with preference for those that have renal excretion represent the best options. Examples include norfloxacin, ciprofloxacin or tazocin. However, local infection control policies should be followed.

PPI Therapy

Shallow ulcers normally occur at variceal banding sites in the oesophagus and occasionally these can bleed. The risk of bleeding is significantly lower in patients given an adequate daily dose of a PPI following band ligation. A loading dose of intravenous PPIs is commonly given after variceal band ligation. Depending on the condition of the patient and other co-morbidities, an intravenous infusion or daily divided doses could be given thereafter [22].

Rescue Therapy for Variceal Bleeding

In around 10%-20% of patients, variceal bleeding continues despite combined pharmacological and initial endoscopic therapy. In a clinically stable patient, repeat endoscopy should be considered. The rescue procedure should be dictated by the patient's general condition, the availability of different modalities of treatment and the experience of the staff attending the patient.

Balloon Tamponade

Balloon tamponade using a Sengstaken-Blakemore tube is indicated if variceal bleeding continues with cardiovascular compromise. Balloon tamponade is also indicated with torrential variceal bleeding where endoscopy fails to identify the source of bleeding or adequately treat bleeding varices. In this setting tamponade is usually used as a bridge to either a further attempt endoscopic treatment or radiological placement of an intrahepatic porto-systemic shunt. Balloon tamponade achieves control of bleeding in around 80% of patients. However, complications occur in as many as 20% including aspiration, tube migration and oesophageal necrosis or perforation.

Trans-Jugular Intrahepatic Porto-Systemic Shunt (TIPSS)

Portal hypertension is present when the HVPG—the difference between the wedged and free hepatic venous pressures—is >5 mm Hg. It is considered clinically significant when it exceeds 10 mm Hg as this usually results in the development of varices. In patients with variceal bleeding, an HVPG of >20 mm Hg is associated with failure to control bleeding, a higher rate of rebleeding and higher 1-year mortality. TIPSS is the percutaneous placement of a radiological stent between the hepatic vein and intrahepatic segment of the portal vein in order to reduce portal pressure [23]. Although a very useful technique to control recurrent variceal bleeding, it can also be placed to reduce other complications of liver failure such as refractory ascites or hepatic hydrothorax. A reduction in HVPG to <12 mm Hg or by 20% from the baseline value reduces the risk of variceal haemorrhage and improves survival. The two most important complications of TIPSS are hepatic encephalopathy due to systemic exposure to toxin-containing blood and heart failure due to the sudden increase in cardiac preload.

Covered Self-Expanding Metal Stents (SEMS)

Small case series have reported on the use of removable or biodegradable SEMS for refractory variceal bleeding. Preliminary data suggest that they are effective in achieving haemostasis. However, SEMS removal followed by conservative treatment is associated with a high rebleeding rate (60% at 9 days), suggesting that this approach should be used as a bridging strategy to more definitive therapy such as TIPSS or liver transplantation.

Secondary Prevention of Variceal Haemorrhage

Without additional therapy, patients with variceal bleeding that survive an index bleed have a 60% chance of rebleeding within 1-2 years with a 33% mortality. Propranolol has been shown to significantly reduce rebleeding and mortality in these patients and should be commenced soon after stabilisation. The combination of β-blockers and nitrates is superior to β-blocker monotherapy but is associated with more side effects and is poorly tolerated [24].

Carvedilol is a non-selective β-blocker with α-(1)-adrenergic blocking activity, which has been shown to have a greater portal hypotensive effect than propranolol alone in patients with cirrhosis. Carvedilol is effective in the primary prophylaxis of variceal bleeding and also effective in patients who fail to reduce HVPG on propranolol. Based on these data, some centres use carvedilol in preference to propranolol.

A programme of periodic surveillance gastroscopy with or without further variceal band ligation has been shown to significantly reduce the median rebleeding rate to around 32%. It is currently best practice for patients to be placed on life-long carvedilol or propranolol and a 'banding programme' of surveillance gastroscopy until variceal obliteration has been achieved. This can be followed by surveillance gastroscopies every 3-12 months depending on the findings. The interval between surveillance endoscopies is still debated and practice varies across specialised centres. Recent data report similar effectiveness (rebleeding rate, variceal recurrence and mortality) between two-weekly or monthly intervals. In those patients unsuitable for surveillance gastroscopy, a combination of non-selective β-blocker and nitrate is recommended. Patients, who rebleed despite optimal pharmacological and endoscopic therapy or those who are intolerant to that approach, can be considered for TIPSS.

CONSENT FOR PUBLICATION

Not applicable.

CONFLICT OF INTEREST

The author declares no conflict of interest, financial or otherwise.

ACKNOWLEDGEMENT

Declare none.

REFERENCES

[1]   Roden D F, Altman K W. Causes of dysphagia among different age groups a systematic review of the literature, otolaryngologic clinics of north america, vol 46, pp 965-+, Dec 2013

[2]   Kumar AR, Katz PO. Functional esophageal disorders: a review of diagnosis and management. Expert Rev Gastroenterol Hepatol 2013; 7(5): 453-61.
[http://dx.doi.org/10.1586/17474124.2013.811028] [PMID: 23899284]

[3]   Sidhwa F, Moore A, Alligood E, Fisichella PM. Diagnosis and treatment of the extraesophageal manifestations of gastroesophageal reflux disease. Ann Surg 2016; (Aug): 5.
[PMID: 27455157]

[4]   Schumpelick V, Steinau G, Schluper I, Prescher A. Surgical embryology and anatomy of the diaphragm with surgical applications, Surg Clin North Am, vol 80, pp 213-39, xi, Feb 2000
[http://dx.doi.org/10.1016/S0039-6109(05)70403-5]

[5]   Leeuwen L, Fitzgerald DA. Congenital diaphragmatic hernia. J Paediatr Child Health 2014; 50(9): 667-73.
[http://dx.doi.org/10.1111/jpc.12508] [PMID: 24528549]

[6]   Naunheim KS. Adult presentation of unusual diaphragmatic hernias. Chest Surg Clin N Am 1998;

8(2): 359-69.
[PMID: 9619309]

[7]   Duranceau A. Massive hiatal hernia: a review. Dis Esophagus 2016; 29(4): 350-66.
        [http://dx.doi.org/10.1111/dote.12328] [PMID: 25789563]

[8]   Oleynikov D, Jolley JM. Paraesophageal hernia. Surg Clin North Am 2015; 95(3): 555-65.
        [http://dx.doi.org/10.1016/j.suc.2015.02.008] [PMID: 25965129]

[9]   Granderath FA, Schweiger UM, Pointner R. Laparoscopic antireflux surgery: tailoring the hiatal
        closure to the size of hiatal surface area. Surg Endosc 2007; 21(4): 542-8.
        [http://dx.doi.org/10.1007/s00464-006-9041-7] [PMID: 17103275]

[10]   Poincloux L, Rouquette O, Abergel A. Endoscopic treatment of benign esophageal strictures: a
        literature review, Expert Rev Gastroenterol Hepatol, pp 1-12, Nov 22 2016

[11]   Kozarek RA. Self-expandable stents for benign esophageal disorders: when do the benefits outweigh
        the risks? J Clin Gastroenterol 2016; 50(5): 357-8.
        [PMID: 26974754]

[12]   Johnson CM, Postma GN. Zenker diverticulum - which surgical approach is superior? JAMA
        Otolaryngol Head Neck Surg 2016; 142(4): 401-3.
        [http://dx.doi.org/10.1001/jamaoto.2015.3892] [PMID: 26914440]

[13]   Andolfi C, Wiesel O, Fisichella PM. Surgical treatment of epiphrenic diverticulum: technique and
        controversies. J Laparoendosc Adv Surg Tech A 2016; 26(11): 905-10.
        [http://dx.doi.org/10.1089/lap.2016.0365] [PMID: 27631419]

[14]   Müller M, Gockel I, Hedwig P, *et al.* Is the Schatzki ring a unique esophageal entity? World J
        Gastroenterol 2011; 17(23): 2838-43.
        [PMID: 21734791]

[15]   Huang J, Yan ZN. Dysphagia caused by esophageal duplication cyst. Clin Gastroenterol Hepatol 2016;
        (Aug): 27.
        [PMID: 27574754]

[16]   Salo J, Sihvo E, Kauppi J, Räsänen J. Boerhaave's syndrome: Lessons learned from 83 cases over
        three decades. Scand J Surg 2013; 102(4): 271-3.
        [http://dx.doi.org/10.1177/1457496913495338] [PMID: 24056135]

[17]   Ellabban MA. The sternocleidomastoid muscle flap: A versatile local method for repair of external
        penetrating injuries of hypopharyngeal-cervical esophageal funnel. World J Surg 2016; 40(4): 870-80.
        [http://dx.doi.org/10.1007/s00268-015-3306-z] [PMID: 26578319]

[18]   Glatz T, Marjanovic G, Kulemann B, Hipp J, Theodor Hopt U, Fischer A, *et al.* Management and
        outcome of esophageal stenting for spontaneous esophageal perforations. Dis Esophagus 2016; (Oct):
        28.
        [PMID: 27790804]

[19]   Laukoetter MG, Mennigen R, Neumann PA, Dhayat S, Horst G, Palmes D, *et al.* Successful closure of
        defects in the upper gastrointestinal tract by endoscopic vacuum therapy (EVT): a prospective cohort
        study. Surg Endosc 2016; (Oct): 5.
        [PMID: 27709328]

[20]   Newton NJ, Sharrock A, Rickard R, Mughal M. Systematic review of the use of endo-luminal topical
        negative pressure in oesophageal leaks and perforations. Dis Esophagus 2016; (Sep): 15.
        [PMID: 27628015]

[21]   Wani ZA, Bhat RA, Bhadoria AS, Maiwall R, Choudhury A. Gastric varices: Classification,
        endoscopic and ultrasonographic management. J Res Med Sci 2015; 20(12): 1200-7.
        [http://dx.doi.org/10.4103/1735-1995.172990] [PMID: 26958057]

[22]   Cabrera L, Tandon P, Abraldes JG. An update on the management of acute esophageal variceal

bleeding. Gastroenterol Hepatol 2016; (Mar): 2.
[PMID: 26948179]

[23]   Lakhoo J, Bui JT, Lokken RP, Ray CE Jr, Gaba RC. Transjugular intrahepatic portosystemic shunt creation and variceal coil or plug embolization ineffectively attain gastric variceal decompression or occlusion: Results of a 26-patient retrospective study. J Vasc Interv Radiol 2016; 27(7): 1001-11.
[http://dx.doi.org/10.1016/j.jvir.2016.02.019] [PMID: 27106732]

[24]   Mandorfer M, Peck-Radosavljevic M, Reiberger T. Prevention of progression from small to large varices: are we there yet? An updated meta-analysis. Gut 2016; (Sep): 30.
[PMID: 27694143]

CHAPTER 7

Gastro-oesophageal Reflux Disease

Aminah Khan and **Sami M. Shimi**[*]

Department of Surgery, Ninewells Hospital and Medical School, Dundee, Scotland, UK

Abstract: Pathological gastro-oesophageal reflux is multifactorial chronic disorder with increasing prevalence. Incompetence of the physiological anti-reflux mechanisms at the gastro-oesophageal junction results in this reflux and the cardinal symptoms are heartburn and regurgitation as well as a host of extra-oesophageal manifestations. Severe chronic GORD results in prolonged oesophageal acid exposure and to the development erosive esophagitis, deep ulcers, strictures and Barrett's oesophagus.

The goal of treatment for GORD is to control symptom control, to heal any oesophagitis and to improve the quality of life. Acid suppression represents the mainstay of medical treatment for GORD. Proton pump inhibitors provide symptomatic relief and healing of erosive oesophagitis in over 80% of patients. Surgical intervention aims to provide a curative reconstruction of the anti-reflux barrier at the GOJ and should be considered in patients with continuing or drug-refractory GORD. Anti-reflux surgery has shown greater resolution of reflux symptoms and oesophagitis compared to medical therapy. Currently laparoscopic total or partial fundoplication is the gold standard for surgical intervention. The most common post-operative complications are gaseous bloating, dysphagia and diarrhoea.

A number of novel therapies, such as the LINX and Esophyx, have shown promise in achieving good symptomatic relief by correcting pathological reflux and possessing a better side-effect profile than surgical fundoplication.

Keywords: GORD, Reflux, Hiatus hernia, Oesophagitis, Oesophageal strictures, pH metry, Impedance, Proton pump inhibitors, Fundoplication, Oesophageal lengthening.

GASTRO-OESOPHAGEAL REFLUX

Gastro-oesophageal reflux is a physiological phenomenon, with small amounts of retrograde flow, of gastric contents into the oesophagus, occurring commonly in the postprandial period. Pathological gastro-oesophageal reflux however, is a multi-factorial chronic disorder. It is the commonest benign disorder of the upper

[*] **Corresponding author Sami M. Shimi:** Department of Surgery, Ninewells Hospital and Medical School, Dundee DD1 9SY, Scotland, UK; Tel: +44 1382 660111; E-mail: s.m.shimi@dundee.ac.uk

Sami M. Shimi (Ed.)

digestive tract and has a high prevalence in the general population. A panel of experts (Montreal consensus, 2006), defined gastro-oesophageal reflux disease as 'troublesome or persistent symptoms and/or complications resulting from the reflux of gastro-duodenal contents' [1]. Gastro-oesophageal reflux disease (GORD) can cause a wide range of both oesophageal and extra-oesophageal symptoms. In up to 70% of patients with typical GORD symptoms, the disease is mild and intermittent with normal endoscopic findings. This is known as non-erosive reflux disease (NERD). In around 10% of patients, however, the reflux is severe and unremitting, leading to the development of erosive oesophagitis. Scarring, ulceration, stricture formation, columnar metaplasia (Barrett's oesophagus) and adenocarcinoma are complications of erosive oesophagitis (Table 1).

Table 1. Clinical manifestations of gastro-oesophageal reflux (Montreal Consensus, 2006 [1]).

Oesophageal Syndromes		Extra-oesophageal Syndromes	
Symptomatic Syndromes	**Syndromes with Oesophageal Injury**	**Established Associations**	**Proposed Associations**
Typical reflux syndrome	Reflux oesophagitis	Reflux cough syndrome	Pharyngitis
Reflux/chest pain syndrome	Reflux stricture	Reflux asthma syndrome	Sinusitis
	Barrett's oesophagus	Reflux laryngitis syndrome	Recurrent otitis media
	Oesophageal adenocarcinoma	Reflux dental erosion syndrome	4. Idiopathic pulmonary fibrosis

Epidemiology

The prevalence of GORD is highest in the western world, affecting around 20-25% of the population in North America compared with just 5-7% of the population of East Asia. Epidemiological studies have shown a worldwide upward trend in the prevalence of GORD that may herald serious societal consequences as GORD conveys a negative effect on health-related quality of life, (HRQoL), and a substantial economic burden. Factors that possibly explain this increase include lifestyle choices such as smoking, alcohol consumption and dietary choices. Neither age nor gender appears to influence the occurrence of symptoms.

The current global obesity 'epidemic' may be fuelling the rise in GORD as evidence suggests a strong association between a high body mass index and an increased risk of GORD, as well as its temporal progression and complications. The eradication of *Helicobacter pylori* infections, whilst dramatically reducing the incidence of peptic ulcer disease, may provoke reflux oesophagitis and the occurrence of GORD. Finally the improvement of diagnostic techniques and routine deployment of endoscopy may also account for the increase in GORD prevalence [2].

Pathophysiology

Physiological gastro-oesophageal reflux is a short-lived phenomenon, which commonly occurs in the post-prandial period, and manifests occasionally by burping. The main driving force is the pressure gradient between the positive pressure of the intra-abdominal cavity and the negative pressure of the intra-thoracic cavity. This promotes the reflux of gastric contents into the lower oesophagus. Homeostasis of this system is maintained by normal anatomy and physiology of the oesophagus and stomach, in particular the competence of the gastro-oesophageal junction. Pathological reflux or GORD is defined as chronic acid and/or bile reflux causing unacceptable symptoms and/or demonstrable pathology, often arising from the imbalance of these physiological factors [3].

Physiological Anti-Reflux Mechanisms

Three main factors contribute to the physiological anti-reflux mechanism. These consist of the competence of the gastro-oesophageal junction, oesophageal clearance and mucosal defence mechanisms [4].

1. Competence of the Gastro-oesophageal Junction

The gastro-oesophageal junction (GOJ), also known as the high-pressure zone, is the natural anti-reflux barrier. Its core structural components are, the lower oesophageal sphincter or distal oesophageal muscle fibres and the sling and clasp fibres of gastric cardia, the diaphragmatic crura and the length of the intra-abdominal oesophagus.

Lower Oesophageal Sphincter: The lower oesophageal sphincter (LOS) is the most important factor maintaining the competence of the GOJ. It is a specialised partial ring of smooth muscle extending along 3 to 4 cm of the distal oesophagus, at the diaphragmatic hiatus. It is kept tonically active by the vagus nerve and generates a myogenic resting pressure greater than intra-abdominal pressure, of around 12-20 mmHg. This is usually enough pressure to prevent reflux, and can be evaluated during oesophageal manometry. The partial ring is known as the semi-circular clasp and reinforced by a condensation of the oblique muscle layer at the gastric cardia, known as the gastric sling. The sling and clasp configuration creates an asymmetrical circumferential profile, as the muscles have differing functional and contractile properties. This results in higher pressures in the left lateral portion of the sphincter (Fig. **1**).

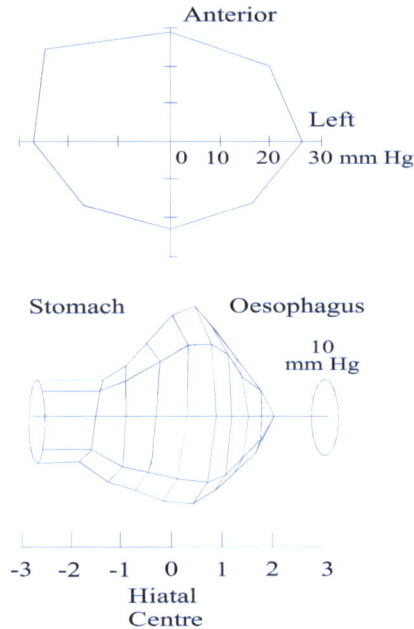

Fig. (1). 3-Dimensional pressure profile of the lower oesophageal sphincter.

The sling muscles also contribute to the oblique angle of HIS, facilitating the abrupt insertion of the oesophagus into the stomach. The resulting small diameter aperture of the distal oesophagus creates a 'flap-valve' like mechanism, which prevents reflux. Distortions in the angle of HIS, such as following partial gastrectomy, are associated with increased symptoms of reflux.

The resting tone of the LOS varies throughout the day and activities such as sleeping will increase it whilst feeding decreases it. Furthermore, the administration of gastrin, cholinergic and alpha-adrenergic agents and prokinetic drugs, like metoclopramide and domperidone, produce an increase in the resting tone of the LOS. Potent reducers of LOS pressure include the hormones secretin, cholecystokinin and glucagon, as well as agents such as nitric oxide, prostaglandins and calcium channel blockers. Dietary agents such as coffee, alcohol, fatty foods and nicotine also lower LOS pressure.

Transient lower oesophageal sphincter relaxations (TLOSR) are the phenomena behind both physiological reflux and in patients with GORD. They are neurally mediated vago-vagal mediated reflexes triggered by mechanoreceptors in the gastric cardia, mostly to gastric distension and are independent of swallowing. TLOSR act as a form of gastric venting, reducing the sphincter pressure to allow belching to occur. The frequency of TLSOR is believed to be the same in both normal and GORD patients, however the occurrence of acid reflux during a TLOSR is greater in patients with GORD.

Crural Diaphragm: The crural diaphragm is seen as the second sphincter component of the GOJ. It wraps around the distal oesophagus as it passes into the abdomen and so acts by compressing the GOJ thereby dramatically increasing the LOS pressure. It is attached to LES by phreno-oesophageal membrane (ligament), so when the striated muscles fibres of the crural diaphragm contract, during inspiration or straining, pressure is exerted on the LES and in turn the GOJ pressure increases. Acting in concert the LES and the diaphragm crura are considered the internal and external sphincters of the GOJ. This union does not work in presence of hiatus hernia and during TLOSR.

Length of Abdominal Oesophagus: The insertion point of the phreno-oesophageal ligament determines the length of the abdominal oesophagus. This ligament is an extension of the visceral peritoneum covering the under surface of the diaphragm. It anchors the GOJ within the abdomen to prevent herniation through the hiatus, thereby maintaining a length of the oesophagus within the positive-pressure environment of the abdomen. Approximately, 2 cm of intra-abdominal oesophagus is needed to maintain the competence of the GOJ. This length can be greatly affected by a hiatus hernia.

2. Oesophageal Clearance

The sequential peristaltic contraction of circular muscle within the oesophageal body generates peristaltic waves to propel an ingested food bolus aborally into the stomach. This propulsive pump works against a pressure gradient of around 12 mmHG, intra-thoracic and 6 mmHg intra-abdominal. Primary peristalsis is centrally mediated and initiated by deglutition whilst, secondary peristalsis is triggered, by local neural reflexes when the oesophageal lumen is distended. The role of the non-peristaltic tertiary contractions, detected during 24-hour manometry investigations, is unclear.

The coordination of peristalsis is through centrally mediated activation of vagal lower motor neurons in the vagal nucleus ambiguous that project onto peripheral, inhibitory and excitatory neurons in the oesophageal myenteric plexus. In addition to transporting swallowed boluses, these peristaltic waves, which reach amplitudes of over 20 mmHg, are important in the clearing of refluxed gastric contents. While oesophageal peristalsis provides volume clearance of up to 95% of an acidic refluxate, chemical clearance also takes place through the neutralisation, of the acid bolus, by the bicarbonate contained in saliva. Finally, it is worth emphasising that oesophageal clearance only shortens the contact time between the injurious refluxate and the oesophageal mucosa.

3. Mucosal Defence

The endogenous defence of the oesophageal mucosa to refluxate occurs in three levels:

Pre-epithelial: The oesophagus is afforded some mucosal buffering by a sparse mucous layer and small bicarbonate secreting glands, however these provide limited protection against the high load of hydrochloric acid contained in the refluxate.

Epithelial: The stratified squamous epithelium has a hydrophobic cell membrane, active membrane-bound ion pumps and tight junctions to provide resistance to trans-mucosal hydrogen ion diffusion. Essentially it acts as a physical barrier to noxious agents attempting to penetrate the cell. Acid refluxate causes epithelial injury by increasing the cell permeability, leading to swelling and cell rupture. This provokes the generation of free radicals and an inflammatory response.

Post-epithelial: The post-epithelial layer has a rich capillary blood supply, which delivers acid neutralising bicarbonate ions, oxygen, inflammatory and phagocytic cells, and disposes of noxious products. Blood flow increases in response to an acid insult, suggesting that post-epithelial defences may be activated rather than impaired in reflux disease.

Contributory Factors for Reflux

The factors that contribute to gastro-oesophageal reflux contradict and negate the physiological anti-reflux mechanisms. Failure of the gastro-oesophageal sphincter competence and a hiatus hernia negate the sphincter function. Abnormal gastric and oesophageal motility contribute to failure to clear the refluxate. The presence of the noxious refluxate together with helicobacter pylori infection negate the mucosal defences.

1. Failure of the GOJ

Reflux occurs when intra-gastric pressure is higher than the LOS pressure, which can be categorised into one of three mechanisms:

A Hypotensive LOS: A LOS with a resting pressure of less than 6 mmHg allows free reflux of gastric contents. This can occur either with a primary weakness of the LOS smooth muscle, such as in scleroderma, or in response to inflammation of the oesophageal mucosa. Inflammatory mediators such as prostaglandins, in particular PDE_2, and nitric oxide cause LOS hypotension by reducing its vagal mediated resting tone.

Inappropriate TLOSR: Most individuals with GORD do not have more frequent TLOSR than healthy subjects, however the occurrence of acid reflux during TLOSR is twice as likely for GORD patients. The estimated 40% of GORD patients that do have more frequent or longer TLOSR are termed to have 'reflex reflux'. Inappropriate TLOSR can occur in obesity, due to the increased sensitivity of the gastric stretch receptors or in diabetes, due to hyperglycaemia. TLOSR are vagally mediated reflexes that are modulated by the neurotransmitter gamma-aminobutyric acid (GABA) *via* $GABA_B$ receptors, and the $GABA_B$ agonist baclofen may have a role in reducing their frequency.

Increased Intra-Abdominal Pressure: A positive gastro-oesophageal pressure gradient facilitates retrograde flow, and is termed stress reflux. Transient pressure rises are seen with abdominal straining, whilst chronically raised intra-abdominal pressures are usually due to a gravid uterus and morbid obesity.

2. Gastric Dysmotility

Abnormalities of gastric emptying increase gastric volume, by prolonging the retention of food, and thereby increase the gastro-oesophageal pressure gradient, the frequency of TLOSR and the volume of the potential refluxate. Delayed gastric emptying can be caused by gastric outlet obstruction, benign or malignant, or by gastroparesis. Although impaired gastric emptying is reported more often in individuals with GORD, than in those without, a clear relationship between delayed gastric emptying and oesophageal acid exposure has not been convincingly demonstrated and as such the significance of it in the pathogenesis of GORD is unclear.

3. Oesophageal Dysmotility

Numerous oesophageal motility abnormalities are associated with GORD, the most common being ineffective primary peristalsis and hypomotility. Patients with GORD that demonstrate peristaltic dysfunction, have prolonged mean duration of the reflux episodes, especially at night as peristaltic frequency is greatly reduced by sleep, and a higher risk of developing oesophagitis. Around 66% of patients with oesophagitis have abnormalities in oesophageal motility, with the proportion of patients having dysmotility increasing with the severity of the oesophagitis. Furthermore, secondary dysmotility can develop from the delay in oesophageal transit and increase in acid exposure times causing mucosal damage. This releases inflammatory mediators that decrease the cholinergic excitation and increase the nitrergic inhibition of the oesophageal muscle body resulting in low amplitude peristaltic waves and ultimately further hypomotility. This vicious cycle leads to potentially irreversible oesophageal myo-neuronal damage, worsening the severity of both the dysmotility and the oesophagitis.

4. Hiatus Hernia

A hiatus hernia disrupts the normal anatomy and physiological mechanisms of the GOJ and facilitates GORD, with approximately 50% of individuals with GORD symptoms having a hiatus hernia. This is an important distinction. Not all patients with a hiatus hernia have gastro-oesophageal reflux. Equally, not all patients with gastro-oesophageal reflux have a hiatus hernia. There is however 50% of people from either group who will have both gastro-oesophageal reflux and a hiatus hernia (Fig. **2**).

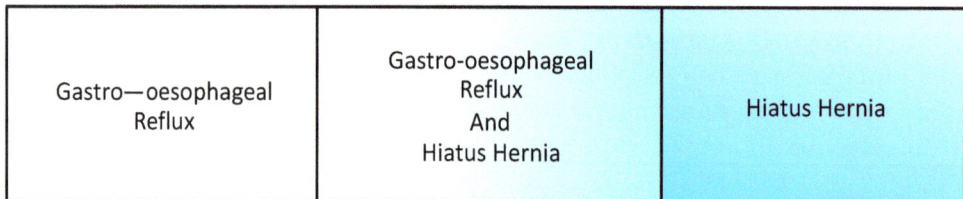

Gastro—oesophageal Reflux	Gastro-oesophageal Reflux And Hiatus Hernia	Hiatus Hernia

Fig. (2). A hiatus hernia does not always cause gastro-oesophageal reflux. A third of patients will have both and they tend to be more symptomatic of reflux.

Those people tend to have more symptomatic reflux and are more likely to develop complications of gastro-oesophageal reflux. Although any type of hiatal hernia may render the GOJ incompetent, it most commonly occurs with Type I (sliding) hiatus hernias. In these the GOJ is no longer maintained in the abdomen, as the crural diaphragm and phreno-oesophageal ligament are disrupted, and as a result the intra-abdominal length and pressure of the LOS are decreased (Fig. **3**). There is also effacement of the LOS through widening of the angle of HIS. Furthermore, the hiatal sac can act as a reservoir, as acid rich refluxate can reside unimpeded in the hernia pocket, termed an acid pocket, above the diaphragmatic crura. From here it can re-reflux into the oesophagus either upon LOS relaxation, for example swallowing, or upon increased intra-abdominal pressure, such as on straining.

The frequency of reflux, in GORD patients with a hiatus hernia, is nearly doubled to those without, resulting in a significantly increased risk of severe oesophagitis. A hiatus hernia greater than 2 cm is associated with a greater incidence of erosive oesophagitis and Barrett's oesophagus. In many patients, however, the LOS function is maintained despite the hiatus hernias and they do not have GORD.

5. The Refluxate

The dominant irritants in gastro-intestinal refluxate are hydrochloric acid and pepsin although bile, pancreatic juice and other components of gastric juice also contribute. Just over 40% of GORD patients experience only gastric acid and pepsin reflux whilst the remainder have mixed reflux of gastric and duodenal juices. Pure alkali reflux is uncommon.

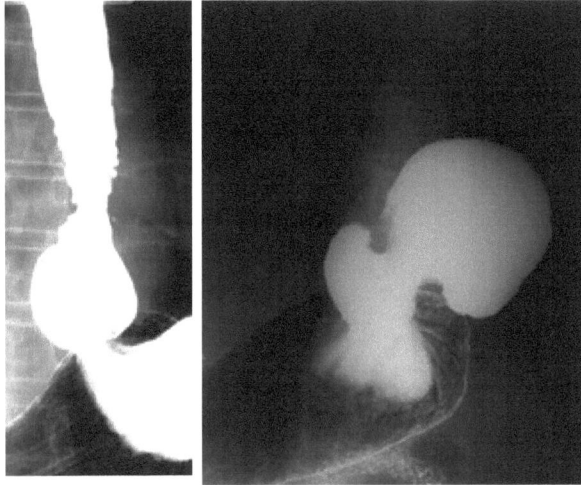

Fig. (3). Sliding (*left*) and rolling (*right*) hiatal herniae demonstrated on double contrast barium meal examination.

The hydrochloric acid in gastric juice is noxious to epithelial cells and damages the oesophageal mucosal barrier. Most GORD patients have similar acid secretory levels compared with control subjects and gastric acid hyper secretion, as found in Zollinger-Ellision syndrome, is the exception rather than the rule. The low pH environment created by the acid activates pepsin enabling it to permeate the mucosal cell membrane, to cause further damage. Bile has also shown synergism with acid, and exposure of the oesophageal mucosa to gastroduodenal juices is associated with the highest grade of mucosal injury. With gastric acid evidently playing the most toxic role, potent acid suppression remains the mainstay of medical therapy.

6. Helicobacter Pylori

Current evidence suggests that *helicobacter pylori (H. pylori)* infection maybe protective against the development of GORD with oesophagitis being less prevalent in individuals infected with the bacterium. This relationship is complex, and depends on the location and burden of infection and any subsequent gastric atrophy. Infection of the pyloric antrum, with *H. pylori* causes antral gastritis leading to increased gastric acid production, whilst proximal gastric involvement results in atrophic gastritis and decreased acid production. The more virulent the strain of *H. pylori*, such as CagA, iceA1 and vacS1, and the greater the extent of *helicobacter* induced atrophic gastritis, with severe corpus gastritis causing profoundly low gastric acid levels, the greater the protective effect conferred against GORD. Furthermore, eradication therapy, leading to the disappearance of *H.pylori*, increases the risk of developing reflux oesophagitis, presumably through resolution of the gastritis and resumption of 'normal' acid secretion. Interestingly the severity of corpus gastritis prior to eradication therapy is an important predictor in the occurrence of the oesophagitis. The available evidence suggests that this phenomenon has no clinical relevance for the treatment of GORD and current guidelines promote the eradication of *H.pylori,* regardless of GORD, due to its increased risk on peptic ulceration and gastric cancer.

CLINICAL PRESENTATION AND DIAGNOSIS

The clinical manifestations of GORD can be divided into oesophageal and extra-oesophageal syndromes, as agreed by the Montreal consensus. The cardinal oesophageal symptoms are heartburn and regurgitation. The heartburn is described as retrosternal and/or epigastric, whilst the regurgitation of gastric contents into the oropharynx or mouth may lead to a sour taste, and is referred to as water brash. Symptoms can be aggravated by posture, large meals and activities that increase the intra-abdominal pressure, such as bending over. Dysphagia can also occur, and may attest to severe GORD in which passage of the food bolus is impaired. This can be due to spasm or oedema of the inflamed lower oesophagus, as a result of a secondary motility disorder or due to chronic reflux induced fibrosis of the lower oesophagus. Persistent dysphagia may indicate stricture formation.

The extra-oesophageal symptoms of GORD include upper aero digestive disease such as voice changes in particular hoarseness sometimes called Cherry Donner syndrome, globus sensation, stomatitis and dental decay due to dental erosions, which is termed reflux dental erosion syndrome. It is also a causative factor in lower respiratory disease such as persistent dry cough, named reflux cough syndrome, and asthma, or reflux asthma syndrome. Other, still debated, manifestations of GORD include pharyngitis, sinusitis and otitis.

A clinically validated scoring system introduced by De Meester is useful for assessing the extent of GORD severity. It is based on the number of reflux episodes and duration of acid exposure in the upright and supine positions (Table **2**).

Severe and longstanding GORD results in prolonged exposure of the oesophageal mucosa to acid and can lead to erosive esophagitis, deep ulcers, strictures and Barrett's oesophagus. Aspiration pneumonia is another potential complication of severe reflux.

Table 2. Johnston DeMeester Score [5]. A normal score is <14.72. Acid exposure times are recorded when the oesophageal pH is <4.

Component of 24 hr. Oesophageal pH Monitoring	95th Percentile
Total Acid Exposure Time (%)	<4.5%
Upright Acid Exposure Time (%)	<8%
Supine Acid Exposure Time (%)	<3%
Number of episodes	<50
Number of episodes lasting > 5 minutes	< 4
Duration of longest episode (minutes)	20

Table 3. Symptoms of Gastro-oesophageal Reflux.

Oesophageal Symptoms	Laryngeal Symptoms	Pulmonary Symptoms
Heartburn	Hoarseness	Cough
Regurgitation	Globus	Wheeze
Epigastric pain	Stomatitis	Shortness of breath
Dysphagia	Dental decay	
Belching	Throat pain	

Oesophagitis:Oesophagitis, or mucosal damage, is present in 30 to 40% of patients undergoing endoscopy for problematic GORD symptoms. Not all patients with oesophagitis are symptomatic and there is no correlation between the severity of GORD symptoms and the presence of oesophagitis, however erosive or ulcerative oesophagitis is considered a marker for severe GORD. Furthermore, oesophagitis can decrease in severity even resolving completely, can persist or can progress to a more severe grade without treatment. A variety of grading systems have been suggested to reflect the severity of the oesophagitis and to help evaluate the impact of treatment. The Los Angeles classification is the most widely used system to correlate the endoscopic appearances with the severity of reflux oesophagitis (Table **3**) [6]. Finally, the likelihood of coexisting oesophageal peristaltic dysfunction appears to increase with the severity of oesophagitis.

Deep Ulceration with Peri-oesophagitis: This complication is usually found in patients with long-standing severe reflux disease. The ulcers can extend beyond the oesophageal submucosa, causing a peri-oesophagitis and extensive mural fibrosis, which can ultimately result in stricture formation. Full thickness penetration may involve the peri-oesophageal arterial plexus and cause massive haemorrhage. However, this complication and overt perforation are rare. Chronic blood loss, however, is a recognised sequel.

Strictures and Webs: Oesophageal strictures and webs are a late complication of severe GORD, occurring in 10 to 20% of patients with ulcerative oesophagitis. Stricture formation is the result of repeated oesophageal damage with fibrosis replacing the muscular coat along a segment of the oesophagus. This submucosal fibrosis can lead to the formation of webs, most commonly found at the lower end or at the level of the aortic arch, and they may cause dysphagia with intermittent solid bolus obstruction. Schatzki's ring is a distinctive circular mucosal ridge situated at the oesophago-gastric junction and tend to occur in association with hiatus hernia, usually without any evidence of oesophagitis (Fig. **4**). They are mostly asymptomatic but those with a ring aperture less than 13 mm cause intermittent dysphagia with sudden episodes of total obstruction, sometimes called 'Steakhouse Syndrome'.

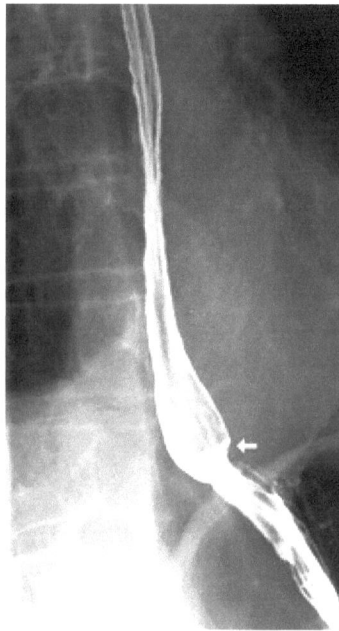

Fig. (4). Schatzki's ring demonstrated on a double contrast barium swallow in a patient with long-standing GORD.

Patients with dysphagia due to oesophageal strictures often require repeated dilatation in spite of optimal medical therapy. Evidence suggests that the initial severity of the stricture is an indicator of the propensity for recurrence after dilatation. Strictures with a luminal diameter of less than 3 mm and a length greater than 3 cm are classified as severe and are both difficult and dangerous to dilate. Surgical management, such as fundoplication, of peptic strictures may be challenging due to concomitant oesophageal shortening, peri-oesophagitis and existence of Barrett's mucosa, increasing the likelihood of fundoplication disruption, slippage or herniation.

Columnar Metaplasia of the Oesophagus (Barrett's Oesophagus): The development of intestinal metaplasia, with characteristic "goblet" cells, in the lower oesophagus occurs in around 10% of patients with severe and chronic gastro-oesophageal reflux. The on-going reflux trauma leads to the accumulation of genetic instability in these areas of intestinal metaplasia and the development of dysplasia. Even a short segment of Barrett's oesophagus has a malignant potential and adenocarcinoma will occur in a proportion of these patients. This condition will be discussed separately.

Diagnostic Investigations

A presumptive diagnosis of GORD can be established in the setting of typical symptoms, which are heartburn and regurgitation. Empirical medical therapy with a proton pump inhibitor is recommended on the basis of this clinical diagnosis. A response to such therapy would ideally confirm the diagnosis; however, this approach may only yield a sensitivity of 78% and specificity of 54%. Diagnostic testing for GORD is advised for three broad situations:

1. To investigate the failure of empirical treatment
2. To identify complications of GORD, e.g. Barrett's oesophagus
3. To identify alternate diagnoses, e.g. peptic ulcer disease

Fortunately, due to its location, the oesophagus is very accessible to endoscopic and physiological investigations, and as such many techniques are available to study its structure and function. Guidelines have been published by specialist societies to guide the clinical communities in investigation and management of patients with both erosive and non-erosive gastro-oesophageal reflux [7, 8].

Endoscopy

Flexible oesophago-gastric endoscopy is not required in the presence of typical GORD symptoms that respond to empirical medical treatment. The primary goals of endoscopy are to detect mucosal damage, in particular Barrett's oesophagus, which can occur in 1 in every 10 GORD patient, and to identify other aetiologies. As such endoscopy is recommended in the following circumstances:

1. Presence of alarm symptoms, especially dysphagia, weight loss, suspected gastrointestinal bleeding and/or persistent vomiting
2. Screening of patients at high risk of complications as clinically indicated, such as high grade erosive oesophagitis, or Barrett's oesophagus
3. Evaluation of patients with extra-oesophageal manifestations

4. Evaluation of patients with persistent or recurrent symptoms despite appropriate medical therapy or after anti-reflux procedures, surgical or endoscopic
5. When other aetiologies such as peptic ulcer disease, gastric malignancy, and eosinophilic oesophagitis are suspected

Endoscopy has a high specificity of 90-95% for discerning the spectrum of histopathological changes that arise in the oesophagus as a complication of GORD. But it suffers from poor sensitivity, as 50% of patients with GORD have normal endoscopic findings. There are several classification systems for grading the endoscopic extent of erosive reflux oesophagitis, and its squeal. The Los Angeles classification is the most widely used validated grading system and it both clinically and functionally correlates the extent of oesophagitis with oesophageal acid exposure, as determined by pH monitoring, and the severity of the reflux (Table **4**).

Table 4. Modified Los Angeles Grading System of oesophagitis.

Grade	Grade Description
A	One (or more) mucosal break, less than 5 mm, that does not extend between the tops of 2 mucosal folds
B	One (or more) mucosal break, more than 5 mm, that does not extend between the tops of 2 mucosal folds
C	One (or more) mucosal break that is continuous between the tops of 2 or more mucosal folds but involves < 75% of the circumference
D	One (or more) mucosal break that involves > 75% of the oesophageal circumference

In addition to visual examination of the mucosa, histological and cytological specimens can be obtained and therapeutic procedures such as stricture dilatation can be performed. Biopsies are advised if there is endoscopic evidence of irregular or deep ulceration, Barrett's oesophagus, presence of a mass lesion or nodularity, an irregular or malignant-appearing stricture, or to rule out other aetiologies. In the case of eosinophilic oesophagitis greater than 5 biopsies are recommended. Endoscopy may also identify a hiatus hernia and point towards the presence of an oesophageal motility abnormality although it is a poor method of investigating muscular functional problems.

Repeat endoscopy for patients with GORD, is reserved for patients whose symptoms failed to respond to medical therapy, those who had severe esophagitis or an oesophageal ulcer, or for those who needed additional biopsy to clarify a diagnosis. Repeat endoscopy is not indicated in patients without Barrett's oesophagus in the absence of new symptoms.

Contrast Radiology

The old role of contrast radiology is now mostly performed by endoscopy. And whilst a barium radiograph should not be performed to establish a diagnosis of GORD, it can be a valuable tool in defining the anatomy and demonstrates the presence of Schatzki rings, oesophageal strictures and the size and type of hiatus hernias. A double-contrast barium study can also reveal classical motility disorders along with the presence or absence of normal propagating contractions. Techniques such as video-fluoroscopy combined with solid and liquid bolus swallows can help in the diagnosis of pharyngeal and upper oesophageal motility disorders.

pH Metry

Prolonged Ambulatory pH Study: Prolonged ambulatory pH monitoring has shown good sensitivity and high specificity in identifying pathological reflux and therefore is regarded as the gold standard in establishing a diagnosis of GORD. It is indicated before consideration of endoscopic or surgical therapy in patients with symptoms but no evidence of oesophagitis on endoscopy, for the evaluation of GORD refractory to acid suppression therapy, and in situations when the diagnosis of GORD is in question, such as in the presence of atypical symptoms.

Ambulatory pH monitoring can be performed over 24 or 48 hours, and requires the patient to discontinue any acid suppression therapy for at least 1 week for the pH monitoring to be accurate. If the patient cannot discontinue the medication, an impedance test should be considered. There are two monitoring devices in widespread use. The first is a trans-nasal placed catheter, which is positioned so that the pH probe lies 5 cm above the LOS (Fig. **5**). A poorly positioned probe will result in inaccurate oesophageal acid exposure times, and if the position of the LOS is uncertain it can be reliably determined by manometry. The probes record periods when the oesophageal pH is below 4 as acid exposure time. The catheter-based pH probes have a reproducibility of only 70-80% and are criticised for interfering with normal daily activities and affecting the reflux episodes. Furthermore, up to 10% of patients cannot tolerate the nasal catheter and report discomfort with gagging, nausea and vomiting. Combined ambulatory manometry and pH metry provides a comprehensive study of the oesophageal acid exposure as well as peristaltic attempts to clear the refluxate over a prolonged period of time (24 Hours) (Fig. **6**)

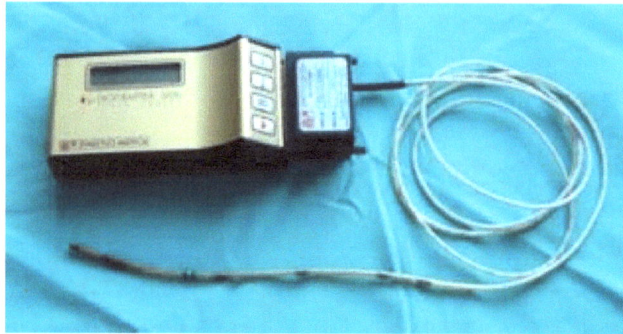

Fig. (5). Ambulatory pH monitoring device which consists of a solid-state catheter with a pH sensor and multiple pressure sensors which connect to a data logger.

The Bravo® pH system (Medtronic, Shoreview, MN, USA) is an innovative, endoscopically placed, wireless pH monitoring system. A radio telemetric capsule is deployed in the oesophageal mucosa 6 cm above the endoscopically identified Z-line, via a trans oral delivery device. Oesophageal pH data are then transmitted to a portable receiver attached to the patient's belt for 48 hours. Prolonged measurement, of up to 96 hours, increase diagnostic reproducibility and sensitivity, especially in patients with intermittent symptoms. Capsules are designed to fall off within 10 days. Although the Bravo® system is better tolerated than catheter-based pH measurement, it is associated with much higher costs.

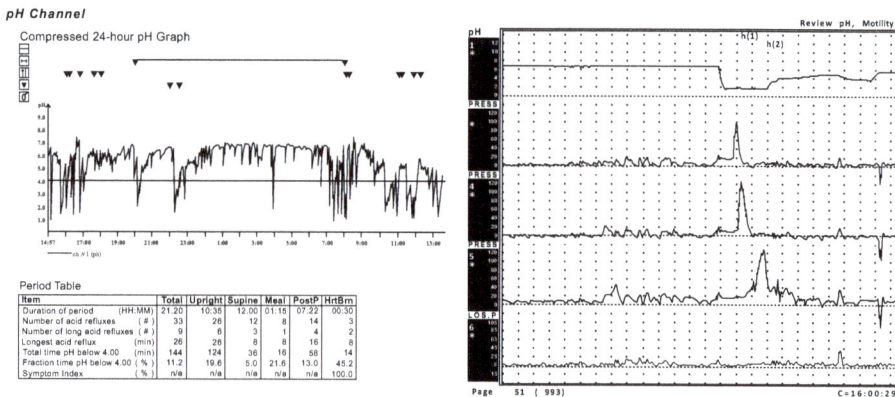

Fig. (6). Recordings from ambulatory pH metry (left) and manometry with pH metry (right).

Ambulatory pH monitoring is the only test that can define the temporal relationship between reflux episodes and symptom association, as it is able to record oesophageal acid exposure times and correlates those episodes to any patient symptoms using an event marker. Computerised software then analyses the recording to produce tables of standard variables that are referenced to known control values. Of these the most widely used system is the revised Johnson-DeMeester score, a convenient, clinically validated system for assessing the severity of reflux disease, based on the number of reflux episodes and duration of acid exposure in the upright and supine positions. As well as stratifying patients according to severity these scores are useful in predicting outcome of any intervention. Patients with a positive relationship between reflux and symptoms and episodes of acid reflux are more likely to respond to conservative or surgical management.

Manometry

The primary aim of manometry is to assess the muscular function of the oesophagus and both its upper and lower sphincters. It will evaluate the resting pressures and length of the lower oesophageal sphincters and oesophageal body, as well as assessing the peristaltic contractions of the oesophageal body for adequate amplitude and duration (Table 5). Consequently, manometry will reliably identify disorders in oesophageal motility, including achalasia, nutcracker oesophagus, diffuse oesophageal spasm and scleroderma that can cause dysphagia and heartburn. As it locates the LOS, manometry can be critical in the accurate placement of the catheter in ambulatory PH monitoring.

Manometry can either be standard or high resolution. Standard manometry is performed after a 4-hour fast using a nasogastric catheter with pressure sensors and transducers linked to a recording device. A pull through technique is used to assess and locate the LOS, whilst wet swallows, around 10 of 5 mls each, evaluate peristalsis. High-resolution manometry uses multiple pressure-recording sensors along the length of the oesophagus to acquire pressure data, and reconstruct it into a visual spatiotemporal plot in real time. It is technically easier but costlier than standard manometry. High-resolution manometry is used to detect focal dysmotility, and yields a more complete pictures of oesophageal motility, as well as depicting LOS function and anatomy in far greater detail.

Table 5. Standardised results for Oesophageal Manometry.

Lower Oesophageal Sphincter	Normal Range	Oesophageal Body Manometry	Normal Range
Distance from Nares	38 – 42 cm	Resting Pressure: Proximal Distal	30 – 140 mm Hg 60 – 180 mm Hg
Length	2 – 5 cm	Peristaltic contractions	> 80%
Resting Pressure	10 – 30 mm Hg	Duration of contractions	< 7 msec
		Velocity	2 – 6 cm/sec

Oesophageal manometry does not have a role in the diagnosis of GORD (other than the localisation of the LOS, for subsequent pH metry) but is recommended for preoperative evaluation. As patients with poor oesophageal motility are more likely to suffer post-operative dysphagia, some surgeons determine the type of surgery necessary, *i.e.* total or partial fundoplication, on the results of manometry.

Multichannel Intraluminal Impedance

Multichannel intraluminal impedance (MII) is a tool used to follow intraluminal bolus movement within the oesophagus, without the use of radiation. It measures the changes in resistance to alternating current, also known as the opposition to current flow (impedance), when a bolus passes by a pair of metallic rings mounted on an intra-oesophageal catheter. In the absence of a bolus, there is low conductivity and high impedance, with the inverse being true when a bolus is present. Measuring impedance at multiple sites (multichannel) can determine the direction of bolus movement and whether it is antegrade, *i.e.* aboral. MII is performed in an ambulatory manner and often combined with manometry or pH sensors for additional information. When combined with manometry, it demonstrates whether the manometrically detected peristaltic contractions result in the actual passage of the bolus. Meanwhile when combined with pH testing, it detects the presence of gastro-oesophageal reflux independent of pH, so both acid and non-acid reflux are recorded. MII also provides greater information on symptom correlation and oesophageal clearance times and is not compromised during the post-prandial period. It can be performed on patients on maximal acid suppression therapy, to evaluate non- acid reflux. Finally, MII can help evaluate dysphagia in GORD patients after anti-reflux surgery.

MANAGEMENT OF GORD

The goal of treatment for GORD is to control the symptoms, heal any oesophageal mucosal injuries, and improve quality of life. Naturally, treatment should be dependent on the severity and persistence of symptoms and the presence of any complications. Given the epidemiology of the disorder, many patients will consult their primary care practitioner with reflux symptoms. The initial focus of management is placed on life-style advice, including weight reduction, avoidance of precipitating factors, elevation of the head of the bed (20-25 cm), avoidance of eating before lying down, smoking cessation and reduction of alcohol intake. However, there is little or no evidence for the efficacy of these interventions. Conversely, there is evidence to suggest that a high BMI is an independent risk factor for the development of GORD, and that the clinical efficacy of medical therapy seems to be hindered by obesity. Subsequently, weight loss is recommended for GORD patients who are overweight, with studies showing a 40% reduction in symptomatic GORD for patients who reduced their BMI by 3.5 or more. Most individuals will benefit from advice on healthy eating. There is little evidence that the routine universal elimination of foods believed to trigger reflux, such as fatty or spicy foods, chocolate, coffee, citrus fruits and juices, tomato, carbonated drinks, and alcohol is effective and hence is no longer recommended. Review of current medication should eliminate or reduce medications that may contribute to reflux or dyspepsia such as theophylline, calcium-channel blockers, NSAIDs, steroids and bisphosphonates. Antacids are also indicated in the initial management of these patients. Antacid use can also serve as an indicator of symptom persistence and severity. It is important to note that conservative measures, such as lifestyle and dietary modifications may benefit some selected patients with GORD, but alone they are almost ineffective in relieving reflux symptoms.

Patients, who continue to experience symptoms despite the initial measures, should be progressed to active medical treatment. At this juncture, it is worth spending some time to evaluate the extent of patient's symptoms and their effect on night sleep, social function and work. Mild symptoms can be managed with increasing antacids with or without additional use of H_2-Receptor blockers. Moderate and severe symptoms and healing of oesophagitis requires the use of proton pump inhibitors (PPIs). An initial course of 4-8 weeks of maintenance therapy using the lowest effective dose to settle symptoms should be followed by either therapy withdrawal, reduction to "per need" or continuation depending on response. Patients with persistent symptoms require endoscopic evaluation. Severe oesophagitis requires high dose PPI therapy for eight weeks followed by maintenance therapy. Patients found to have Barrett's epithelium require long-term maintenance therapy. Given the natural history of the disease, patients on maintenance therapy may intermittently require dose escalation for 4 weeks to settle symptoms before resumption of the maintenance dose. It is important to emphasise that some patients may have symptoms of GORD that interfere with their activities of daily life, despite no objective evidence of oesophagitis at endoscopy. These patients have what is termed 'non-erosive reflux disease'. Provided they are not proven to have any other aetiology; every attempt should be made to manage their symptoms.

Patients with persistent symptoms or inflammation despite maximal doses of PPIs, may benefit from combination treatment with H_2-receptor blockers and PPIs with the addition of pro-kinetic agents (particularly in the presence of a hiatus hernia) or baclofen. Persistence of symptoms or inflammation after these measures warrants referral for surgery.

Several studies have shown that fundoplication, both open and laparoscopic, provides better acid suppression and control of reflux symptoms compared to optimal medical therapy both in the short and long term [9]. Surgery is also associated with greater resolution of oesophagitis, with the endoscopic findings showing around a 10% therapeutic gain in patients who have undergone anti-reflux surgery, even in those who had good symptom control on pharmacologic therapy. Finally, patients report greater satisfaction and larger improvements in health related quality of life (HRQL) following surgical treatment then they do with medical therapy. The curative rate of anti-reflux surgery is estimated at 85-93% of cases.

The main risks associated with anti-reflux surgery are due to the creation of a one-way valve by fundoplication. The tight wrap may cause dysphagia, which is severe enough to require dilatation in about 6% of patients undergoing anti-reflux surgery. Patients also find they cannot belch leading to increased intra-abdominal gas, distension, and flatulence. Similarly, patients may not be able to vomit. Although studies show that surgery significantly improves GORD symptoms, namely heartburn and regurgitation, a substantial proportion of patients still need anti-reflux medication post-operatively. Finally, by reducing the gastric capacity patients may find they have early satiety and subsequent weight loss. Not all patients will regard weight loss as a negative outcome.

Medical Treatment

Medical treatment is indicated for persistent GORD. The medications can be broadly divided into two mechanisms of actions; either neutralisation and/or suppression of gastric acidity to render the refluxate less harmful to the oesophageal mucosa or the improvement of oesophageal clearance, to minimise exposure time to the refluxate. Of the two, acid suppression represents the mainstay of medical treatment for GORD and the current consensus is that empirical therapy with these agents is appropriate initial management for GORD. Therapy other than acid suppression, including prokinetic agents and/or baclofen, should not be used without diagnostic evaluation. It is interesting to note that the placebo response in some GORD clinical trials has been up to 20%, although this is lower in trials comparing proton pump inhibitors efficacy.

Antacids

Antacids are readily available over the counter and are well tolerated, safe and effective in providing fast-acting symptomatic relief in mild cases, though this may be short lived. Antacid – alginate mixtures, such as Gaviscon® provide effective symptom control by forming a viscous solution which floats on top of the gastric contents. This theoretically provides a barrier between the oesophageal mucosa and the refluxate. They are, however, less effective in controlling non-acid reflux and regurgitation and do not heal existing oesophagitis.

H_2 Receptor Antagonists

Drugs that block the H_2 receptor on the parietal cell, leading to decreased gastric acid secretion, include cimetidine, ranitidine and famotidine. Given in divided doses, they may be effective in the symptomatic control and endoscopic healing of oesophagitis in patients with less severe forms of GORD. However, H_2 receptor antagonists have shown lower efficacy than proton pump inhibitors in suppressing acid levels, and their continuous use is associated with the development of tolerance, limiting their long-term use. There is evidence that the addition of a bedtime dose of H_2 receptor antagonist, alongside twice-daily proton pump inhibitor therapy, can be beneficial in selected patients with objective evidence of nocturnal reflux, but again the development of tachyphylaxis may occur after several weeks of use. The H_2 receptor antagonists are generally well tolerated with adverse drug reactions being rare.

Proton Pump Inhibitors

Proton pump inhibitors are the most potent inhibitors of gastric acid secretion available and act by inhibiting the enzyme H^+/K^+-ATPase required for the formation of hydrochloric acid within the parietal cell. An 8-week high dose empiric treatment regimen with a proton pump inhibitor (PPI) is universally advised for patients with symptoms suggestive of GORD. Symptomatic relief and healing of erosive oesophagitis is seen in around 80-85% of patients treated empirically and is considered diagnostic. Furthermore, PPI therapy is associated with superior healing rates and faster symptom control (12% per week) compared with H_2 receptor antagonists (6% per week) and placebo (3% per week) for patients with erosive esophagitis. There are currently six clinically used PPIs, of which two (omeprazole and lansoprazole) can be obtained over the counter, whilst the remaining four (rabeprazole, pantoprazole, esomeprazole and dexlansoprazole) are available only by prescription. Meta-analyses have not shown any major differences in efficacy between the various drugs.

PPI therapy should be initiated with once daily dosing, before the first meal of the day for maximal pH control. In patients with partial response to PPI therapy, increasing the dose to twice daily or switching to a different PPI may provide additional symptom relief. Although data supporting the use of higher-dose PPIs is weak, the pharmacodynamics of the drugs logically supports twice daily dosing and as such makes that a reasonable upper limit for empirical therapy. Non-responders to PPI should be referred for evaluation. In some patients with non-erosive oesophagitis PPIs can be discontinued but for the vast majority of GORD patients' recurrence is universal unless maintenance therapy is administered indefinitely. Maintenance therapy is best used regularly on a daily basis rather than on demand when symptoms occur. There is evidence that the addition of a H_2 receptor agonist to PPI maintenance therapy can establish substantial acid release suppression but is limited by the development of tachyphylaxis.

Generally speaking, PPIs are safe to use, including in pregnant patients if clinically indicated. The risks associated with PPI use include vitamin B12 and calcium deficiencies due to a reduction in the gastric acid. Whilst the former is a theoretical risk not proved in clinical trials, the deficiency in calcium may lead to osteoporosis and fractures of the hip, wrist or spine. The current advice is that concern for hip fractures and osteoporosis should not affect the decision to use PPIs long-term except in patients with other risk factors for hip fractures. PPI therapy may increase the short-term risk of community-acquired pneumonia and enteric infections with *Clostridium difficile* or *Salmonella* and whilst, it is advised, PPI therapy should not be withheld, it should be used with care in patients at particular risk of these infections. Finally, there was a theoretical concern that activation of the antiplatelet agent clopidogrel *via* CYP 2C19 may be impeded by PPIs as they use the same pathway for their metabolism. Clinical studies however have not shown an increased risk for adverse cardiovascular events and as such PPI therapy does not need to be altered in patients with concomitant clopidogrel use.

Prokinetic Agents

The use of prokinetic agents as monotherapy or add-on therapy is not recommended for the routine management of GORD. Oesophageal and gastric motility abnormalities however are relevant in the pathogenesis of GORD and patients with impaired peristaltic function or LOS function may benefit from augmentation of these. As such prokinetic agents are advocated in the management of selected patients, in conjunction with acid suppression therapy, in an effort to reduce oesophageal exposure time. Prokinetic agents such as metoclopramide and domperidone can produce improvements of symptoms but do not heal any underlying oesophagitis.

Metoclopramide works by increasing the pressure at the GOJ, enhancing oesophageal peristalsis and increasing gastric emptying. There is currently limited clinical data showing any additional benefit of metoclopramide to PPI therapy, and in the absence of gastroparesis there is no clear role for it. In a small number of patients, less than 1%, metoclopramide can have serious central nervous system side effects, including drowsiness, agitation, depression, dystonia and tardive dyskinesia. The peripherally acting dopamine agonist domperidone has an efficacy that is similar to that of metoclopramide for gastric emptying and may be used as an alternative prokinetic. Prior to treatment, the patient should be monitored for a prolonged QT due to a small risk of domperidone causing ventricular arrhythmias and sudden cardiac death.

Baclofen

The neurotransmitter GABA modulates the frequency of TLOSR and baclofen is a $GABA_B$ agonist that has shown to reduce both their frequency and subsequent reflux episodes. It may have a role as an alternative for patients with GORD symptoms refractory to PPIs, in which case a trial of baclofen at a dosage of 5-20 mg up to three times day can be initiated. Currently, however, as there is limited data regarding the efficacy of baclofen in GORD, its use is not licensed. The side effects of the drug include dizziness, constipation and somnolence.

ANTI-REFLUX SURGERY

Most patients with GORD will find that their symptoms are adequately controlled with changes in lifestyle and/or pharmacological agents. Around 15% of patients however will experience 'failure of medical treatment', defined as on-going reflux symptoms despite acid suppression therapy, of adequate dosage, for a minimum period of 3 months. Within this group, patients intolerant of medical therapy either due to troublesome side effects to multiple agents or patients who are unable to comply with medical therapy should be considered for surgical treatment. Furthermore, whilst medical therapy treats the symptoms of reflux, the underlying reflux problem is not corrected and so treatment will often be continued indefinitely. Surgical management on the contrary aims to provide a curative reconstruction of the anti-reflux barrier at the GOJ and achieve effective control of gastro-oesophageal reflux [10]. Subsequently, surgical intervention should be considered in patients with continuing symptoms while on medical therapy or drug-refractory GORD [11]. In addition, surgical treatment should be considered for patients who develop complications of GORD while on medical therapy.

Indications for Surgery

1. *Failed Medical Management:* Surgery for GORD is indicated in situations where the patient has tried optimal dosage drug therapy and it has either failed to control the symptoms or caused unacceptable side effects, or when the patient is poorly compliant with the medication regimen. This category also includes cases where the disease has continued to progress despite best medical therapy. Patients with reflux symptoms due to the presence of a hiatus hernia (stress reflux), rendering the LOS incompetent, are also candidates for surgical intervention.

2. Severe Disease: The complications of GORD include ulcerative oesophagitis, strictures, columnar metaplasia and secondary motility disorders of the oesophagus. If the patient is fit enough to withstand surgical intervention, then it should be considered, although many patients who develop complications are elderly, frail with multiple co-morbidities for whom surgery would be inappropriate. The extra-oesophageal complications of GORD arise from the probable overspill of the refluxate into the respiratory tree and acid suppression therapy alone will not reduce the volume of the refluxate. Anti-reflux surgery is indicated in those patients who can tolerate surgery. Another scenario where anti-reflux surgery gives better symptom control compared to acid suppression alone is in Barrett's oesophagus, possibly due to the role of alkaline reflux, and as such anti-reflux surgery is preferable.

3. Individual Choice: Some people, especially younger ones, may not wish to take continuous and lifelong acid-suppression medication. In these cases, an individualised assessment of the risk to benefit ratio of anti-reflux surgery should be undertaken. Ideally this should also consider socio-economic implications, both for the state and the individual. It is estimated that the cost of maintenance therapy, in the form of PPIs, over the course of 10 years far exceeds the costs of anti-reflux surgery.

Contra-indications to Surgery

The absolute contra-indications to anti-reflux surgery are the presence of oesophageal cancer and Barrett's mucosa with untreated high-grade dysplasia. The relative contra-indications include elderly patients with significant comorbidities, due to the unacceptable high risk of cardiopulmonary complications in this group, and patients with functional heartburn and no objective evidence of gastro-oesophageal reflux as anti-reflux surgery will not benefit this group and may even make the symptoms worse.

Objectives of Surgery

The first surgical approach to managing GORD focused on hiatal hernia repair. Unsurprisingly, this approach was unsuccessful and attention shifted on to augmentation of the GOJ. The aim of current anti-reflux surgery is to restore the GOJ below the diaphragm and achieve an adequate length of intra-abdominal oesophagus. In addition, the competency of the LOS is restored and any existing hiatal herniae are repaired, with crural approximation. Fundoplication was first introduced in 1956, by Rudolph Nissen, and since then fundoplication, whether it be Nissen's total fundoplication or one of its modifications, has become the most commonly performed anti-reflux operation in the world. In fundoplication, the lower oesophagus is mobilised and then the fundus of the stomach is either totally or partially wrapped around it. A range of partial fundoplication procedures have been described of which the two most enduring are Toupet's posterior 270° and Dor's 180° anterior approaches. The Belsey Mark IV repair is an anterior partial fundoplication performed via thoracic access whilst a Collis gastroplasty is performed, in the presence of a short oesophagus, to construct a tension free fundoplication.

It is postulated that fundoplication works by

i. Creating a floppy one-way valve so that an increase in intra-gastric pressure causes increased compression of the lower oesophagus and increased LOS pressure and tone
ii. Exaggerating the angle of HIS and preventing effacement of the lower oesophagus, during gastric distension, thereby strengthening the LOS
iii. Reducing the frequency of TLOSR and rendering swallowing induced relaxations incomplete
iv. Decreasing gastric capacity and improving transit times

In addition, the reduction of any hiatal hernia, and restoration of anatomy, during anti-reflux surgery improves oesophageal clearance, enhances crural and diaphragmatic function and increases the LOS pressure.

Pre-operative Considerations

The proper selection of patients for anti-reflux surgery optimises its outcomes. All patients must undergo a thorough history and physical assessment and it is critical to have objective evidence demonstrating that pathological reflux exists.

Diagnostic Tests: Current advice is that all patients undergoing anti-reflux surgery should have pre-operative endoscopy, manometry and ambulatory pH studies to obtain objective evidence of reflux [12]. Pre-operative endoscopy is the most essential, and will confirm the presence of any oesophagitis or length of Barrett's. It can also identify a hiatus hernia, which may need concurrent repair, and be used to dilate existing strictures prior to anti-reflux surgery. Ambulatory 24-hour pH monitoring is essential in NERD patients and is particularly useful if there are atypical symptoms, as it confirms the presence of increased distal oesophageal acid exposure and establishes if the symptoms are associated with reflux events. Prolonged ambulatory pH monitoring is currently the gold standard for establishing a diagnosis of pathological acid reflux. Manometry evaluates peristaltic function pre-operatively and if there is any oesophageal dysmotility then some surgeons advocate a partial fundoplication. Finally, impedance testing maybe performed in selected patients to distinguish between acid and non-acid reflux. A word of caution, none of these tests, however, is individually sufficiently reliable to base *all* preoperative decisions on its outcome.

Strictures and Rings: In patients with long-standing GORD the chronic mucosal inflammation leads to the formation of reflux associated strictures, which are pathognomonic for severe disease. Strictures can cause significant dysphagia, with weight loss and malnutrition. They are also associated with oesophageal shortening making it difficult to mobilise an adequate length of intra-abdominal oesophagus for fundoplication. When detected on endoscopy they should be dilated, preferably with a balloon dilator, prior to attempting fundoplication. Ambulatory pH monitoring becomes unnecessary as the presence of a tight stricture may prevent reflux of acid, resulting in a false-negative pH study.

Schatzki's rings may also cause dysphagia in GORD patients, but unlike strictures they are submucosal fibrotic bands and not pathognomonic for GORD. Whilst they can be dilated on endoscopy using pneumatic balloon dilators (Fig. 7), abnormal distal oesophageal acid exposure must be documented, *via* ambulatory pH monitoring, prior to performing anti-reflux surgery.

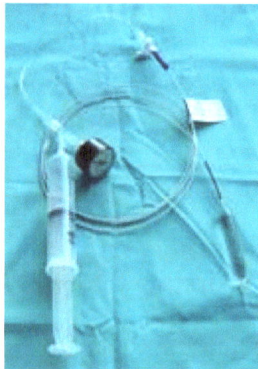

Fig. (7). Pneumatic balloon dilator.

Hiatus Hernia: Hiatus hernias disrupt the crural diaphragm thereby affecting the competence of the LOS and the length of the intra-abdominal oesophagus. It is prudent that they are detected pre-operatively, through endoscopy or radiology contrast studies, as it is necessary to repair them at the time of the fundoplication, to ensure a satisfactory outcome from the subsequent anti-reflux surgery.

Obesity: The prevalence of GORD increases linearly with BMI as obesity raises intra-abdominal pressure, lowers LES pressure, and leads to more frequent TLOSR. Obese patients with GORD pose a challenge to surgeons, and whilst laparoscopic anti-reflux surgery can be performed safely, studies have shown a higher rate of surgical failure compared to normal weight patients. A laparoscopic Roux-en-Y gastric bypass is the most durable method of weight loss and control of obesity-related GORD, with short-term results showing the resolution of reflux symptoms in 94% of patients. In morbidly obese patients, serious consideration should be given to performing a laparoscopic Roux-en-Y gastric bypass instead of a fundoplication. Ultimately, this decision must include a careful balance of the patients' interest in bariatric surgery, presence of other medical comorbidities, and availability of a surgeon with adequate experience.

Surgical Anti-reflux Procedures

Anti-reflux surgery, usually laparoscopic fundoplication, is effective at reducing all forms of reflux and is the best treatment for patients with a hiatus hernia. It works best in those with documented reflux and a PPI response. The choice of which anti-reflux surgery to perform is largely dictated by the surgeon's individual preference and experience. Nonetheless most general surgeons prefer the laparoscopic trans-abdominal route and use the Nissen procedure or one of its modifications. Fundoplication may however be difficult in obese patients, those with dense adhesions from previous abdominal surgery or those with a narrow barrel-shaped chest. Evidence evaluating anti-reflux surgery over the last few decades suggests that a systemisation of the key operative steps, irrespective of fundoplication type, may help ensure operative success. There is no longer a common place for the Belsey Mark 4 repair in the general surgical community although some thoracic surgeons continue to practice this repair. Oesophageal lengthening procedures are very rarely required.

Total (Nissen) Fundoplication

Total fundoplication is designed to create a circumferential wrap of gastric fundus around the mobilised abdominal oesophagus, and is associated with excellent long-term outcome. In this procedure, the distal oesophagus is extensively mobilised in the posterior mediastinum to bring the GOJ at least 3 cm intra-abdominally, reducing any hiatal hernias simultaneously. The vagal trunks are preserved and so are the vagal branches to the liver that run through the pars flaccida. Adequate mobilisation of the fundus may entail division of the upper short gastric vessels, the posterior gastric artery and adhesions between the posterior surface of the upper stomach and the pancreas. Crural repair is performed posteriorly with interrupted sutures. The posterior fundus is passes behind the oesophagus and brought forward, to encircle it. This fundoplication is fixed using 3 or 4 interrupted sero-muscular sutures, which must also anchor the oesophageal wall and the anterior margin of the diaphragmatic hiatus to prevents slippage of the wrap. The classic fundoplication described by Nissen was a 360° wrap that was around 5 cm in length and created using a 32F bougie in the oesophagus (Fig. **8**).

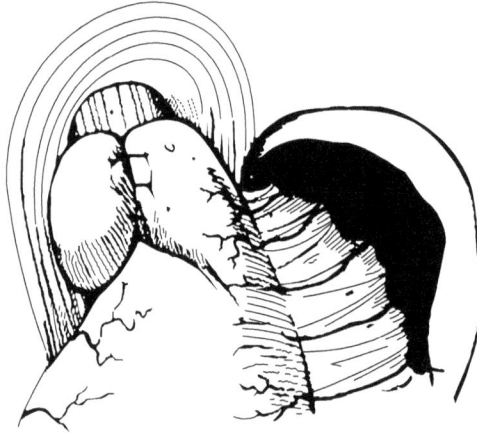

Fig. (8). Nissen fundoplication.

Notably, Nissen did not repair the crura or divide the short gastric vessels in his original description. It resulted in a super competent sphincter, which did not permit belching, or vomiting, and lead to dysphagia and gas bloat syndrome in an unacceptable proportion of patients. He subsequently modified the procedure, the **Nissen-Rosetti**, by dividing the short gastric vessels, using the anterior gastric fundus alone to create the wrap and by adding a gastropexy to prevent slippage.

Further modifications to the original procedure, to create a loose or floppy wrap, were made by Donahue and Bombeck, who recommended the use of a larger 50F bougie and using a shorter length of intra-abdominal oesophagus. They emphasised the role of this 'short floppy cuff' in avoiding post-operative dysphagia and dehiscence. These recommendations were supplemented by DeMeester, who advocated the use of a larger 60F bougie, division of the short gastric vessels to allow sufficient fundal mobilisation and shortening the length of the fundoplication to 2 cm using three interrupted sutures. This procedure is called a **Floppy Nissen** fundoplication and when properly constructed post-operative dysphagia is usually transient.

Another modification is the **Rosetti-Hell**, which was advocated for obese and difficult patients. This procedure creates a smaller wrap using the anterior wall of the fundus only, preserving the short gastric vessels and simplifying both the fundal and oesophageal mobilisation. Crural repair is also optional. The Rosetti-Hell has shown good results and does have its advocates but is rarely used in practise.

Partial Fundoplication

These procedures have become popular in order to minimise the problems of dysphagia and the gas bloat syndrome frequently encountered after a complete wrap. The two procedures that provide good reflux control comparable to that achieved by the Floppy Nissen fundoplication are the Toupet (posterior) partial fundoplication and the Dor (anterior) partial fundoplication. In addition, the Belsey Mark IV repair is an anterior partial fundoplication.

Toupet Posterior (270°) Partial Fundoplication.

After full mobilisation of the abdominal oesophagus and gastric fundus, including division of the short gastric vessels if necessary, the gastric fundus is passed behind the oesophagus. A posterior (270°) wrap is created by anchoring the right hemi-fundus, to the right pillar of the diaphragm and oesophageal wall, using one of the stitches to also fix the gastric fundus to the median arcuate ligament. Similarly, the left hemi-fundus is sutured to the left oesophageal wall and left crura. The fixation of the partial wrap to the crura is important as it prevents herniation through the hiatus and abolishes tension on the oesophageal sutures. Crural approximation to close the diaphragmatic hiatus is also performed. The procedure is thought to result in less post-operative dysphagia but its efficacy is thought to be short lasting.

Dor Anterior (180°) Partial Fundoplication

This procedure does not require extensive mobilisation of the posterior oesophageal attachments. The fundus is wrapped in front of the anterior 180° aspect of the oesophagus and sutured to both the gastro-oesophageal junction and the right crus. Any hiatal defects are also suture closed. The overall effect is to accentuate the angle of His and anchor 3-5 cm of oesophagus in the abdomen. The Dor fundoplication is frequently used in combination with a Heller myotomy for achalasia. This procedure is also thought to result in less post-operative dysphagia but its efficacy is thought to be short lasting.

Belsey Mark IV Repair

This entails a 270° anterior partial fundoplication performed through a left postero-lateral thoracotomy at the level of the sixth rib. Through the hiatus, the gastric fundus is mobilised and wrapped around a length of 3-5 cm of the anterior two-thirds (or 270 degrees) aspect of the distal oesophagus. A crural repair is considered an essential component of the operation. Whilst it has shown good results, its thoracic approach is associated with significant morbidity and with the advent of minimal access anti-reflux surgery has fallen from favour. However, it can still be used in patients who have had a previous abdominal fundoplication with significant post-operative adhesions.

Oesophageal Lengthening Procedures

The length of the intra-abdominal oesophagus is integral for a successful fundoplication, and a length greater than 3 cm is deemed adequate. If the GOJ lies at the oesophageal hiatus then the length of oesophagus is usually sufficient. However, patients with long-standing large hiatal herniae or scarring from chronic reflux disease may have a significantly shortened oesophagus. Mobilisation of the posterior mediastinum to the level of the inferior pulmonary veins or, in some cases, selected vagotomy may add 1-2 cm of additional length. Failing that, the oesophagus can be lengthened by means of a **Collis Gastroplasty,** to allow construction of a tension free fundoplication. The Collis gastroplasty entails fashioning a 'neo-oesophagus' from a tube of the gastric lesser curvature to substitute for the intra-abdominal segment of oesophagus. A partial or complete fundoplication may then be performed around the neo-oesophagus. The Collis gastroplasty can be performed via both the open or laparoscopic approaches. Stapling devices are commonly used to construct the neo-oesophagus (Fig. **9**).

It is important to emphasise that oesophageal lengthening procedures are very rarely required nowadays. The reasons for this are not clear. Some surgeons believe that the adequate mobilisation of the lower oesophagus or remnants of the hernia sac adhesions by laparoscopy have allowed the oesophagus to reach the abdomen easily. Whilst some surgeons do not believe that a shortened oesophagus entity exists other than a congenital short oesophagus. A minority of surgeons believe of the existence of this entity and believe that it is responsible for severe dysphagia or early recurrence post-operatively. Surgical dogma apart, when the oesophago-gastric junction could not reach the infra-diaphragmatic abdomen, a lengthening procedure is required. In this circumstance, the procedure becomes more complex and lengthy and requires expertise.

A number of additional anti-reflux procedures, such as the **ligamentum teres cardiopexy** and the **Hill posterior gastropexy,** have been described by enthusiasts citing good results. However, these seem to be only practiced by a diminishing number of surgeons today with limited dissemination of post-operative outcomes. Finally, the insertion of the **Angelchick prosthesis,** a gel filled silastic prosthesis, around the GOJ has also been rendered obsolete due to significant complications and an unacceptably high rate of surgical revision.

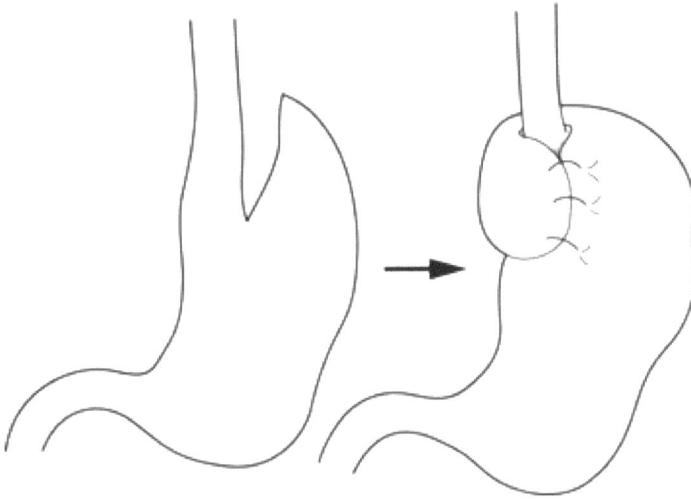

Fig. (9). Collis gastroplasty (left) and fundoplication (right).

Choice of Anti-Reflux Operation

The choice of which anti-reflux surgery to perform is largely dictated by the surgeon's individual preference and experience. Nonetheless most general surgeons prefer the laparoscopic trans-abdominal route and use the Nissen procedure or one of its modifications. Fundoplication may however be difficult in obese patients, those with dense adhesions from previous abdominal surgery or those with a narrow barrel-shaped chest. Evidence evaluating anti-reflux surgery over the last few decades suggests that a systemisation of the key operative steps, irrespective of fundoplication type, may help ensure operative success.

Open or Laparoscopic: Minimal access anti-reflux and hiatal hernia surgery has become increasingly established throughout the world, but it does require significant operative experience and skills in complex laparoscopy [13]. Currently the laparoscopic, trans-abdominal approach for a fundoplication is the gold standard for surgical intervention in patients with GORD. Both laparoscopic total fundoplication and laparoscopic partial fundoplication have shown excellent and comparable clinical outcomes [14, 15]. Laparoscopic fundoplication confers a reduction in peri-operative morbidity, of 65%, compared with open surgery. Whilst the operative times with minimal access surgery are longer, patients undergoing a laparoscopic fundoplication have shorter hospital stays. The minimal access route has further benefits of reduced post-operative pain, wound infections and abdominal wall hernias. Finally large cohort long-term (20 year) studies have shown excellent efficacy of laparoscopic anti-reflux surgery with regards to symptom control, PPI use and objective evaluation of reflux control [16].

Robotic Surgery: The use of robotic anti-reflux surgery, in the form of da Vinci Surgical System (Intuitive Surgical, Sunnyvale, CA), may be a viable and safe option. The results from short-term studies show robotic fundoplication has comparable clinical efficacy, morbidity and length of hospital stay to laparoscopic surgery, though there are no studies suggesting its superiority. It does have advantages for the surgeon, such as improved ergonomics, visualisation and comfort. However, its use maybe limited due to higher costs and longer operating times.

Total or Partial Fundoplication: The evidence available remains conflicting on whether there is a significant difference between partial and total fundoplication [17]. Studies comparing the anterior Dor wrap to a Nissen showed less dysphagia in those undergoing a Dor, however the Dor appeared less effective than a Nissen in controlling the symptoms of reflux and had higher re-operation rates. Similarly, when compared to the posterior Toupet wrap, the Dor again demonstrated less dysphagia but higher prevalence of post-operative heartburn and PPI use. On the other hand, the Toupet and Nissen both demonstrate a high level of reflux control and seem comparable in efficacy on long term follow up studies. The Toupet partial fundoplication has been advocated by some studies as a more physiological repair compared to a Nissen's with reduced morbidity, 8.5% versus 13.5% respectively, with regards to post-operative dysphagia, bloating or flatulence.

The tailored approach in patients with GORD and oesophageal dysmotility, which promoted a partial over a total fundoplication, has long been discredited. Studies have failed to demonstrate a difference between patients undergoing partial versus total fundoplication, in terms of reflux control and improved peristalsis. With inconsistent data on which fundoplication gives the most durable control of reflux symptoms and the best side effect profile, the decision to employ a partial versus a total wrap currently appears to be based on local cultures and practices [18].

Division of Short Gastric Vessels: In his original fundoplication Nissen did not divide the short gastric vessels. Since then much debate has arisen on this topic with some advocating division of the short gastric vessels to achieve full fundal mobilisation, enabling a tension free fundoplication and better post-operative outcomes. To date, however, evidence suggests that the division of the short gastric vessels does increase the length of the operation but does not affect post-operative complications nor the clinical outcome of anti-reflux surgery [19]. It may not, therefore, be routinely necessary. It is necessary if the gastric fundus could not be placed without tension to fashion the fundoplication.

Predictors of Operative Success

Certain aspects of the preoperative work up may help predict operative success.

Of these an abnormal 24-hour ambulatory pH study is the strongest predictor of success, followed closely by the presence of typical symptoms of GORD. In patients with typical symptoms of GORD the long-term success rates of laparoscopic Nissen fundoplication is 85% compared to 41% in those with atypical symptoms. A clinical response, albeit partial, to acid suppression therapy is also a predictor of operative success. The combination of all three of these aforementioned predictors will lead to symptomatic improvement in over 90% of patients after anti-reflux operations.

Operative considerations, which are key to maximising the success of any fundoplication include adequate mobilisation of the mediastinal oesophagus, to achieve an intra-abdominal oesophageal length of at least 3 cm, and recognising a short oesophagus. A short oesophagus is rare but should be suspected if there is a long-standing, large non-reducible hernia, or a long segment of Barrett's or multiple peptic strictures. In these situations, oesophageal lengthening procedures such as the Collis gastroplasty should be considered. In additional the gastric fundus should be mobilised fully, and division of the short gastric vessels should be considered to facilitate this. The fundoplication should be loose, (formed around a bougie) and it should be secured intra-abdominally. The length of the wrap also appears to determine the quality of reflux control with a 2 cm wrap yielding better patient outcomes than a 5 cm wrap. Finally, crural closure is imperative.

In contrast, several factors are classed as being indicative of operative failure. These factors include large hiatal hernias, reflux that predominately occurs during the daytime and in the upright position, severe oesophageal dysmotility disorders, such as achalasia or scleroderma, or the presence of functional gastrointestinal disorders or chronic pain problems. Patients with failure or poor response to PPI therapy preoperatively also show poor resolution of reflux symptoms after surgery, with long-term success rates of laparoscopic Nissen fundoplication being 77% in patients that responded to pre-operative acid suppression therapy compared with 56% in the poor response category.

Post-operative Recovery

The majority of patients, without pre-existing cardiopulmonary co-morbidities can be managed post-operatively in a surgical ward. The length of hospital stays ranges from 1 to 4 days, and in some centres anti-reflux surgery is performed as a day case procedure. Initially patients are started on a clear fluid diet after the operation with a view to progressing to a free fluid diet by day 1 post-operatively. Patients can be considered for discharge once they have established a diet that allows them to maintain their hydration and nutrition levels, have adequate pain control on oral analgesics and are voiding their bladder without the use of a urinary catheter. Following discharge patients are advised to introduce soft foods into their diet slowly. They should expect to return to normal daily activities in 2 weeks and to be able to resume a diet without limitations in about 4 to 6 weeks. Before discharge, patients should be given dietary advice on which foods to avoid in order not to have dysphagia.

Complications of Anti-Reflux Surgery

All surgical procedures carry risks of complications or adverse outcomes. Fortunately for anti-reflux surgery these risks are rare, in large part due to its elective setting and minimal access approaches. In particular the 30-day post-operative risk of mortality is below 1% and morbidity is 5-15%, whilst the rate of converting a laparoscopic fundoplication to an open one is around 2.5% [10, 20]. The common post-operative complications are gaseous bloating, dysphagia and diarrhoea (Table **6**). For most patients these symptoms will improve with conservative management within 3-6 months.

Table 6. Complications arising from anti-reflux surgery [10, 20].

Complication	Frequency
Mortality (commonly from gastric necrosis, GI perforation or haemorrhage or from cardiopulmonary complications *e.g.* PE)	<1%
Gastrointestinal Perforation	0-4%
Bleeding +/- Splenic Injury	0-2%
Pneumothorax	0-2%
Severe nausea and vomiting	2-5%
Gas Bloat Syndrome and Flatulence	12-85%
Dysphasia	3-24%
Diarrhoea	18-33%

Gastrointestinal Visceral Perforation: Perforation of any hollow viscus can rarely occur, with oesophageal or gastric perforations being the commonest. Perforation rates range from 0-4% and the rates are similar in both laparoscopic and open approaches and are higher in re-do fundoplications. They can arise from trocar introduction, bougie placement, through excessive traction or during adhesiolysis. If not discovered and repaired immediately at the time of the primary surgery, they can cause considerable morbidity and be life threatening.

Bleeding and Splenic Injury: Bleeding can arise from many causes, but the two pertinent to fundoplication are from division of the short gastric vessels and from capsular tears of the spleen. The incidence of splenic parenchymal injury that results in bleeding is around 2%, with concurrent splenectomy being needed on rare occasions. The advent of laparoscopic fundoplication has significantly reduced the rate of concurrent splenectomy during anti-reflux surgery. Patients that do require an emergency splenectomy, however, have increased rates of post-operative morbidity and mortality. Early mobilisation of the gastric fundus, using left crus first approach, may visualize the spleen and short gastric vessels sooner and help prevent splenic injuries. In addition, a tension free wrap reduces the tension on short gastric vessels that may bleed.

Pneumothorax: Tearing of the left pleura can occur during mediastinal dissection, in around 2% of cases, and is more likely in patients with large hiatal hernias. Violation of the pleura should be identified intra-operatively and sutured. As the underlying lung is not injured, the lung will re-expand rapidly and a chest drain may not be necessary. However, a post-operative chest radiograph should be obtained in all patients as an ongoing pneumothorax may necessitate the placement of a chest drain.

Post-operative Nausea and Vomiting (PONV): PONV usually arises in around 5% of patients from the use of anaesthetic medications. Vomiting early on in the post-operative period, such as in recovery, can lead to disruption of the crural closure or herniation of the fundoplication. Consequently, patients with persistent PONV should undergo contrast swallow imaging to assess the integrity of the fundoplication, as soon as feasible as a delay can lead to increased morbidity, and increase the complexity of re-do surgery, such as from the presence adhesions.

Gas Bloat Syndrome and Flatulence: The recreation of a functional GOJ, via fundoplication, can lead to a super competent LOS and an inability to belch. This can lead to gaseous distension of the abdomen and increased flatulence, known as gas bloat syndrome, in a wide range, around 12-85%, of post-operative patients. The true risk of this complication is uncertain, partly as it is poorly defined and often self-reported by way of questionnaire (recall bias) in many studies. Generally, though these symptoms are worse after a total fundoplication as opposed to a partial one. Remedies for gas bloat syndrome include dietary modifications, especially the elimination of carbonated beverages from the diet, stopping smoking and taking prokinetic medication. Accidental vagotomy is a risk of fundoplication, and as such patients with debilitating symptoms should be investigated for delayed gastric emptying.

Dysphagia: An element of dysphagia is expected, as the oesophageal tissues are hypersensitive and oedematous from handling. Most dysphagia resolves in 2-3 months with some dietary modifications. However, 3-24% of patients report ongoing dysphagia. This can be due to a tight fundoplication or crural closure, or from unidentified achalasia or strictures. Dysphasia persisting beyond 3 months and/or dysphagia to liquids will warrant investigation, either by OGD, manometry or contrast studies. If the fundoplication is intact, dilatation may be attempted and in two thirds of cases the dysphagia responds to this maneuver. If, however there is a slipped fundoplication, para-oesophageal hernia or failure to dilatation than re-do surgery may need to be considered.

Diarrhoea: For most patients post-operative diarrhoea is mild, low volume and settles within 6 weeks post-operatively. The cause for this diarrhoea is uncertain and maybe due to inadvertent vagal injury or a form of dumping syndrome. In any case the management is largely empirical.

Failed Anti-reflux Surgery

The predictors of a favourable surgical outcome have been discussed. Patients not meeting these criteria or those with atypical symptoms should receive pre-operative counselling that anti-reflux surgery may have a higher risk of symptomatic failure and/or that the complications of surgery may be more common. Alternative explanations for their symptoms should be aggressively pursued by adequate investigations of their symptoms taken individually and collectively, prior to embarking on anti-reflux surgery. It is important to note that up to 50% of patients can be on acid suppression therapy within 5 years after surgery. In the absence of anatomical disruption of the wrap in the majority of patients, the reasons for this are not clear.

The rate of failure for anti-reflux surgery can be as high as 15%, whereby the patient has a recurrence of their reflux symptoms necessitating a return to acid suppression therapy and an abnormal 24-hour pH monitoring and/or oesophageal manometry. Failures usually occur within two years of the operation and can be physiological, usually due to poor patient selection, or anatomical from disruption of the fundoplication [21]. Anatomical failures tend to fit into 5 main categories:

Herniation of the Fundoplication into the Chest (Type Ia)

This is the commonest failure reported, between 30-80%, and leads to the displacement of the GOJ into the chest. These usually result from disruption of the crural repair or failure to perform a tension free wrap. Ensuring at least 2-3 cm of tension free intra-abdominal oesophagus below a clearly identified GOJ can help avoid these types of failures (Fig. **10**).

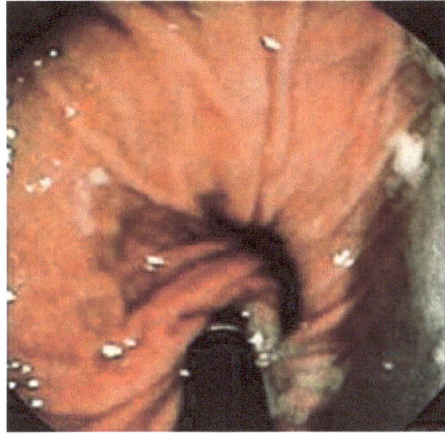

Fig. (10). Herniation of the fundoplication in to the chest (Type Ia) seen through an endoscopic view.

Slipped Fundoplication (Type Ib)

This occurs in 15-30% of failures either through slipping of the stomach through the fundoplication or incorrect positioning of the wrap around the stomach at the time of operation, leaving a part of the stomach above and below the wrap (Fig. **11**).

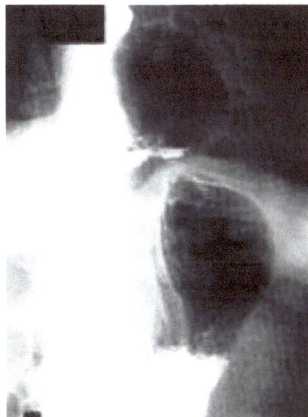

Fig. (11). Slipped fundoplication with recurrent hiatus hernia (Type Ib) as seen on a double contrast barium meal.

Para-oesophageal Herniation (Type II)

Accounting for up to 20% of failures, these arise from inadequate hiatal closure or a redundant wrap, with the excess wrap leading the formation of the hernia. Ensuring the wrap is not twisted or redundant and positioned appropriately on the distal oesophagus may help prevent this (Fig. **12**).

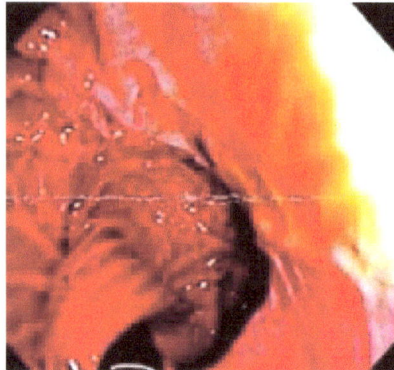

Fig. (12). Para-oesophageal herniation after a Nissen's fundoplication seen endoscopically.

Malpositioned Fundoplication (Type III)

This leads to the formation of a bilobed stomach and occurs in around 10% of failures, with patients presenting with abdominal pain and worsening regurgitation.

Tight Fundoplication

In these cases, the wrap may be appropriately positioned but generated too much resistance leading to failure of the oesophageal pump. The deployment of pre-operative manometry to identify underlying oesophageal peristaltic problems, the use of an intra-operative bougie (52-56°F) or performing a floppy or partial wrap may help prevent this.

Corrective Surgery

Re-do operations for fundoplication should only be undertaken by experienced upper GI surgeons after careful review of the patients' pre-operative work-up. The key principles for a successful re-do fundoplication are restoring the original anatomy by completely taking down the old fundoplication and the recognition and management of oesophageal shortening. Re-do operations can be performed laparoscopically but have higher conversion rates to open surgery. Furthermore, in comparison to the initial operation, re-do surgery has longer operation times and higher complication and mortality rates and lower likelihood of successfully controlling the GORD symptoms.

NOVEL THERAPIES OF GORD

Several endoscopic anti-reflux techniques have been developed, with varying success over the last two decades [22, 23]. As they potentially offer a less invasive curative procedure they have been applied with enthusiasm in some parts of the world. The current endoscopic therapies showing clinical promise are Stretta®, which utilises radiofrequency energy, and Esophyx™ procedure which involves endoscopic fundoplication. A new laparoscopic procedure, the magnetic scarf LINX™, has been introduced more recently. This uses a ring of linked magnetic beads to reinforce the lower oesophageal sphincter and initial clinical experience has produced promising results, though the follow up is limited.

Some of the previously available endoscopic procedures, such as Endocinch™ suturing, the Enteryx injection and the NDO plicator have not survived, due to limited effectiveness and/or severe complications. As a word of caution, most novel procedures appear to be reserved for patients who have documented symptomatic GORD, with positive oesophageal pH studies, and have shown some response to acid suppression medication. Patients with evidence of pulmonary disease, Barrett oesophagus, large hiatal hernias, obesity, severe medical comorbidities, or oesophageal dysmotility disorders have largely been excluded from feasibility studies using these novel therapies.

The Stretta® Procedure

Stretta® (Mederi Therapeutics Inc., Norwalk, CT) was first approved for use by the FDA in 2000. This purpose built device consists of a flexible catheter attached to a balloon and fitted with four sharp titanium electrodes to deliver radiofrequency energy, via a 4-channel generator, into the oesophageal wall and LOS (Fig. **13**). Tissue temperatures are constantly monitored and the device can simultaneously irrigate the overlying mucosa to prevent thermal injury. Delivery of radiofrequency energy causes neurolysis and tissue necrosis leading to contraction and fibrosis of the sphincter. This leads to tightening of the LOS and fewer TLOSR, and ultimately should reduce oesophageal acid exposure thereby improving reflux symptoms. The Stretta® procedure has been reported as being safe, with few recorded adverse events, and can be performed on an outpatient basis with conscious sedation. However, patients with high-grade oesophagitis, Barrett's oesophagus and a hiatus hernia greater than 2 cm have been deemed unsuitable for this procedure.

Clinical data on Stretta® have shown heterogeneous results with regards to oesophageal acid exposure, symptom control, health related quality-of-life (HRQL) and DeMeester scores. There are a number of randomised control trials with poor methodological quality showing debatable benefits of Stretta® over sham therapy, whilst some long-term follow up studies demonstrate an initial improvement in reflux symptoms and HRQL scores that seemingly tails off on follow-up a few years later. Furthermore, there is no evidence to suggest that Stretta® results in higher LOS pressures, or improved outcomes as compared to surgery. Some professional organisations however have found that Stretta® has an acceptable safety profile, with some long-term improvement in reflux symptoms. A few current clinical guidelines, list Stretta® as appropriate therapy for patients with GORD symptoms, of greater than 6 months' duration, who have not responded to medical treatment and have declined fundoplication.

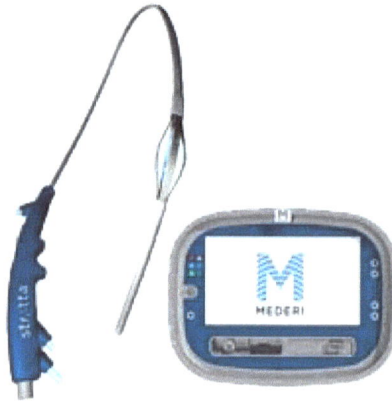

Fig. (13). Stretta device showing the flexible catheter balloon and the 4-channel generator.

Esophyx™ Plication

The Esophyx™ (EndoGastric Solutions, San Mateo, CA) device allows creation of an incision-less 270° anterior partial fundoplication, of 2-3 cm, by using proprietary tissue manipulating apparatus and approximately 12 full-thickness polypropylene H-fasteners (Fig. **14**). The procedure is performed endoscopically under general anaesthesia and visualised via a flexible video endoscope passed down the device. This trans-oral incision-less fundoplication (TIF), procedure mimics the principles of surgical fundoplication by elongating the intra-abdominal oesophagus, reducing any hiatal hernias, approximating the fundus around the distal oesophagus and restoring the distal high pressure zone. The manufacturers claim that as a partial wrap, the TIF provides a more physiological repair than a full 360° degree wrap and that the 'over shaft' construction technique prevents excessively tight fundoplication and subsequent dysphagia or gas bloat. Finally, the incision less and dissection free approach may result in less discomfort, faster recovery times and eliminate the risk of intra-abdominal adhesions.

Clinical evaluation of the Esophyx™ device has shown some promise. The TIF procedure appears to be effective, improving about 80% of typical and 65% of atypical symptoms of GORD in short term follow up studies. It has also shown improved symptom outcomes as measured by GORD-HRQL and DeMeester scores. Patients are advised to remain on PPIs for 2 weeks post procedure, and then to discontinue usage, with evidence suggesting the reduced need for long term PPIs. Follow up at 2 years post TIF has shown around 70% of patients had remained completely PPI free. Complications that have arisen post TIF include mediastinal abscesses, haemorrhages, pneumothorax, oesophageal perforations and dysphagia. Overall failure rate requiring alternate intervention was around 10% with particularly low efficacy in patients with large hiatus herniae or oesophageal dysmotility.

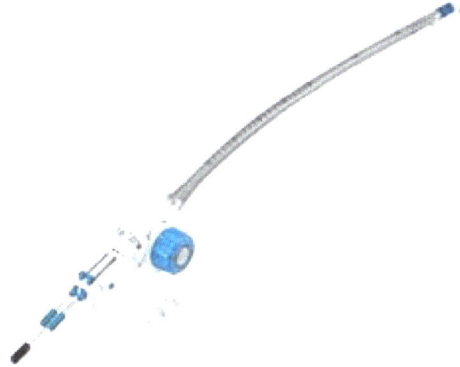

Fig. (14). The Esophyx plication device.

The current recommendation is that Esophyx™ may be effective in patients with small hiatal herniae with typical and atypical GORD symptoms. However, there is insufficient long-term data to define appropriate patient selection criteria, and to fully evaluate the device's efficacy and safety.

LINX™

The LINX™ (Torax Medical Inc., Shoreview, MN) procedure entails placing a ring of magnetic beads laparoscopically at the LOS to augment the sphincter. The beads are linked to each other via magnetic bonds and titanium wires, so that they cannot separate but can move independently, thus reducing the compressive forces at the oesophageal sphincter and allowing swallowing, belching and vomiting to occur unimpeded (Fig. **15**). The procedure requires less dissection than a Nissen fundoplication, so it is hoped to have a shorter learning curve and will allow patients to re-establish a solid diet earlier than after a traditional fundoplication procedure. It is not suitable for patients with metal allergies, pacemakers or defibrillators and patients cannot undergo magnetic resonance imaging after the procedure.

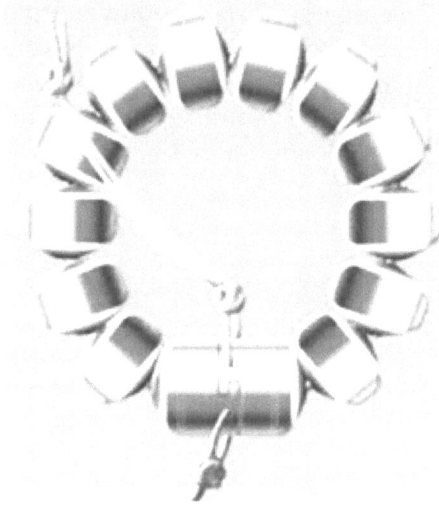

Fig. (15). The magnetic beads LINX device.

The LINX™ procedure was granted FDA approval in 2012, for patients with symptomatic GORD, with documented abnormal pH recordings, and those who have symptoms despite acid suppression therapy and do not want to undergo fundoplication. The clinical evidence supporting its use comes from non-randomised small cohort studies, of 100 patients or less, with no control groups for comparison. Nonetheless this data has shown an acceptable safety profile, with no migration or erosion of the beads into the oesophagus, and some improvement in oesophageal acid exposure and HRQL, as well as a decreased need for acid suppression therapy. The main complication of the procedure is dysphagia occurring in up to 68% of patients. The current opinion is that LINX™ has reasonable assurance of efficacy, although clearly there is a need for longer follow up studies.

CONSENT FOR PUBLICATION

Not applicable.

CONFLICT OF INTEREST

The authors declare no conflict of interest, financial or otherwise.

ACKNOWLEDGEMENT

Declare none.

REFERENCES

[1]   Vakil N, van Zanten SV, Kahrilas P, Dent J, Jones R. The Montreal definition and classification of gastroesophageal reflux disease: a global evidence-based consensus. Am J Gastroenterol 2006; 101(8): 1900-20.
[http://dx.doi.org/10.1111/j.1572-0241.2006.00630.x] [PMID: 16928254]

[2]   El-Serag HB, Sweet S, Winchester CC, Dent J. Update on the epidemiology of gastro-oesophageal reflux disease: a systematic review. Gut 2014; 63(6): 871-80.
[http://dx.doi.org/10.1136/gutjnl-2012-304269] [PMID: 23853213]

[3]   Boeckxstaens G E, Rohof W O. Pathophysiology of gastroesophageal reflux disease, gastroenterology clinics of north america, vol 43, pp 15-+, Mar 2014
[http://dx.doi.org/10.1016/j.gtc.2013.11.001]

[4]   Mikami D J, Murayama K M. Physiology and pathogenesis of gastroesophageal reflux disease, surgical clinics of north america, vol 95, pp 515-+, Jun 2015
[http://dx.doi.org/10.1016/j.suc.2015.02.006]

[5]   Johnson LF, DeMeester TR. Development of the 24-hour intraesophageal pH monitoring composite scoring system. J Clin Gastroenterol 1986; 8 (Suppl. 1): 52-8.
[http://dx.doi.org/10.1097/00004836-198606001-00008] [PMID: 3734377]

[6]   Dent J. Endoscopic grading of reflux oesophagitis: the past, present and future. Best Pract Res Clin Gastroenterol 2008; 22(4): 585-99.
[http://dx.doi.org/10.1016/j.bpg.2008.01.002] [PMID: 18656818]

[7]   Vela MF, Gerson LB, Katz PO. Non-Erosive reflux disease is more complex than negative endoscopy only response. Am J Gastroenterol 2013; 108: 1658-9.
[http://dx.doi.org/10.1038/ajg.2013.284] [PMID: 24091512]

[8]   Katz PO, Gerson LB, Vela MF. Guidelines for the diagnosis and management of gastroesophageal reflux disease (vol 108, pg 308, 2013). Am J Gastroenterol 2013; 108: 1672-2.
[http://dx.doi.org/10.1038/ajg.2013.314]

[9]   Yates RB, Oelschlager BK. Surgical treatment of gastroesophageal reflux disease. Surg Clin North Am 2015; 95(3): 527-53.
[http://dx.doi.org/10.1016/j.suc.2015.02.007] [PMID: 25965128]

[10]   Wileman SM, McCann S, Grant AM, Krukowski ZH, Bruce J. Medical versus surgical management for gastro-oesophageal reflux disease (GORD) in adults. Cochrane Database Syst Rev 2010; (3): CD003243.
[PMID: 20238321]

[11]   Rickenbacher N, Kotter T, Kochen MM, Scherer M, Blozik E. Fundoplication versus medical management of gastroesophageal reflux disease: systematic review and meta-analysis (vol 28, pg 143, 2014). Surgical Endoscopy and Other Interventional Techniques 2014; 28: 2002-2.
[http://dx.doi.org/10.1007/s00464-014-3473-2]

[12]   Jobe BA, Richter JE, Hoppo T, *et al.* Preoperative diagnostic workup before antireflux surgery: an evidence and experience-based consensus of the Esophageal Diagnostic Advisory Panel. J Am Coll Surg 2013; 217(4): 586-97.
[http://dx.doi.org/10.1016/j.jamcollsurg.2013.05.023] [PMID: 23973101]

[13]   Fuchs KH, Babic B, Breithaupt W, *et al.* EAES recommendations for the management of gastroesophageal reflux disease. Surg Endosc 2014; 28(6): 1753-73.
[http://dx.doi.org/10.1007/s00464-014-3431-z] [PMID: 24789125]

[14]   Broeders JA, Roks DJ, Ahmed Ali U, *et al.* Laparoscopic anterior 180-degree versus nissen fundoplication for gastroesophageal reflux disease: systematic review and meta-analysis of randomized clinical trials. Ann Surg 2013; 257(5): 850-9.
[http://dx.doi.org/10.1097/SLA.0b013e31828604dd] [PMID: 23470572]

[15]   Broeders JAJL, Mauritz FA, Ahmed Ali U, *et al.* Systematic review and meta-analysis of laparoscopic Nissen (posterior total) versus Toupet (posterior partial) fundoplication for gastro-oesophageal reflux disease. Br J Surg 2010; 97(9): 1318-30.
[http://dx.doi.org/10.1002/bjs.7174] [PMID: 20641062]

[16]   Engström C, Cai W, Irvine T, *et al.* Twenty years of experience with laparoscopic antireflux surgery. Br J Surg 2012; 99(10): 1415-21.
[http://dx.doi.org/10.1002/bjs.8870] [PMID: 22961522]

[17]   Kim D, Velanovich V. Surgical treatment of GERD where have we been and where are we going?, gastroenterology clinics of north america, vol 43, pp 135-+, Mar 2014

[18]   Moore M, Afaneh C, Benhuri D, Antonacci C, Abelson J, Zarnegar R. Gastroesophageal reflux disease: A review of surgical decision making. World J Gastrointest Surg 2016; 8(1): 77-83.
[http://dx.doi.org/10.4240/wjgs.v8.i1.77] [PMID: 26843915]

[19]   Markar SR, Karthikesalingam AP, Wagner OJ, *et al.* Systematic review and meta-analysis of laparoscopic Nissen fundoplication with or without division of the short gastric vessels. Br J Surg 2011; 98(8): 1056-62.
[http://dx.doi.org/10.1002/bjs.7519] [PMID: 21560121]

[20]   Rantanen TK, Oksala NK, Oksala AK, Salo JA, Sihvo EI. Complications in antireflux surgery: national-based analysis of laparoscopic and open fundoplications. Arch Surg 2008; 143(4): 359-65.
[http://dx.doi.org/10.1001/archsurg.143.4.359] [PMID: 18427023]

[21]   Richter JE. Gastroesophageal reflux disease treatment: side effects and complications of fundoplication. Clin Gastroenterol Hepatol 2013; 11(5): 465-71.
[http://dx.doi.org/10.1016/j.cgh.2012.12.006] [PMID: 23267868]

[22]   Hopkins J, Switzer NJ, Karmali S. Update on novel endoscopic therapies to treat gastroesophageal reflux disease: A review. World J Gastrointest Endosc 2015; 7(11): 1039-44.
[http://dx.doi.org/10.4253/wjge.v7.i11.1039] [PMID: 26322157]

[23]   Hummel K, Richards W. Endoscopic treatment of gastroesophageal reflux disease, surgical clinics of north america, vol 95, pp 653-+, Jun 2015
[http://dx.doi.org/10.1016/j.suc.2015.02.016]

CHAPTER 8

Barrett's Oesophagus

Michael Wilson[*]

Department of Surgery, Ninewells Hospital and Medical School, Dundee, Scotland, UK

Abstract: Barrett's oesophagus (BE) is a metaplastic change of the oesophageal mucosa from squamous to columnar mucosa (with intestinal metaplasia). The condition is recognized endoscopically as pink salmon extensions in the lower oesophagus. It is an acquired condition arising as a result of chronic gastro-oesophageal reflux disease (GERD) and is regarded as a premalignant condition of the oesophagus leading to oesophageal adenocarcinoma. Patients typically present with symptomatic GERD, but the condition also occurs in asymptomatic individuals. The diagnosis of BE is made endoscopically and confirmed histologically. BE is a common problem with prevalence rates ranging from 5% to 15% in the general population. The condition is associated with an increased risk of oesophageal adenocarcinoma (OAC), approximately 0.5% per patient per year. This translates to an estimated lifetime risk of cancer development of 5-8%. There is growing acceptance of the metaplasia, dysplasia, adenocarcinoma sequence in the development of adenocarcinoma of the oesophagus. A small but significant proportion of patients with Barrett's metaplasia will develop dysplastic change. Those who progress from low-grade dysplasia (LGD) to high-grade dysplasia (HGD), have a 10% annual risk of developing adenocarcinoma and the 5-year survival for these patients is of the order of 12%. Treatment is dependent upon the degree of dysplasia, and for cancer, the depth of invasion and the presence of lymphovascular invasion. Endoscopic surveillance is warranted for those with low-grade dysplasia (LGD), followed by endoscopic mucosal resection and ablative therapy in those with HGD limited to the mucosa. Surgical resection is reserved for those with established submucosal disease and a high likelihood of lymphovascular invasion.

Keywords: Barrett's oesophagus, Metaplasia, Dysplasia, Oesophageal adenocarcinoma, Surveillance, Endoscopic resection, Radio-frequency ablation, Chemoprevention, Prague classification, Paris Classification, Vienna classification, Seattle biopsy protocol, Guidelines.

OESOPHAGEAL METAPLASIA

To make a diagnosis of Barrett's oesophagus two criteria should be met. First,

---

[*] **Corresponding author Michael Wilson:** Department of Surgery, Ninewells Hospital and Medical School, Dundee DD1 9SY, Scotland, UK; Tel: +44 1382 660111; E-mail: michaelwilson3@nhs.net

Sami M. Shimi (Ed.)

endoscopy should show upward extension of the salmon pink mucosa above the true oesophago-gastric junction (Fig. **1**).

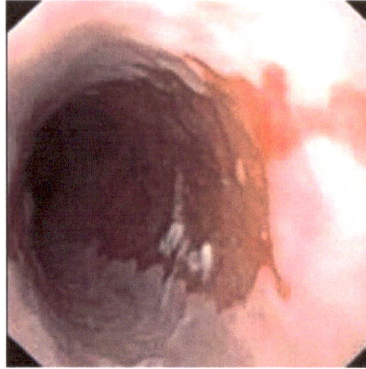

Fig. (1). Endoscopic view of a segment of Barrett's oesophagus. It is pink-salmon coloured in contrast to the paler grey-pink appearance of the native squamous epithelium.

In other words, the squamo-columnar junction is displaced upwards. Normally, the squamo-columnar junction should coincide with the most distal extent of the tubular oesophagus and just above the rugal folds of the stomach. The intersection of the squamous epithelium of the tubular oesophagus and the columnar epithelium of the stomach is termed the Z line (because of its jagged appearance). There is difficulty in accurately depicting the location of the oesophago-gastric junction between surgeons and gastroenterologists. However, the point of cessation of the gastric rugal folds should be taken as the line separating the oesophagus from the stomach. Usually, the Z line separates two types of epithelia: normal squamous epithelium of the lower oesophagus is white or very light pink, whereas columnar epithelium of the stomach is salmon-pink. In Barrett's oesophagus, salmon-coloured epithelium projects into the tubular oesophagus. These projections might present as tongues of tissue, or as circumferential involvement of the mucosa, or both. The second criterion for diagnosis is metaplasia of the epithelium, (containing goblet cells), in a biopsy specimen of mucosa above the oesophago-gastric junction [1]. Metaplastic tissue with or without goblet cells has been termed columnar lined epithelium. Whether identification of goblet cells in the metaplastic epithelium is necessary for diagnosis is debatable. All guidelines require endoscopy showing columnar epithelia (metaplasia) lining the esophagus [2, 3], but the US guidelines require the additional finding of intestinal metaplasia on biopsy to confirm the diagnosis (Fig. **2**).

The need for intestinal metaplasia with identification of goblet cells on biopsy samples, for a diagnosis of BE continues to be the main point of controversy, particularly between American and European gastroenterology societies. Evidence of an increased risk of progression to EAC in subjects exhibiting columnar metaplasia with goblet cells (a marker of intestinal differentiation) compared to those without goblet cells is robust, with large population based cohort studies showing substantially different progression risks amongst these two histologic types. Nevertheless, there is some evidence of comparable molecular abnormalities found in columnar esophageal metaplasia with and without goblet cells associated with neoplastic risk in cross sectional studies of Barrett's patients. Moreover, sampling error and/or a patchy distribution of these cell types may account for a variable appearance of goblet cells on biopsy.

British Society of Gastroenterology
BE is defined as an oesophagus in which any portion of the normal distal squamous epithelium lining has been replaced by **metaplastic columnar epithelium***, which is clearly visible endoscopically ≥1 cm above the gastroesophageal junction and confirmed histopathlogically from oesophageal biopsies.*

American College of Gastroenterology
BE should be diagnosed when there is an extension of salmon coloured mucosa into the tubular oesophagus extending ≥1 cm proximal to the gastroesophageal junction with biopsy confirmation of **intestinal metaplasia***.*

Fig. (2). Contrasting definitions of BE from the British Society of Gastroenterology (BSG) [2] and the American College of Gastroenterology (AGC) [3].

The length of the columnar epithelium above the oesophago-gastric junction should be measured during endoscopy: longer than 3 cm is termed long-segment Barrett's oesophagus; 3 cm or shorter is termed short-segment Barrett's oesophagus. Some investigators have suggested that short segments are not clinically significant, but others have shown an increased cancer risk in even short-segment disease compared with the general population.

Prevalence and Risk Factors

Although Barrett's oesophagus is highly prevalent in the general population, it is much higher in patients undergoing upper GI endoscopy to investigate chronic reflux symptoms, at 5-15%. In interpreting prevalence estimates it is important to take account of the definitions used in prevalence studies. The clinically diagnosed prevalence is around 5% in patients having endoscopy for chronic reflux symptoms. There is less data on patients without reflux symptoms, but it is estimated that about 0.5% of such people in the general population having Barrett's oesophagus. The older (more than 60 years of age) general population have a higher prevalence of around 1%. There is no reliable data on the incidence of Barrett's oesophagus, but the available data suggests very little change in the incidence of this entity despite the apparent increase in the incidence of oesophageal adenocarcinoma. The risk of oesophageal adenocarcinoma in patients with Barrett's oesophagus is low, about 0·5% per patient-year, and most die with the disorder, not as a result of it. However, patients with high-grade dysplasia might have cancer rates of 10% or greater per patient-year

The risk and segment length of Barrett's oesophagus increase with the amount of acid exposure in the distal oesophagus, and are both associated with the presence and size of hiatal hernias. A number of risk factors have been positively associated with an increased risk of Barrett's (Table **1**).

Table 1. Recognised risk factors for BE.

Risk Factors
• Increasing age
• Male gender
• Obesity (visceral)
• Caucasian ethnicity
• Cigarette smoking
• History (and duration) of GERD
• Family history of BE or OAC

In addition to the classic risk factors of gastroesophageal reflux, male gender and Caucasian race, other BE risk factors recently identified include obesity, specifically central obesity, metabolic syndrome, and obstructive sleep apnea. These factors may contribute to the risk of BE which is independent of their additive effects on gastroesophageal reflux.

The association with male gender may be linked to higher BMI and differences in the function of the lower oesophageal sphincter at the cellular level. In females, BE tends to occur later in life than in men. The risk of developing BE increases with each decade of life, and is greater if the onset of GERD symptoms occurs at a young age. This suggests that the development of BE is associated with the duration of GERD symptoms.

The onset of BE is often at a younger age in those with a positive family history and is the subject of current research. Genetic factors, which contribute to BE have also been published. Two recent genome wide association studies have identified polymorphisms which is associated with an increased risk of BE and OAC. Associations have been found in 19p13 in CRTC1, whose aberrant activation has been associated with oncogenic activity, as well as 9q22 in

BARX1, which encodes a transcription factor, which is important in esophageal specification.

Obesity is not directly linked to an increased risk of BE, but may play an indirect role by promoting GERD. The link is strongest in those with a greater degree of visceral obesity. Cigarette smoking and alcohol consumption are also thought to increase the risk of BE and OAC and for smoking, the increase has been found to correlate with the number of pack years.

An inverse relationship between *Helicobacter pylori* (*H. pylori*) and BE has been noted in some observational studies, with significant heterogeneity between studies. A recent meta-analysis focused on four methodologically robust studies, found a relative risk of 0.46 (95% CI: 0.35-0.60) for the development of BE among persons infected with *H. pylori*. A subgroup analysis showed that the inverse effect was stronger for infection with CagA-positive strains.

Other associated factors that are the subject of current research and debate include: diabetes mellitus, obstructive sleep apnoea, metabolic syndrome, low birth weight and the use of oral bisphosphonates. Each of the identified risk factors may increase the risk of BE and OAC in isolation or in a synergistic manner.

Pathogenesis

The risk of both Barrett's oesophagus and oesophageal adenocarcinoma has long been known to be related to body-mass index (BMI). There are several theories as to how central obesity might contribute to the development of Barrett's oesophagus. However, the initiating event is probably related to an episode of erosive oesophagitis denuding the oesophagus of normal epithelium and allowing it to become repopulated with columnar epithelium. As a result of synergy between acid and bile, continued epithelial exposure and injury (chronic reflux) appears to stimulate oxidative stress and DNA damage. These alterations seem to underlie the development of Barrett's oesophagus and ultimate progression to cancer in a subgroup of patients.

The diminishing prevalence of *H. pylori* infection (with associated decrease in intra-gastric acidity) in developed countries is temporally associated with an increased incidence of GERD complications, including Barrett's oesophagus. The molecular changes underlying the morphological change of Barrett's oesophagus are still being elucidated.

It is widely accepted that carcinogenesis in BE occurs in a stepwise manner from metaplasia to low-grade dysplasia, HGD, early adenocarcinoma, and, finally, metastatic carcinoma. Briefly, this has been termed the metaplasia-dysplasia adenocarcinoma sequence (MDAS) [4]. This makes it an excellent model system for investigation of the multistep nature of carcinogenesis. A specific combination of genomic, transcription, and epigenetic changes is responsible for this multistep transformation of normal squamous esophageal epithelium to BE, dysplasia, and adenocarcinoma. A number of genes involved in a wide range of biological pathways have been implicated, including: DNA repair (*TP53*), cell cycle (*TP53*, *CDKN2A*), signaling (*CTNNB1*), cell adhesion (*CDH1*), and detoxification (*GPX3*, *NOX5*). Progression of BE to EAC is thought to be an unpredictable process, and the time of progression is variable, most likely because a number of unrelated mechanisms are involved in carcinogenesis.

In metaplastic cells exposed to an acidic environment, the natural protective mechanism against reactive molecules is blocked by down regulation of GPX3 and upregulation of NOX5. Acid-stimulated NOX5 is a source of overproduction of ROS in BE that leads to increased accumulation of mutations in general and, in particular, in *TP53*. It prevents cell apoptosis due to DNA damage, and, as a consequence, clones with altered *TP53* get an evolutionary superiority in survival. Another side effect of NOX5 upregulation is hyper methylation of the *CDKN2A–p16INK4A* promoter and, as a consequence, enhanced proliferation. An incompletely understood mechanism of CDH1 down regulation leads to the remarkable cell shape change and release of β-catenin into the cytoplasm and eventually to its nuclear accumulation. This (together with CDKN2A elimination/ablation) leads to the abnormal proliferation through expression of MYC and CCND1. The presence of one or several of these mechanisms is sufficient for cell progression and dysplastic changes.

All the involved genes accumulate genomic, transcription, and/or proteomic alterations in a large subpopulation of OAC patients, and this accumulation correlates well with progression. It attests that each of the genes plays a certain role in BE progression. In addition, all involved genes are functionally interrelated, serving as an essential core for BE progression.

However, most BE patients never progress to OAC in their lifetime. This indicates that the progression mechanism of BE to cancer is complex and involves more than one genomic alteration to initiate cancer. Inevitably, there are a number of additional factors that might influence the time and/or the steps of progression, including inflammation *via* activation of NF-κB, deregulation of telomerase expression through TERT upregulation, enhanced angiogenesis *via* VEGFA upregulation, apoptosis prevention *via* BCL2 overexpression, and cell signaling disruption through genomic alterations in SMAD4, among others. In addition, aneuploidy, clonal expansion, and genomic instability will play a role in this progression. Incorporation of all these (and possibly other unknown) factors will enhance our understanding of BE progression [5].

Biomarkers

Several biomarkers have shown promise as objective adjunct tests to improve risk stratification of patients with BE. Panels of immunohistochemical stains including α-methylacyl-CoA racemase (AMACR), β-catenin, cyclin D1, and p53 show promise in separating grades of dysplasia and in distinguishing true neoplastic progression from reactive changes.

Other biomarkers which test for DNA abnormalities have been evaluated in cross-sectional or retrospective studies. The detection of aneuploidy, increased tetraploidy, and loss of heterozygosity (LOH) for chromosome 17p in patients with no dysplasia or low-grade dysplasia on biopsy has been shown to have good predictive value for neoplastic progression. These studies utilized flow cytometry to detect DNA content abnormalities in fresh frozen tissue, which may not be practical in clinical practice. Fluorescence in situ hybridization can theoretically be used to detect these same abnormalities in fixed tissue and most initial studies show promising results [6].

Presentation

Patients may be entirely asymptomatic, or more typically present with symptoms of longstanding gastroesophageal reflux disease (GORD). Heartburn or acid regurgitation has been reported to be present for more than ten years in up to 98.6% of patients. Symptoms commencing at a younger age are linked to the development of BE and thought to be associated with the duration of GORD.

DIAGNOSIS AND SCREENING

The present gold standard diagnostic tool for BE is standard white-light endoscopy. This is usually sufficient for the diagnosis of metaplasia. More importantly however, is the diagnosis of dysplasia. High-resolution white light endoscopy combines endoscopes with large numbers of pixels (600,000 to 1,000,000), magnification devices, and high-definition screens to optimize visualization of the esophageal mucosa. It has shown greater sensitivity in the detection of early neoplastic lesions when compared to standard endoscopy. Although the primary diagnostic procedure may involve the use of standard white-light endoscopy, patients found to have metaplasia should undergo a further procedure with high-resolution endoscopy. Chemoendoscopy involves the application of chemicals that selectively react with and highlight various mucosal features, theoretically improving the detection of abnormalities. Methylene blue,

Lugol's iodine and indigo carmine have all been examined for detection of dysplasia in BE segments. However, they have not been shown to increase the detection of dysplasia beyond that of high-resolution endoscopy.

Electronic chromoendoscopy includes optimal band imaging which involves post-processing to accentuate the contrast between columnar and squamous epithelia and narrow band imaging (NBI) which uses optical filters to highlight vascular patterns on the mucosal surface. A comparison of NBI to high resolution white light endoscopy showed no significant difference in the detection of BE or dysplasia.

Autofluorescence imaging utilizes differences in the endogenous fluorophores found in normal and neoplastic epithelia. While the technique has good sensitivity for the detection of high grade dysplasia, studies have shown poor specificity with high false positive rates.

Light scattering spectroscopy and diffuse reflectance spectroscopy use algorithms to analyze light scattered back to the sensing device by the tissue. This spectroscopic information has been able to distinguish neoplastic from non-neoplastic tissue with both good sensitivity and specificity in a few small trials. Optical coherence tomography uses variations in the reflectance of near-infrared light from different tissues to create a high-resolution cross-sectional image of the mucosa. Some studies have shown good sensitivity and specificity in identifying high-grade dysplasia.

While many of these endoscopic techniques show promise, there is currently no definitive evidence that they provide additional information beyond careful examination using high-resolution white light endoscopy. Also, most require specialized equipment and/or training that may not currently be available outside of specialty centers.

Endoscopic Assessment

Traditionally, BE is termed long segment if the tongues are 3 cm or more in length, short segment BE when less than 3 cm, and ultra-short segment BE when less than 1 cm. The key to ensuring an accurate visual diagnosis is reliant upon accurate identification of the gastro-oesophageal junction (GOJ). The GOJ is located at the proximal limit of the gastric folds, or alternatively at the distal end of the palisade vessels. When identified, an assessment of disease extent should be undertaken prior to the commencement of any biopsy protocol.

The importance of assigning the category of length to the metaplastic mucosa in the oesophagus was due to the perceived differences in cancer progression rates amongst the different length segments. Some investigators found a larger increase in the rate of cancer progression with short segment Barrett's in comparison to longer segment Barrett's. Others have found a similar increase in cancer progression rates in both groups. However, most investigators have found an increased rate of cancer progression in the presence of specialised intestinal metaplasia (SIM). In addition, patients with low-grade dysplasia have a higher risk of progression to cancer than those without dysplasia.

The extent of the disease may be measured in centimetres using the Prague C&M criteria [7]. The Prague C and M criteria assess the circumferential (C) and maximum (M) extent of the endoscopically visualised Barrett's oesophagus segment, above the gastro-oesophageal junction, assessed with minimum insufflation (Fig. **3**).

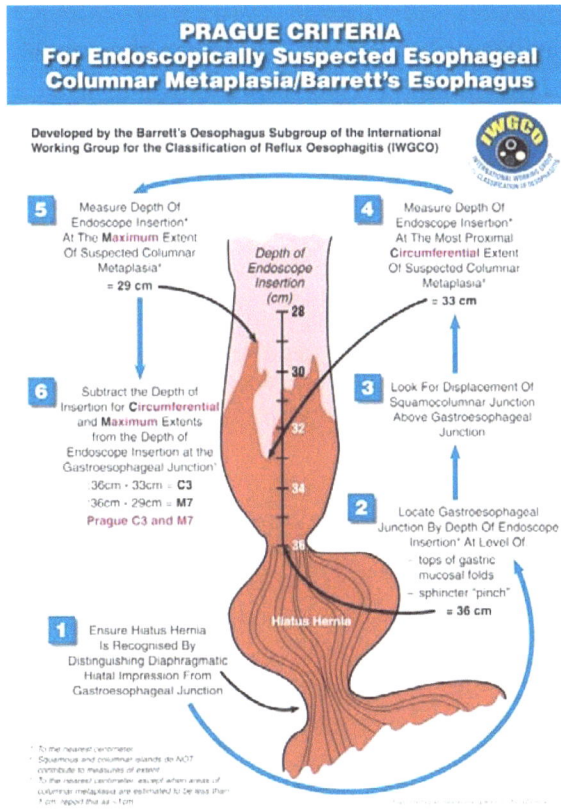

Fig. (3). The Prague classification to assess the extent of BE, Reproduced with permission from the International Working Group for the Classification of Reflux Oesophagitis, available at http://www.iwcgo.net.

The presence of separate islands above the most proximal segment should also be documented. The first step in assessing the extent of the disease is to accurately define the location of the GOJ, and confirm that the squamo-columnar junction lies ≥1 cm above the GOJ. The distance from the GOJ to the level of the most proximal Circumferential (C) segment of suspected BE should be noted. Thereafter a measurement of the length of the Maximum (M) extent of the segment of BE should be made, also taking note of any separate islands of BE.

As an example in Fig. (**3**), if the GOJ is located at 36 cm with the most proximal Circumferential extent at 33 cm, and the Maximal extent of the macroscopically suspected segment of BE at 29 cm, then the Prague C&M is documented as C3 (36 cm-33 cm), M7 (36 cm-29 cm).

Having assessed the extent of the suspected segment of BE macroscopically, the next step is to obtain biopsies for histopathological analysis. Some suggest that eight random biopsies should be taken to enhance the probability of identifying intestinal metaplasia. The Seattle biopsy protocol describes a standardised protocol for maximising the diagnostic yield of dysplasia in a segment of BE [8]. The protocol includes:

1. The use of a therapeutic endoscope to enable larger biopsies using 'jumbo forceps' to be taken.

2. Initial visualisation of the entire length of the Barrett's mucosa with targeted biopsies of any mucosal lesions due to the clear association with underlying OAC.

3. Four quadrant biopsies every 2 cm along the full length of the Barrett's segment.

To prevent the endoscopic view being obscured by bleeding, biopsies should be taken distally and extend proximally. The diagnostic yield of BE increases with the number of biopsies taken and maximises the likelihood of diagnosing IM. Therefore, at least 8 biopsies should be taken in segments >2 cm. If the segment of Barrett's is >3 cm, then this should be considered long segment BE. Long segment BE is an independent risk factor for the development of OAC and this cohort of patients warrant interval endoscopic screening. The endoscopic report should also contain information regarding the position of the GOJ, diaphragmatic hiatus and squamo-columnar junction.

Following pathological analysis the BSG advocates three descriptive terms:

• BE with gastric metaplasia only
• BE with IM

• No evidence of BE

Screening

Standard endoscopic screening for BE in an unselected population is currently neither feasible nor cost effective for the general population. However, most guidelines agree that in a high-risk group for BE including Caucasian men aged 50 and above with chronic reflux symptoms and with other coexisting risk factors such as central obesity and history of smoking should be screened. Conventional endoscopy for screening is expensive, not widely available and is usually performed by a trained endoscopist, which makes it more expensive in time and resource. A possible alternative is ultrathin nasal endoscopy, which avoids the additional costs of sedation, personnel, recovery time and requirement for time off work. Another alternative screening method involves the use of an ingestible sampling device (*e.g.* cytosponge). This device consists of an ingestible gelatin capsule containing a compressed sponge attached to a string. The gelatin dissolves in the stomach leaving the exposed expanded sponge. Withdrawing the string allows the expanded sponge to obtain brushings from the GOJ and oesophagus. The brushings obtained by the device are analyzed with an immunological assay for trefoil factor 3, a marker for columnar epithelium with intestinal metaplasia. This device is currently being evaluated in terms of sensitivity, specificity and cost effectiveness [9]. However, in males with chronic GORD and at least three risk factors, endoscopic screening should be considered, particularly if there is a family history of BE or OAC in a first-degree relative.

Table 2. The Vienna classification of dysplasia in BE.

	Type of Dysplasia	Features
1	Negative for dysplasia	No dysplastic features seen.
2	Indefinite for dysplasia	Suspicious of high-grade dysplasia, but with insufficient findings to support the diagnosis.
3	Low-grade dysplasia	Cytological atypia, but glandular architecture is preserved
4a	High-grade dysplasia	Nuclear atypia with architectural changes.
4b	Intramucosal carcinoma (and suspected invasive carcinoma)	Neoplastic cells have penetrated the basement membrane and entered the muscularis mucosa or lamina propria, without invading the submucosa.
5	Submucosal invasion by adenocarcinoma	Neoplastic cells have invaded the submucosa or beyond.

Table 3. Classification of superficial oesophageal adenocarcinoma

Class		Description
T1a	m1	Carcinoma *in situ*
	m2	Invasion into the lamina propria
	m3	Invasion into the muscularis mucosa
T1b	sm1	Invasion into the upper third of the submucosa
	sm2	Invasion into the middle third of the submucosa
	sm3	Invasion into the lower third of the submucosa

Although a number of potential screening modalities have been described and are currently available, they remain largely as research tools and continue to be evaluated for sensitivity, specificity, cost-effectiveness and tolerability. To date no single modality has been incorporated into BE management guidelines (Table **4**). Ultra-thin nasal endoscopy has produced relatively high sensitivity and specificity and a number of institutions have adopted this modality for screening in clinical practice. The addition of this modality to existing endoscopy adds little capital outlay and may be a reasonable way for screening.

Table 4. Candidate novel screening modalities and a summary of the findings to date.

Screening Modality	Summary of Evidence
Video capsule endoscopy	77% sensitivity and 86% specificity but currently not cost-effective due the need for confirmatory standard endoscopy.
Ultrathin nasal endoscopy	98% sensitivity and 100% specificity. Comparable acceptability, yield and quality to standard endoscopy.
Cytosponge	90% sensitivity and 93% specificity for BE segments >2 cm. Cost effective for screening in selected high-risk groups. Non-invasive.

Adjuncts to Endoscopic Screening

High-resolution endoscopes should be used when screening for BE, or in those undergoing surveillance with known dysplasia. Chromoendoscopy uses dyes to enhance the mucosal architecture with the aim of improving the diagnostic yield of IM from oesophageal biopsies. A number of agents have been reported in the literature; methylene blue, indigo carmine and acetic acid.

Other imaging adjuncts, referred to as 'virtual chromoendoscopy' have also been reported in the literature. These do not use dyes, but instead employ light filters (*e.g.* NBI) or post image acquisition processing (*e.g.* i-scan). Finally, autofluorescence imaging (AFI) has also been shown to increase the yield of IM, but with a high false positive rate. Endoscope based confocal laser endomicroscopy (eCLE), is a probe-based technique, which has resolution to yield close to a histologic view of the epithelium. The use of such techniques may allow for targeted rather than random biopsies but experience is currently limited to tertiary centers with expert endoscopists. More recently techniques using optical coherence tomography are being developed to allow comprehensive assessment of the BE segment with assessment of the sub epithelial layers making this an intriguing technique to study sub-squamous BE.

Overall, the current evidence base for adjuncts to endoscopic screening are either impractical or lack efficacy in comparison to those of standard white light endoscopy and are therefore not routinely recommended for use at present.

CANCER PROGRESSION

BE is a relatively common metaplasia that confers a significant risk for the development of OAC. The prevalence of BE in Western countries is estimated at 1.6% (95% CI 0.8–2.4) in the adult population aged 20–80 years. This means that, in the Western world, 16 adults out of every 1000 people are at risk of OAC. Although the rate of BE progression to cancer is very low (approximately 0.22% of BE cases will progress to OAC per year), the 5-year survival rate of those who develop OAC is poor (22%) and the overall median survival is short (10 months).

Increased risk of progression to OAC is associated with the presence of IM, male gender, smoking and long segment BE. On the basis of the current evidence, the most sensitive discriminators of progression are the presence of IM and long segment (>3 cm) BE. In the absence of intestinal metaplasia, the risk of progression to OAC is considerably reduced.

Dysplasia and Early Cancer

The presence of dysplasia is stratified according to the Vienna classification, (Table **2**). The critical distinction is between low-grade dysplasia (LGD) and high-grade dysplasia (HGD) and is made on the basis of glandular architecture; preserved in LGD and altered in HGD. This is sometimes difficult on the basis of biopsy samples and relies on the expertise of specialist GI pathologists. Frequently, the consensus opinion of two specialist GI pathologists is required to label a biopsy to have LGD or HGD.

Patients with 'indefinite' for dysplasia should have maximal anti-reflux therapy and repeat endoscopy six months later. Those with LGD should undergo endoscopic surveillance and biopsies every 6 months. In those with HGD, high-resolution endoscopy is indicated to fully assess the changes and to map out any visible lesions prior to any subsequent endoscopic therapy.

Classification of superficial oesophageal adenocarcinoma (OAC)

In those with evidence of OAC, specimens should be further sub-classified according to the Paris classification (Table 3 & Fig. 4).

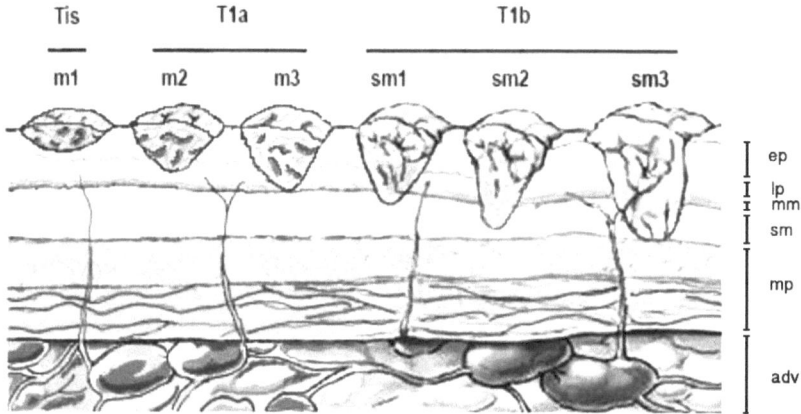

Fig. (4). A schematic diagram illustrating the layers of the oesophageal wall and the T classification of superficial tumours with different levels of invasion into the wall of the oesophagus. ep: Epithelium, lp: Lamina propria, mm: Muscularis mucosa, mp: Muscularis propria, adv: Adventitia.

The depth of invasion and the presence of lymphovascular invasion are essential prognostic indicators and should be included in the pathology report. Lesions confined to the mucosa (T1a) have a low rate of lymhovascular invasion (0-2 per cent) and would therefore be amenable to endoscopic therapies with curative intent. Lesions with invasion into the mid or deep submucosa (T1b sm2 or sm3) have significantly higher rates of lymphovascular invasion (up to 20 per cent) and are therefore not amenable to endoscopic therapies with curative intent [10]. Surgical resection is indicated in this cohort of patients followed by adjuvant therapies. Lesions of the superficial submucosa (T1b sm1) require careful consideration due to the conflicting reports of the likelihood of lymphovascular invasion. Each case of T1b sm1 OAC should be considered carefully on its merits. Surgery remains the primary treatment of choice, but in those considered at high risk for surgery then endoscopic therapy may be indicated.

The important consideration is for accurate alignment of endoscopic resection material (ESD and EMR) biopsies and careful histological observation and reporting by experienced specialist pathologists. This should be followed by careful consideration of each individual patient at the local multi-disciplinary cancer meeting to determine the risks and benefits of different therapies for each individual patient on the basis of available information from diagnostic modalities as well as performance status. Only then can each patient be given options of management which they can choose from.

MANAGEMENT

Barrett's oesophagus is associated with a decreased quality of life compared with the general population mainly due to misunderstanding and overestimation of the associated cancer rates. Most patients with Barrett's oesophagus do not progress past transient low-grade dysplasia and fewer than 10% of patients progress to high-grade dysplasia or cancer. The consensus in guidelines is that patients with non-dysplastic disease or low-grade dysplasia should be managed conservatively in the first instance, with periodic surveillance endoscopy determined by the risk profile of existing pathology. Patients with High-grade dysplasia merit intervention due to the increased risk of progression to cancer. Three strategies are in common use: observation with frequent surveillance endoscopy, endoscopic therapy and surgical oesophagectomy. The best management for Barrett's oesophagus with high-grade dysplasia is dependent on the patient's characteristics and preferences, and local expertise. In patients with multiple comorbidities, endoscopic ablation or endoscopic surveillance might result in the best life expectancy. In young patients with extensive, multifocal high-grade dysplasia, surgical intervention or endoscopic therapy might be preferable to intensive endoscopic surveillance.

Endoscopic Surveillance for BE

Currently surveillance is recommended for all patients with BE at intervals depending on the grade of dysplasia. The aim of endoscopic surveillance in those with BE is to diagnose early progression to dysplasia and OAC. Historically, the annual cancer conversion rate for BE was quoted as 0.5% per annum, but more recent studies suggest a lower figure of 0.33% [11]. The risk of conversion to OAC increases with the degree of dysplasia. In LGD the annual risk of developing OAC is 0.5%, or 1.7% for developing HGD or OAC [12]. In those with HGD the annual risk is 7% on a recent meta-analysis but has been shown to be higher in other studies [13].

At screening endoscopies, adequate representative biopsies should be obtained at various levels of the Barrett's segment(s) particularly at raised areas or nodules. Due to inter-observer variability, experienced pathologists should examine screening biopsies. Two experienced, specialist pathologists should confirm the presence of dysplasia in biopsy material. The presence of dysplasia is the most sensitive biomarker for risk of progression to OAC.

Surveillance Intervals

In order to be considered for endoscopic surveillance a patient should be fit enough to undergo serial endoscopic procedures and therapies. When available, high-resolution endoscopy should be the minimum standard of assessment for patients entering a Barrett's surveillance programme. Staining for aberrant p53 over-expression may help corroborate the presence of dysplasia and has now been recommended as an adjunct to standard histopathological examination in some guidelines

The frequency of endoscopic surveillance should be guided by the presence and grade of dysplasia. In the absence of dysplasia current best practice is surveillance at 3 to 5 yearly intervals, unless there is long segment BE when the endoscopic screening interval is generally 2 - 3 years. In those categorised as indefinite for dysplasia, maximal acid suppression therapy should be commenced with repeat endoscopic assessment and biopsies within 6 months.

In those with LGD, a second experienced pathologist should confirm the diagnosis. Maximal acid suppression therapy should be instituted followed by endoscopic reassessment to confirm the diagnosis. Thereafter, surveillance every 6 months with four quadrant biopsies every 1 cm until there have been two negative examinations for dysplasia. Ablative therapy is not currently recommended, but results from further studies are awaited.

A diagnosis of HGD (or T1 intramucosal cancer), should be confirmed by a second experienced pathologist. The patient should then undergo high-resolution endoscopy by an experienced endoscopist. The overall aim is to closely inspect the BE mucosa for any visible abnormalities and assess suitability for endoscopic resection. In the context of HGD, all visible mucosal abnormalities should be considered neoplastic until proven otherwise. If no visible abnormalities are found, then standard four quadrant biopsies should be taken.

Biopsies taken at surveillance should follow the same protocol as at diagnosis. This involves four quadrant biopsies, but at 1 cm intervals in screening patients. Any mucosal abnormalities should also be biopsied due to their clear association with underlying OAC. There is a correlation between the increased detection of early precancerous lesions and the number of biopsies taken.

Guidelines on Management

A large, systematic literature review has evaluated all the available literature on this topic worldwide. Using a Delphi consensus analysis, practical clinical recommendations have been produced [14]. For the management of Barrett's oesophagus with HGD or early adenocarcinoma, the following is a summary of these recommendations:

- Endoscopic Mucosal Resection (EMR) specimens are better than biopsies for staging visible lesions within a Barrett's segment.
- Careful mapping of areas of visible dysplasia is important.
- Patients that receive ablative or resection treatment require follow-up.
- High-resolution endoscopy is essential for accuracy.
- Endoscopic intervention is preferred to surveillance for HGD.
- Endoscopic intervention for HGD is preferred to surgery.
- Combination EMR/Radio Frequency Ablation (RFA) is the most effective therapy.
- Following EMR of HGD lesions, all areas of Barrett's should be ablated.

The role of radio-frequency ablation (RFA) has recently been extended to selected patients with persistent LGD. The recently published 'SURF' trial, which compared surveillance versus RFA in patients with LGD, was terminated early when the RFA treatment group demonstrated a significantly reduced progression to HGD or adenocarcinoma after two years of follow-up. As a result, NICE recommendation of RFA therapy in high-grade dysplastic Barrett's has been extended to include selected Barrett's patients with persistent LGD.

Assessment of the Barrett's Segment

In order to identify those patients with Barrett's metaplasia who are progressing to dysplasia and neoplasia, a comprehensive endoscopic assessment of the metaplastic segment is essential. The optimal situation is to have a dedicated Barrett's surveillance programme with experienced endoscopists in Barrett's assessment, employing a modern high-resolution white-light endoscopy system to scrutinise the mucosa for nodularity and areas of visible dysplasia. Some endoscopists employ narrow-band imaging as an adjunct, to highlight hyper-vascular areas (indicating possible dysplasia) but this modality is not essential. Acetic acid can also be employed to highlight suspicious areas.

A standardised method of describing the Barrett's segment is optimal. This documentation of the characteristics of the segment allows for communication between endoscopists and assessment of change in an individual patient. The accepted method is to employ the 'Prague criteria' to define metaplastic segment size and morphology. If there are no nodular or other areas suspicious of dysplasia, then a standardised biopsy protocol of the metaplastic segment is undertaken (Fig. **5**).

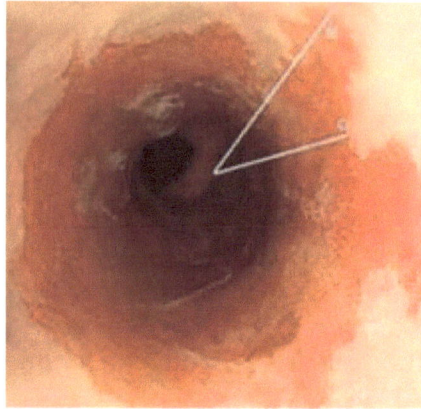

Fig. (5). Documentation of the metaplastic segment size and morphology using the Prague criteria. The length of the segment is measured from the oesophago-gastric junction using the endoscope markers, C: Circumferential extent, M: Maximum extent.

The 'Seattle protocol' involves taking a biopsy from each of the four quadrants of the endoscopic field of view at recorded distances from the mouth guard. This should start at the apparent Z-line, (top of the gastric mucosal folds) and repeated at 1 cm or 2 cm intervals of gastroscope withdrawal, (depending on the intensity of histological 'mapping' required) until the top of the circumferential component is reached. When a tongue is present, this protocol continues, with a number of biopsies taken at each level dependent on the breadth of the tongue. The biopsies from each level are placed in separate formalin pots, marked with the distance from mouth guard, and sent for histological analysis.

Assessment of a Nodule

The presence of a nodule within the Barrett's segment is highly suggestive of dysplasia or early neoplasia. The size, distance from mouth guard, and position on the 'clock face' (of the endoscopic field of view) of any nodular area within the metaplastic area is recorded. This allows easier location of nodules at subsequent therapeutic sessions. The morphology of a nodule can help predict dysplasia or early neoplasia. The 'Paris Classification' is the accepted method of characterising the morphological features of a nodule [15]. Using this classification enables a better analysis of lesions that would be suitable for EMR (Fig. **6**).

Ultimately, the EMR specimen will be the staging biopsy as it is known that intra-mucosal adenocarcinoma or involvement of the submucosa no deeper than 500µ is associated with a low risk of nodal metastases and can be considered therapeutic. The patient can then undergo ablative therapy to the rest of the Barrett's segment once the resection site has healed. If the involvement is deeper than 500µ, lymphovascular invasion is more likely and further staging and consideration of surgery or other management strategies is required.

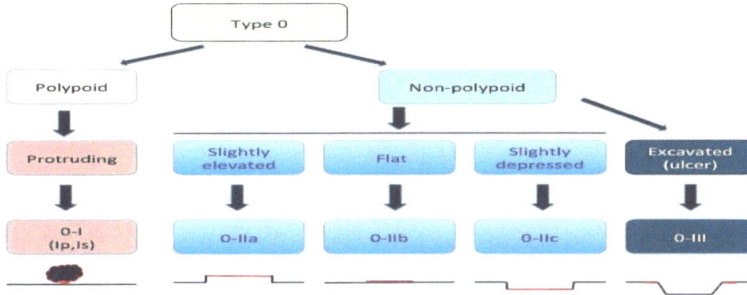

Fig. (6). Superficial neoplastic lesions in the upper digestive tract (Paris Classification).

Endoscopic Therapy

Endoscopic therapy is indicated for BE with focal HGD or mucosal (T1a) adenocarcinoma over endoscopic surveillance or oesophagectomy. There is debate about the precise role of endoscopic therapy in those with T1b sm1 OAC (Fig. 7). Initial studies have demonstrated that endoscopic therapy results in similar disease free survival, lower morbidity and short-term mortality with better cost-effectiveness when compared to surgical resection [16]. The aim of endoscopic therapy should be to resect all visible abnormalities, as this provides superior staging information in terms of differentiating between deep invasive cancer and mucosal cancer in early Barrett's neoplasia when compared to standard biopsies. Endoscopic therapy should always incorporate both mucosal resection and ablative therapies with the aim of eradicating the BE segment.

In those with LGD, ablative therapy has been shown to reduce the risk of progression to both HGD and OAC and this may well result in increased uptake of ablative therapy in this cohort. In those with no dysplasia, endoscopic therapy is not presently indicated due to the perceived greater risk of endoscopic complications versus the low rate of histological progression. However, there is debate about whether targeted ablative therapy should be offered to those deemed at high risk of progression to OAC

Endoscopic therapy should only be offered in centres that have the surgical expertise to deal with any complications that arise, and the aim should be to resect all visible lesions. The most common complication from endoscopic therapy is bleeding, often noted at the time of the procedure and usually managed with conventional haemostatic endoscopic techniques. Oesophageal perforation is also a recognised, but rare complication of endoscopic therapy and indicates the need for specialist management and surgical opinion. Oesophageal perforations secondary to endoscopic therapy may be managed by the placement of a covered oesophageal stent, or the defect may be clipped endoscopically and supported by the placement of endoloops beneath the mucosal defect. In the most severe cases of oesophageal perforation then prophylactic antibiotics, oesophageal tube placement, acid suppression therapy and nil by mouth are indicated. If this fails, then emergency surgery may be required.

Resection Techniques

There are two recognised techniques for endoscopic resection: *cap and snare* and *band ligation*. Both are considered to be equally effective with equivocal complication rates and depth of resection. With both techniques, the target area is initially mapped out with a diathermy device.

Cap and snare: involves submucosal injection of the target resection site, with suction of the specimen into a transparent cap placed on the distal end of the endoscope before it is removed using a snare.

Band ligation: does not require lifting of the specimen with submucosal injection. A transparent cap with rubber bands and a snare are placed on the distal end of the endoscope. The target area is sucked in to the cap and secured with application of the rubber bands to create a pseudo polyp. This can then be excised using a snare.

Endoscopic Ablative Therapy

Ablative therapy is indicated in cases with HGD and T1a adenocarcinoma when there are no visible lesions after thorough endoscopic assessment. Additionally, after EMR of any nodules that are present, an ablative procedure is then necessary for the dysplastic segment. This is usually carried out 6-12 weeks after any prior EMR procedure.

Ablation therapy to the remaining segment of BE following endoscopic resection reduces the risk of later metachronous lesions. An increasing number of centers refer patients to undergo endoscopic ablative therapy for BE. Techniques include thermal ablation with radio-frequency ablation (RFA), cryotherapy (freezing of BE tissue) with liquid nitrogen, PDT (photodynamic therapy) or endoscopic mucosal resection (EMR). RFA, liquid nitrogen spray cryotherapy and EMR all have acceptable success rates for eliminating HGD and IM in the short to medium term. The criteria for measuring success of these procedures include efficacy (complete eradication of dysplasia) and durability (complete remission from intestinal metaplasia without recurrence). On the basis of the current evidence, RFA has the best tolerability and side-effect profile [17].

All ablative therapies rely on the replacement of BE with neosquamous epithelium but the durability and functional characteristics of this tissue are less clear. It is also important to note the existence of "sub squamous" intestinal metaplasia in up to 30% of patients undergoing ablation, which may lead to neoplasia. For these reasons, ongoing surveillance despite successful ablation is recommended until the long term behavior and durability of the neosquamous epithelium has been delineated. Follow up at 3 monthly intervals for a year and annually thereafter with standard biopsies of the previous BE segment is recommended.

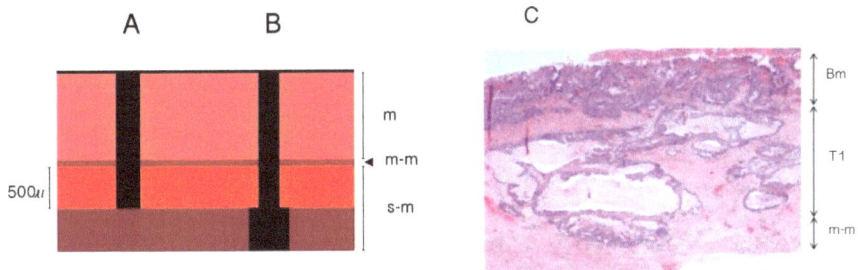

Fig. (7). Left: (A) - Lesions that are limited to the mucosa (m) and first 500μ of the submucosa (s-m) are candidates for curative EMR. (B): lesions penetrating 500μ or deeper to the muscular mucosae (m-m) at EMR should be considered for surgical or oncological management. **Right**: (C) Histology of a T1 EMR biopsy. Ulcer slough and dysplastic Barrett's mucosa are evident (Bm) overlying a T1 intramucosal adenocarcinoma (T1) which abuts, but does not breach the muscular mucosae (m-m).

Surgical Management of Barrett's Oesophagus with Dysplasia

Given the advances in endoscopic and ablative therapy for HGD and T1a adenocarcinoma, surgical resection should no longer be considered as first line therapy. The surgery itself should include resection of the BE segment and include full surgical lymphadenectomy. Surgical management remains the treatment of choice for adenocarcinoma that has extended into the submucosa (T1b) on account of the increased risk of lymph node metastases, particularly in those extending into the middle and distal third of the submucosa (sm2 and sm3) (Figs. 4 & 7). There is debate as to whether T1b sm1 disease can be managed with curative intent endoscopically due to the risk of lymphovascular invasion and the results of further studies are awaited. A recent study reporting data from NHS England has demonstrated that oesophagectomy remains the most common treatment for early OAC (T1 disease), with one in four cases managed endoscopically with curative intent. 5-year survival figures were broadly similar when comparing oesophagectomy to the endoscopic cohort [18].

Oesophagectomy for HGD or early OAC is associated with an operative mortality of <5% and 30-day mortality of 2%. This is comparable with mortality rates following oesophagectomy for any cancer. However, surgical resection is associated with significant short-term morbidity. When compared to endoscopic therapy for HGD or T1a OAC there is significantly lower morbidity following endoscopic therapy with similar survival. It is clear that in those with OAC that extends into the submucosa (T1b), surgical resection should be performed in high volume, specialist centres where patient outcomes are known to be better. The type of resection should be made on an individual case basis with consideration paid to the expertise of the centre and surgeon performing the surgery. There is no clear benefit of one surgical procedure over another. However, there is a trend towards laparoscopic or minimally invasive oesophagectomy and the results of a randomised controlled clinical trial comparing minimally invasive to open oesophagectomy are awaited. The perceived benefits of a minimally invasive approach include less pulmonary complications but long-term outcome data is awaited.

BE has been shown to recur in patients who have undergone surgical resection for BE [19]. There is no clear consensus as to whether formal endoscopic surveillance is indicated in this cohort of patients, but endoscopy is indicated in those with symptoms suggestive of GERD.

Both the ACG and BSG agree, that on the basis of current evidence there is no role for anti-reflux surgery in the prevention of OAC for patients with BE. The indications for anti-reflux surgery in the context of BE should be the same as for those with GERD *i.e.* chronic symptoms that are not managed by conventional medical therapy.

CHEMOPREVENTION

Chemoprevention is proposed to halt the progressive environmental and genetic changes in the oesophageal epithelium. The ideal agent would achieve this without harming healthy cells or causing untoward side effects. Given that the genetic changes take several years to manifest, the chemo-preventive agent would need to be taken throughout the period even in the absence of symptoms. Given also that gastro-oesophageal reflux is such a common condition, it would be impractical to recommend a chemoprevention agent to all such afflicted patients. However, it seems reasonable to recommend such agents to the "high risk" subset of patients and only after the diagnosis of metaplasia. The high-risk group includes Caucasian male patients especially with a family history of OAC, early progression to metaplasia, obese patients (obesity measured by a high waist/hip ratio) and cigarette smokers. Chronicity of GORD and the presence of a hiatus hernia have also been described as risk factors.

Biomarkers (epigenetic, cellular and biochemical) could be used to compliment histological assessment as strong predictors of genetic progression. These include abnormal ploidy, loss of heterozygosity of p53, overexpression of cyclin D1, Mcm2, NF –κB, cytosolic phospholipase and COX-2 amongst other targets.

There have been conflicting reports on the type of diet, which can be used in chemoprevention. Diets high in fruit, vegetable and fibre should be recommended for all patients who strive for a healthy life style. However, there is no clear evidence that these diets convey a chemo preventive effect. Replacement of low levels of deficient vitamins and micronutrients is indicated for their general effect on health. However, no specific vitamin or micronutrient has evidentially been labelled as a chemo preventive agent. Polyphenols (green tea), Folic acid and berries have all been suggested as chemo preventive agents for OAC. There are no randomised trials to substantiate their efficacy as chemo preventive agents.

Numerous studies have incriminated acid exposure for driving the genetic changes through metaplasia, dysplasia and neoplasia in the oesophagus. However, there is no universal consensus on the role of prophylactic acid suppression medication in the prevention of the development of dysplasia or OAC in Barrett's. In addition, it is unknown whether standard doses of PPIs achieve normalisation of the oesophageal pH in everyone. It is well established that effective acid suppression favours differentiation and reduces proliferation. For this effect to manifest, acid suppression needs to be complete and sustainable. Acid suppression is advocated in patients for symptomatic relief of reflux symptoms with proton pump inhibitors providing the best symptomatic control and an exceptional safety record. Recent data from observational studies found that PPI use is associated with a reduction in risk of high-grade dysplasia. Thus, PPIs, which are already universally prescribed to BE patients, may have a significant chemo protective effect and further randomized trials are warranted. Anti-reflux surgery is not superior to acid suppression therapy for the prevention of neoplastic progression of BE, but should be considered as an adjunct in those with on-going symptoms of reflux despite maximal acid suppression therapy.

Most cancers evolve *via* a process of progressive changes in molecular pathways including COX-2, Wnt-b-catenin, MAP kinase, cytokine and growth factor signaling. Agents that block these pathways concurrently would be attractive as chemo protective agents as long as they did not have unacceptable side effects. Aspirin is hydrolysed to salicylate in the gut wall which inhibits prostaglandin E2 thereby inhibiting COX-1 and also modifies the enzymatic activity of COX-2. COX-2 is increasingly expressed when progressing from Barrett's oesophagus to dysplasia to adenocarcinoma. Aspirin also hampers β-catenin signaling and NF-κB transcription. Although the exact role of COX-2 in neoplastic progression is not clear, aspirin has received high publicity as a chemo preventive agent. In a similar mechanism, other Non-Steroidal Anti-inflammatory Drugs (NSAIDs) indomethacin and piroxicam inhibit chemically induced oesophageal cancers. There is presently insufficient evidence to advocate the use of aspirin or NSAIDs for the prevention of OAC but the publication of the results of the ASPECT trial are awaited in 2018. This is a pragmatic, multi-centre, phase III, randomised, open, factorial trial. The main aim of the trial is to investigate the benefits of acid suppression with low or high dose esomeprazole with or without aspirin in reducing the risk of cancer in Barrett's oesophagus. Although the trial has reached its target sample size, follow-up data on mortality and conversion from Barrett's metaplasia to HGD or OAC is accumulating.

Similarly, statins may also prevent development of OAC through inhibition of proliferation and induction of apoptosis among esophageal cancer cells. A recent meta-analysis of observational studies found a 28% reduction in the risk of esophageal cancer among patients who took statins [20]. The number needed to treat with statins to prevent one case of EAC in BE patients was 389. This adds further weight to the potential chemo protective role of statins, although no data from a randomized controlled trial are currently available.

In addition to acid reflux, bile reflux has been proposed to promote the progression of BE to OAC sequence. Bile acids, especially in an acidic milieu, increase expression of homeobox gene transcription factor CDX-2. Hydrophobic bile acids, such as deoxycholic acid (DCA), significantly upregulate vascular endothelial growth factor mRNA expression, causing oxidative DNA damage and activating NF-κB. Conversely, hydrophilic bile acids, such as ursodeoxycholic acid (UDCA), protect against DCA-induced injury. Unfortunately, the highly attractive and protective effect of UDCA in preventing damage of esophageal epithelium by DCA has not been effectively translated into the clinical setting.

Oxidative damage has been linked to mucosal damage of the gastrointestinal tract and their consequent carcinogenesis. However, there is no evidence that the use of antioxidants halts or reverses the damaging effect of noxious agents on the oesophageal mucosa.

In conclusion, based on current data regular use of PPIs, NSAIDs, statins, and UDCA to reduce the risk for BE development and prevent the emergence of OAC in patients with BE cannot be recommended because of lack of evidence. Since the vast majority of patients with BE have associated GORD symptoms, PPIs should be given to control GORD and doses should be adjusted to achieve adequate control of GERD-related symptoms. Presently, NSAIDs, aspirin, statins, and bile acid sequestrants should not be prescribed routinely to patients with BE.

CONSENT FOR PUBLICATION

Not applicable.

CONFLICT OF INTEREST

The author (editor) declares no conflict of interest, financial or otherwise.

ACKNOWLEDGEMENT

Declare none.

REFERENCES

[1]   Shaheen NJ, Richter JE. Barrett's oesophagus. Lancet 2009; 373(9666): 850-61.
        [http://dx.doi.org/10.1016/S0140-6736(09)60487-6] [PMID: 19269522]

[2]   Fitzgerald RC, di Pietro M, Ragunath K, *et al.* British society of gastroenterology guidelines on the
        diagnosis and management of barrett's oesophagus. Gut 2014; 63(1): 7-42.
        [http://dx.doi.org/10.1136/gutjnl-2013-305372] [PMID: 24165758]

[3]   Shaheen NJ, Falk GW, Iyer PG, Gerson LB. ACG clinical guideline: Diagnosis and management of
        barrett's esophagus (vol 111, pg 30, 2016). Am J Gastroenterol 2016; 111: 1077-7.
        [http://dx.doi.org/10.1038/ajg.2016.186] [PMID: 27356842]

[4]   Fléjou JF. Barrett's oesophagus: from metaplasia to dysplasia and cancer. Gut 2005; 54 (Suppl. 1): i6-
        i12.
        [http://dx.doi.org/10.1136/gut.2004.041525] [PMID: 15711008]

[5]   Kalatskaya I. Overview of major molecular alterations during progression from Barrett's esophagus to
        esophageal adenocarcinoma. Ann N Y Acad Sci 2016; 1381(1): 74-91.
        [http://dx.doi.org/10.1111/nyas.13134] [PMID: 27415609]

[6]   Booth CL, Thompson KS. Barrett's esophagus: A review of diagnostic criteria, clinical surveillance
        practices and new developments. J Gastrointest Oncol 2012; 3(3): 232-42.
        [PMID: 22943014]

[7]   Sharma P, Dent J, Armstrong D, *et al.* The development and validation of an endoscopic grading
        system for Barrett's esophagus: the Prague C & M criteria. Gastroenterology 2006; 131(5): 1392-9.
        [http://dx.doi.org/10.1053/j.gastro.2006.08.032] [PMID: 17101315]

[8]   Reid BJ, Blount PL, Feng Z, Levine DS. Optimizing endoscopic biopsy detection of early cancers in
        Barrett's high-grade dysplasia. Am J Gastroenterol 2000; 95(11): 3089-96.
        [http://dx.doi.org/10.1111/j.1572-0241.2000.03182.x] [PMID: 11095322]

[9]   Gupta M, Iyer P G. Screening for barrett's esophagus, gastroenterology clinics of north america, vol
        44, pp 265-+, Jun 2015
        [http://dx.doi.org/10.1016/j.gtc.2015.02.003]

[10]   Leers JM, DeMeester SR, Oezcelik A, *et al.* The prevalence of lymph node metastases in patients with
        T1 esophageal adenocarcinoma a retrospective review of esophagectomy specimens. Ann Surg 2011;
        253(2): 271-8.
        [http://dx.doi.org/10.1097/SLA.0b013e3181fbad42] [PMID: 21119508]

[11]   Desai TK, Krishnan K, Samala N, *et al.* The incidence of oesophageal adenocarcinoma in non-
        dysplastic Barrett's oesophagus: a meta-analysis. Gut 2012; 61(7): 970-6.
        [http://dx.doi.org/10.1136/gutjnl-2011-300730] [PMID: 21997553]

[12]   Singh S, Manickam P, Amin A V, Samala N, Schouten L J, Iyer P G, *et al.* Incidence of esophageal

adenocarcinoma in Barrett's esophagus with low-grade dysplasia: a systematic review and meta-analysis, Gastrointest Endosc, vol 79, pp 897-909 e4; quiz 983 e1, 983 e3, Jun 2014
[http://dx.doi.org/10.1016/j.gie.2014.01.009]

[13] Rastogi A, Puli S, El-Serag HB, Bansal A, Wani S, Sharma P. Incidence of esophageal adenocarcinoma in patients with Barrett's esophagus and high-grade dysplasia: a meta-analysis. Gastrointest Endosc 2008; 67(3): 394-8.
[http://dx.doi.org/10.1016/j.gie.2007.07.019] [PMID: 18045592]

[14] Bennett C, Vakil N, Bergman J, *et al.* Consensus statements for management of Barrett's dysplasia and early-stage esophageal adenocarcinoma, based on a Delphi process. Gastroenterology 2012; 143(2): 336-46.
[http://dx.doi.org/10.1053/j.gastro.2012.04.032] [PMID: 22537613]

[15] The Paris endoscopic classification of superficial neoplastic lesions: esophagus, stomach, and colon: November 30 to December 1, 2002. Gastrointest Endosc 2003; 58(6) (Suppl.): S3-S43.
[http://dx.doi.org/10.1016/S0016-5107(03)02159-X] [PMID: 14652541]

[16] Boger PC, Turner D, Roderick P, Patel P. A UK-based cost-utility analysis of radiofrequency ablation or oesophagectomy for the management of high-grade dysplasia in Barrett's oesophagus. Aliment Pharmacol Ther 2010; 32(11-12): 1332-42.
[http://dx.doi.org/10.1111/j.1365-2036.2010.04450.x] [PMID: 21050235]

[17] Phoa KN, van Vilsteren FG, Weusten BL, *et al.* Radiofrequency ablation *vs* endoscopic surveillance for patients with Barrett esophagus and low-grade dysplasia: a randomized clinical trial. JAMA 2014; 311(12): 1209-17.
[http://dx.doi.org/10.1001/jama.2014.2511] [PMID: 24668102]

[18] Chadwick G, Riley S, Hardwick RH, *et al.* Population-based cohort study of the management and survival of patients with early-stage oesophageal adenocarcinoma in England. Br J Surg 2016; 103(5): 544-52.
[http://dx.doi.org/10.1002/bjs.10116] [PMID: 26865114]

[19] Wolfsen HC, Hemminger LL, DeVault KR. Recurrent Barrett's esophagus and adenocarcinoma after esophagectomy. BMC Gastroenterol 2004; 4: 18.
[http://dx.doi.org/10.1186/1471-230X-4-18] [PMID: 15327696]

[20] Singh S, Singh AG, Singh PP, Murad MH, Iyer PG. Statins are associated with reduced risk of esophageal cancer, particularly in patients with Barrett's esophagus: a systematic review and meta-analysis. Clin Gastroenterol Hepatol 2013; 11(6): 620-9.
[http://dx.doi.org/10.1016/j.cgh.2012.12.036] [PMID: 23357487]

SUBJECT INDEX

A

Abdominal oesophagus 149, 174, 193, 217
Ability, functional 9, 10, 63
Acid suppression 189, 208, 212, 255, 256
Acid suppression therapy 203, 210, 211, 212, 221, 224, 230, 252, 255
Acute kidney injury (AKI) 48, 49, 50
Adenocarcinoma 86, 92, 93, 95, 96, 97, 98, 99, 190, 201, 238, 243, 249, 251, 252, 253, 255
Adenomas 101, 139, 140
Agents 63, 71, 182, 183, 208, 210
  pharmacologic 182, 183
  prokinetic 63, 71, 208, 210
Anaemia 80, 152, 153, 170
Anaesthetic techniques 1, 14, 18
Anaesthetist 3, 5, 11, 18, 20
Analgesia 1, 3, 17, 35, 40, 43, 44, 45, 63, 141, 143
  adequate 43, 44, 45, 63
  systemic patient-controlled 40
Anastomosis 15, 16, 28, 30, 79, 114, 120
Antacids 176, 207, 208
Antibiotic prophylaxis 1, 28
Antibiotics 27, 28, 78, 148, 177, 178, 184
Anti-reflux surgery 14, 189, 206, 208, 211, 212, 213, 214, 215, 217, 219, 220, 221, 222, 223, 224, 254, 255
  centres 221
  current 212
  evaluating 215, 219
  minimal access 217
  performing 214
  robotic 220
Appetite, reduced 54, 63, 66, 69, 82, 83
Arterial blood gasses (ABGs) 43, 46
Assessment 1, 3, 9, 37
  basic anaesthetic 3
  pre-operative 1, 9, 37
Atelectasis 42, 43

Atrial fibrillation 32, 36, 46, 47
Axial reformat 123, 124, 133, 134, 138

B

Baclofen 207, 208, 211
Band ligation 182, 183, 252
Bariatric surgery 172, 215
Barium meal 110, 197, 225
Barium swallows 113, 167, 168, 170
Barrett's oesophagus Evaluation of patients 201
Barrett's oesophagus Reflux 190
Barrett's segment 242, 247, 249, 250
Basal metabolic rate (BMR) 60
Benign smooth muscle tumours 106
Bi-level positive airway pressure (BIPAP) 44
Blood glucose levels 68, 76, 77, 78
Body mass index (BMI) 5, 6, 7, 14, 54, 56, 57, 58, 190, 207, 214, 237
Boerhaave syndrome 152, 175, 176
Bone scans 130, 140
British society of gastroenterology (BSG) 235, 242, 254

C

Cancer 3, 54, 55, 60, 121, 126, 130, 137, 138, 139
  oesophageal and gastric 55, 60, 126, 137
  oesophago-gastric 3, 54, 55, 121, 130, 137, 138, 139
Cancer cachexia 52, 53, 55, 62
Cancer progression rate 240, 241
Cancer staging 110
Cancer surgery 14
Carbohydrates 60, 61, 62, 68, 73, 75, 77, 81
Carcinogenesis 86, 92, 99, 237, 238
Cardia, gastric 138, 191, 192
Cardiac output (CO) 13, 16, 30, 32, 39, 46, 47, 48

Herniation 155, 156, 158, 165, 193, 201, 217, 223, 224, 225

Hiatal hernia 159, 161, 162, 166, 167, 168, 170, 175, 176, 196, 213, 215, 228, 236

Hiatus hernia 113, 114, 132, 152, 160, 164, 172, 189, 193, 196, 200, 202, 203, 207, 211, 213, 214, 215, 227, 254

High calorie fluids 63, 67, 83

High-grade dysplasia (HGD) 91, 132, 233, 236, 237, 243, 245, 247, 248, 249, 251, 252, 253, 254, 255, 256

High-risk surgeries 8, 11, 14, 28

Hounsfield Units (HU) 116

Hypovolaemia 47, 48, 81, 176

Hypoxaemia 18, 22, 23, 43, 45

Hypoxic pulmonary vasoconstriction (HPV) 18, 23

I

Image targeted biopsy 110

Immunohistochemistry 98, 99, 102, 103, 104, 106

Immunonutrition 79

Increased metabolic activity 122, 124, 126

Incremental Shuttle Walk Test (ISWT) 10, 11

Infection 26, 27, 28, 32
  pulmonary 26, 27, 32
  surgical site 26, 27, 28

Infection and anti-microbials 1

Intensive care unity (ICU) 25, 29, 36, 38, 41, 45

Intestinal metaplasia 89, 90, 91, 93, 201, 233, 234, 235, 243, 245, 252

Intra-abdominal oesophagus 149, 157, 191, 193, 212, 214, 216, 218, 228
  adequate length of 212, 214

Intramural hematoma 175, 177

Intra-thoracic stomach 162, 163

Invasion, lymphovascular 233, 246, 251, 253

L

Lamina propria 101, 135, 136, 149, 163, 171, 243, 244, 246

tumour invades 136

Laparoscopic anti-reflux surgery 105, 214, 219

Lesions 63, 104, 121, 123, 124, 126, 127, 128, 129, 130, 132, 133, 135, 136, 139, 140, 141, 142, 172, 175, 246, 249, 250, 251, 252, 253
  obstructing 63, 142
  primary 123, 124, 139
  smaller 105, 127, 129, 139, 140
  visible 246, 249, 251, 252

Liver disease 148, 181, 182

Liver dysfunction 75, 78

LOS pressure 192, 193, 194, 213

Loss, chronic blood 152, 160, 161, 199

Lower oesophageal sphincter (LOS) 191, 192, 194, 196, 203, 205, 206, 211, 212, 214, 223, 227, 229, 236

Lower oesophagus 92, 95, 163, 171, 191, 198, 201, 212, 213, 218, 233, 234

Low-grade dysplasia (LGD) 91, 92, 98, 233, 237, 239, 241, 243, 245, 247, 248, 249, 251

Lumen, endobronchial 20, 21, 22

Lungs, patient's 23

Lung Ventilation 18, 19

Lymph nodes, regional 100, 101, 137

Lymphoid tumours 86, 106

M

Magnetic resonance imaging (MRI) 110, 115, 116, 124, 125, 126, 127, 129, 139, 140, 144, 145, 158, 229

Maintenance therapy 207, 209, 210, 212

Major UGI resection surgery 23, 24, 28, 29, 30

Major upper GI surgery 16, 17, 30, 32, 39, 40, 42

Malnutrition 52, 54, 55, 56, 57, 58, 62, 78, 214
  developing 56, 57
  diagnosis of 54
  risk of 54, 56, 57, 58

Manifestation, extra-oesophageal 189, 201

Mechanical ventilation 36, 44, 45, 46

www.ingramcontent.com/pod-product-compliance
Lightning Source LLC
Chambersburg PA
CBHW050817220326

41598CB00006B/235

* 9 7 8 1 6 8 1 0 8 6 5 8 3 *